212

PLACE **IN RETURN BOX** to remove this checkout from your record.
TO AVOID FINES return on or before date due.
MAY BE RECALLED with earlier due date if requested.

DATE DUE	DATE DUE	DATE DUE

6/01 c:/CIRC/DateDue.p65-p.15

THE IMAGE AND APPEARANCE
OF THE HUMAN BODY

THE IMAGE AND APPEARANCE OF THE HUMAN BODY

Studies in the constructive energies of the psyche

BY

PAUL SCHILDER, M.D. PhD.

Research Professor of Psychiatry, New York University;
Clinical Director, Bellevue Psychiatric Hospital, New York;
a.o. Professor of Psychiatry, University of Vienna.

INTERNATIONAL UNIVERSITIES PRESS, Inc.

New York   New York

TABLE OF CONTENTS

5

PREFACE

The problems with which this book deals have for many years attracted my attention. Clinical observations on brain lesions which provoked difficulties in the differentiation between left and right started my interest. These researches came to a preliminary conclusion in a little study on the 'Körperschema' (schema of the body), published in 1923. I tried there to study those mechanisms of the central nervous system which are of importance for the building up of the spatial image which everybody has about himself. It was clear to me at that time that such a study must be based not only on physiology and neuropathology, but also on psychology. I wrote: "It would be erroneous to suppose that phenomenology and psycho-analysis should or could be separated from brain pathology. It seems to me that the theory of organism could and should be incorporated in a psychological doctrine which sees life and personality as a unit". I therefore used the insight psycho-analysis has given to us with its psychic mechanisms for the elucidation of problems of brain pathology. The study of the mechanisms of the brain in perception and action helped to a deeper understanding of psychological attitudes. I have always believed that there is no gap between the organic and the functional. Mind and personality are efficient entities as well as the organism. Psychic processes have common roots with other processes going on in the organism. I found out later that this attitude corresponds closely with the best traditions of American psychiatry, as they appear in the work of Adolph Meyer, William A. White, and Smith Ely Jelliffe. The same attitude is also inherent in the doctrine of psycho-analysis. Psychology under such an aspect is necessarily psychobiology (Adolph Meyer's term) and can also be termed 'Naturwissenschaftliche Psychologie'. It seems to me also that the basic position of the gestalt psychologists is a similar one. For the gestalt psychologist, the gestalt is in the outside world, and is also in the physicochemical processes, which are correlated to the psychic processes in which the gestalt principles appear.

A psychology of this kind necessarily places emphasis on the action and does not consider the organism in its psychic and somatic aspects as a theoretical entity with merely perceptive qualities (perceptions, imaginations, and thoughts). Perception and action, impression and expression, thus form a unit, and insight and action become closely correlated to each other. Human action, badly misjudged in the philosophy of Bergson, and artificially separated by Kant into practical reasoning and pure reasoning, is thus restored to its full dignity. It is easy to see that the pragmatism of James and the instrumentalism of John Dewey express the same principle in a philosophic way. I have come, in this respect also, in my previous formulations (e.g. in my *Ideen zur Naturphilosophie*) nearer to the trend of American philosophy than I realized at that time. Such a biologic, organismic philosophy and psychology takes its starting-point from a naïve realistic attitude and is not concerned with doubts about the reality of the external world. Its exponents feel amply justified in taking up this standpoint not only by philosophic speculation and reasoning, but also by the concrete approach to the innermost problems of human behaviour.

In Germany, philosophic thinking took another direction. Many of the German philosophers and psychologists have felt that there exists a psychology which is not 'Naturwissenschaftlich', a much more important so-called 'Geisteswissenschaftliche' psychology, which deals with the central problems of history, ethics, and human personality in general. But I cannot see any fundamental difference between the insight into personality problems and human behaviour and the insight into the structure of nature. The typical entities and the typical sequences have to be found in both, and science tries, in the one sphere as well as in the other, to find the essential entities, their structure, their genesis, and their more or less typical connections. In nature, new qualities, new entities, new configurations emerge continually. Every new chemical compound displays qualities which could not be foreseen completely and form a new unit or gestalt. In the organismic world, C. Lloyd Morgan has drawn attention to the emergent evolution, pointing to the continual creation of unforeseen organismic entities. A creation in this respect is a general quality of existence, and this creation takes place continually in the inanimate world as well as in the animate.

This book attempts to achieve a deeper insight into the nature of the creative process and emphasizes the constructive psychic effort by which new entities are created. Emergent evolution and gestalten in the psychic sphere are not merely data which are given to us as a present; they have to be obtained by struggling. They are not 'Gegebenheiten' but 'Errungenheiten'. It accords with this point of view that philosophy and psychology should be considered as essentially identical, except that philosophy has the further task of correlating the other data of experience with the data of psychology.

It follows out of this general attitude that the author has tried to solve problems by the careful study of facts, of brain pathology, and psychology. His method is completely empirical, or, to use a word which has become discredited, psychologistic. But psychology in our sense means truthful observation of the empirical data of psychic life, and no intuition and reasoning can go beyond this limit. Psychology also correlates the experiences concerning the outside world and the body with the inner experiences. A psychology which does not utilize the enormous enlargement of the horizon which Freud and psycho-analysis has achieved, neglects an innumerable number of important experiences. This statement does not imply the acceptance of psycho-analytic theory as a whole. I do not think that Freud's basic attitude that our desires try to lead us back to a previous state and merely lead us back to a state of rest is a true description of inner and outer experiences. I insist upon the constructive character of the psychic forces and refuse to make the idea of regression the centre of a theory of human behaviour. It seems to me, also, that Freud has been inclined to neglect the principles of emergent evolution, or, as I would prefer to say, of constructive evolution, which leads to the creation of new units and configurations.

It is clear that the foregoing remarks are merely a programme for further research. The author does not believe that the limited scope of this book can show more than the way in which he thinks the solution of the problem could be sought. The book is merely an empirical investigation concerning the 'image' of the human body. This is certainly one of the central problems of psychology. Wernicke saw this when he spoke of 'somato-psyche', but he distinguished two other spheres of orientation, the orientation about the outer world (allopsyche) and the orientation about our inner self (autopsyche). Autopsyche and allo-psyche are not the objects of this investigation. Even a preliminary attempt to solve the general problem cannot be made when the two other spheres of human experience are not carefully investigated. This book declares itself, therefore, as an incomplete attempt. It approaches only one part of the great realm of empiric psychology and philosophy.

In view of the general tendencies of this book it was necessary to go through empirical material out of the sphere of brain pathology and psychology. I have attempted to make the book digestible also to the reader who is not thoroughly acquainted with the facts of neuropathology and psycho-analysis, and I have added a short interpretation of the basic facts which are utilized in this book. I hope that thus the book will be understandable also to those who are outside the closer circle of neurologists, psychologists, and philosophers, to whom this book is primarily addressed.

P. S.

New York, January 1935.

THE IMAGE AND APPEARANCE OF
THE HUMAN BODY

INTRODUCTION

The image of the human body means the picture of our own body which we form in our mind, that is to say the way in which the body appears to ourselves. There are sensations which are given to us. We see parts of the body-surface. We have tactile, thermal, pain impressions. There are sensations which come from the muscles and their sheaths, indicating the deformation of the muscle; sensations coming from the innervation of the muscles (energy sense, von Frey); and sensations coming from the viscera. Beyond that there is the immediate experience that there is a unity of the body. This unity is perceived, yet it is more than a perception. We call it a schema of our body or bodily schema, or, following Head, who emphasizes the importance of the knowledge of the position of the body, postural model of the body. The body schema is the tri-dimensional image everybody has about himself. We may call it 'body-image'. The term indicates that we are not dealing with a mere sensation or imagination. There is a self-appearance of the body. It indicates also that, although it has come through the senses, it is not a mere perception. There are mental pictures and representations involved in it, but it is not mere representation. Head writes: "But, in addition to its function as an organ of local attention, the sensory cortex is also the storeroom of past impressions. These may rise into consciousness as images, but more often, as in the case of special impressions, remain outside of central consciousness. Here they form organized models of ourselves, which may be termed 'schemata'. Such schemata modify the impressions produced by incoming sensory impulses in such a way that the final sensation of position, or of locality, rises into consciousness charged with a relation to something that has happened before. Destruction of such 'schemata' by a lesion of the cortex renders impossible all recognition of posture or of the locality of a stimulated spot in the affected part of the body".

Previously he had stated: "But in both cases the image, whether it be visual or motor, is not the fundamental standard against which all postural changes are to be measured. Every recognizable change enters into consciousness already charged with its relation to something that has happened before, just as on a taximeter the distance is represented to us already transformed into shillings and pence. So the final product of the tests for the appreciation of posture or passive movement rises into consciousness as a measured postural change.

"For this combined standard, against which all subsequent changes of posture are measured before they enter consciousness, we propose the word 'schema'. By means of perpetual alterations in position we are always building up a postural model of ourselves, which constantly changes. Every new posture or movement is recorded on this plastic schema, and the activity of the cortex brings every fresh group of sensations evoked by altered posture into relation with it. Immediate postural recognition follows as soon as the relation is complete.

"One of our patients had lost his left leg some time before the appearance of the cerebral lesion which destroyed the power of recognizing posture. After the amputation, as in so many similar cases, he experienced movements in a phantom foot and leg. But these ceased immediately on the occurrence of the cerebral lesion; the stroke which abolished all recognition of posture destroyed at the same time the phantom limb.

"In the same way, recognition of the locality of the stimulated spot demands the reference to another 'schema'; for a patient may be able to name correctly, and indicate on a diagram or on another person's hand, the exact position of the spot touched or pricked, and yet be ignorant of the position in space of the limb upon which it lies. This is well shown in Hn. (case 14), who never failed to localize the stimulated spot correctly, although he could not tell the position of his hand. This faculty of localization is evidently associated with the existence of another schema or model of the surface of our bodies, which also can be destroyed by a cortical lesion. The patient then complains that he has no idea where he has been touched. He knows that a contact has occurred, but he cannot tell where it has taken place on the surface of the affected part.

"It is to the existence of these 'schemata' that we owe the power of projecting our recognition of posture, movement, and locality beyond the limits of our own bodies to the end of some instrument held in the hand. Without them we could not probe with a stick, nor use a spoon unless our eyes were fixed upon the plate. Anything which participates in the conscious movement of our bodies is added to the model of ourselves and becomes part of these schemata: a woman's power of localization may extend to the feather in her hat".

When a leg has been amputated, a phantom appears; the individual still feels his leg and has a vivid impression that it is still there. He may also forget about his loss and fall down. This phantom, this animated image of the leg, is the expression of the body schema.

What apparatus of the brain is the basis of these phenomena? What is the physiological basis of the knowledge of our body? Our discussion will show that we have to do with a complicated apparatus. There will arise the general problem of the way in which the body-image reflects the structure of the body. What is the relation between anatomy and the postural model and knowledge of our body? It might be that there is in our body-image more than we consciously know about the body.

But the body has not only an outside. It has also an inside. What do we know about the inside of our body?

What is the psychological structure of our knowledge of the body? Here we have a unit and a very natural one. What is given by experience in this unit? And what is a gestalt, a shape that is given from the very beginning? Is the postural model built up by sensations and memories, or is there something beyond the sensations? Has any sensation any inner meaning without being brought in connection with the postural model of the body? Modern psychology formulates this problem by contrasting the whole which is more than the sum of the single parts, with the "und-" connection of parts which are added to each other. Melody is more than the separate sounds of which it is composed.

In the words of Köhler: "The definite impression of an optic figure, the specific character of a musical motive, and the sum of a sentence with meaning contains more than the sum of coloured points, sound sensations, and word connotations. The same spatial gestalt (shape, configuration) can appear in other colours and in another place, the same musical motive in different heights of tone. Therefore the absolute elements do not constitute the specific nature of the total structure. . . . Such structures as have specific qualities as wholes and can therefore justly be considered as units are meant by the term gestalt" (p. 1).

"On this point the postulate is unavoidable, to let participate organic functions that correlate to higher psychic functions on the characteristic functional qualities of psychic experience and therefore to consider organic processes as Gestalten. . . . Koffka has recently emphasized this thought and has asked with Wertheimer that central psychic processes should not be considered as the sum of single irritations, that is to say, as and-connections, but as shaped total processes." Gestalt is thus an immediate experience, and is, according to Wertheimer, Köhler, and Koffka, perfect and complete in its inner necessity, which is based on mere perception and born like Athene out of the head of Zeus. Köhler even goes so far as to assume that there are physical gestalten and has tried to show that there exist characteristic qualities of total systems in the realm of physics also. "When the partial pressures of two solutions of some types of ions are different, the two solutions form (when there is an osmotic communication) a whole with a characteristic electric system quality, which cannot be deducted out of the qualities of the parts, but determines in reverse the electric qualities of the parts (an additive constant excepted)." We may expect to learn something about this fundamental problem of psychology by studying the human Gestalt, the body-image in the sense formulated above. This is a central problem of psychology.

When one studies the problem of the postural model there arises immediately the old psychological question, "In what way do we determine the localization of our sensations?" How do we bring the single impression in connection with this whole, with this unit, of our body?

Our study is primarily a study of the body-image which lies on the impressive side of our psychic life. But there are no impressions which are not directional and do not find at the same time an expression. There are no perceptions without actions. Every impression carries with it efferent impulses. Even this formulation does not emphasize sufficiently that impression and expression form a definite unit which we can separate in its parts only by artificial analysis. What is the relation between the postural model and the action?

We have also disposed of the idea that there are impressions which are independent from actions. Seeing with an unmoved eye when inner and outer eye muscles are out of function would not be real seeing and would not be seeing at all, if the body were completely immobilized at the same time. If the eye is unmoved, then the head moves, and, should both be paralysed, the body moves. In the case of a total paralysis, there would still be impulses to move as long as life is present. Perceptions are only formed on the basis of the motility and its impulses. We have to expect, therefore, that changes in the motility in its broadest sense will be of determining influence on the structure of the postural model.

In studying the body-image, we must approach the central psychological problem of the relation between the impressions of our senses and our movements and motility in general. When we perceive or imagine an object, or when we build up the perception of an object, we do not act merely as a perceptive apparatus. There is always a personality that experiences the perception. The perception is always our own mode of perceiving. We feel inclined to answer with an action or actually do so. We are, in other words, emotional beings, personalities. And personality is a system of actions and tendencies to such. We have to expect strong emotions concerning our own body. We love it. We are narcissistic. The topography of the postural model of the body will be the basis of emotional attitudes towards the body. Our knowledge will be dependent on the erotic currents flowing through our body and will also influence them. The erotic zones will play a particular part in the postural model of the body.

Is the postural model of the body a fixed static entity, or is it a changing, growing, and developing one? I hope to show that the postural model of the body is in perpetual inner self-construction and self-destruction. It is living in its continued differentiation and integration. Studying it, we shall study the meaning of the idea of development for psychic structures.

Experiences in pathology show clearly that when our orientation concerning left and right is lost in regard to our own body, there is also a loss of orientation in regard to the bodies of other persons. The postural model of our own body is connected with the postural model of the bodies of others. There are connections between the postural models of fellow human beings. We experience the body-images of others. Experience of our body-image and experience of the bodies of others are closely interwoven with each other. Just as our emotions and actions are inseparable from the body-image, the emotions and actions of others are inseparable from their bodies. The postural image of the body must be studied, if we desire to gain a deeper insight into social psychology.

It is a wide range of problems that we have to study. The solution of these problems is a task beyond the reach of the single worker. I do not believe that psychological and philosophical problems can be solved by *a priori* methods. We need the continual contact with the inexhaustible world of reality. One may approach this reality with theories and thoughts which will prove their value in leading to new aspects and to new facts. When a set psychological assumption leads us to these results, its relative value will be proved. But whenever it leads into reality it will come out of this reality changed and enriched and should again lead to new attempts. Theories and thoughts, therefore, can only be passing phases in the asymptotic approach to reality.

PART I

THE PHYSIOLOGICAL BASIS OF THE
BODY-IMAGE

(1) *Postural and tactile impressions in relation to the body-image*

As quoted above, Head emphasizes that even when the visual image is preserved and the sense of posture is impaired, the individual will, if tactile localization is preserved, show the spots where he has been touched, though in the place of the previous posture of the arm and not on the arm, when it is removed to another place, because the movement of the arm has not come to his knowledge. Head therefore regards the postural impression as the basis for the postural model of the body. There is a standard of postures, against which all new incoming perceptions are measured. Head brings the hypotonia, the flaccidity observed in cortical lesions, leading to a disturbance of the sensibility, in immediate connection with a disturbance of the postural model of the body.

I can verify by my own experience Head's observations that there are cases in which the patient can localize the touch and know which particular spot of the arm has been touched, but is unable to determine the position of the arm in space. But I cannot follow his argument that this proves that the postural model is based on posture. I would say on the contrary that this observation proves that an optic image of the body is now present to which the perception is brought in connection. These very observations show the importance of the optic part of the postural model of the body.

I may here draw attention to an observation I published some years ago.[1] The patient suffered from an apoplexy on a luetic basis. She had a serious right-sided hemiplegia of predilection type. She had unimportant spasms and peculiar disturbances of the sensibility of the right side. There were paraesthesias in the

---

[1] Cf. the case report in the Appendix (case a).

face. The sensibility to thermal stimuli, tickling, faradic current, and the sense of posture, were impaired. In contrast to this, she appreciated weights quite well. There was a tendency to hallucinatory experiences; for instance, the patient might feel her hand moved without objective basis. In the tactile sphere there was also a tendency to hallucination. The patient showed polyaesthesia (multiplication of sensations) in this part of the body for tactile, thermal, and pain sensations. One stimulus was felt there several times, at least twice. She localized the various sensations which were provoked by one stimulus in points which were nearer to the end of the body (more distal) than the irritated spots. The interval was between 4 and 10 seconds. The ensuing sensations were very often indefinite sensations of touch. The deep-sensibility also showed a tendency to polyaesthesia. Sensations of the otherwise healthy part of the body were transferred after an interval of from 4 to 10 seconds to the impaired side. The quality of the sensations did not change during the transfer. In this way there might appear warm sensations on the right side, which the patient could not get in any other way. This sensation on the right side of the body, which was transferred from the left side, was followed by one or several after-sensations. The discrimination (differentiations of two simultaneous touches) was good on the right side, whereas the localization showed serious disturbances which were not quite constant and were also very dependent on fatigue.

The patient could not recognize objects placed in her right hand. She probably had a lesion, which went from the capsula interna towards the cortex of the gyrus centralis posterior and of the parietal lobe. The thalamus was probably only very slightly impaired. In this case the warm sensation of the healthy left side was transferred unchanged to the right side, which in itself was not capable of feeling any heat. The patient therefore transferred sensations to symmetrical parts of her body under the lead of the unimpaired optic parts of the postural model of the body. We meet here for the first time the interesting phenomenon of Allochiria or Alloaesthesia, first described by Obersteiner. Sensations of the left side were transferred to the right side and *vice versa*. Our patient felt touches on the left side correctly, but this sensation was followed by one on the right side. There was an actual transfer of sensations from the left (healthy) side to the right (affected) side. It is true that there were sometimes spontaneous tactile-kinaesthetic sensations on the right side (hallucinations), but they were irregular and there was never a thermal hallucination on the right side. The left-side sensation provoked the right-side sensation. Only in two other cases (Brown-Séquard and Hammond) was the sensation transferred, as in our case, from the healthy side to the sick side. In most of the other cases the sensation was transferred from the sick side to the healthy side.

There is a good reason for the transference of the left-side sensation to the symmetrical spot of the right side of the body. According to Brown and Stewart, the sensation when a special point is touched is different from the sensation in other parts of the body 'character'. According to them, all touches of one point must have a particular individuality, which the pain and temperature sensations of the same point have in common with them. But even if the touch of one point provoked a sensation different from all other sensations and similar to all previous touches of the same point, the correct localization of this point on the surface of the body would not be warranted. Every touch must also have a special topical position on the surface of the body. This may be called a position factor. One may not be convinced that the differentiation of individuality and character are necessary; but there is no question that the position factor is absolutely different from the factors of individuality and character. Individuality and character of symmetrical points on the surface of the body are certainly very similar to each other. We may suppose that symmetrical points are very closely connected with each other physiologically. I shall comment later on the experimental proof offered by the interesting findings of Dusser de Barenne. But there is at any rate a close psychological relation between symmetrical spots on the body. Volkmann has proved that when one exercises one side of the body the contralateral parts of the body improve in their faculty of localization. We know that every touch provokes a mental image of the spot touched. These optic images are certainly of very great importance for the localization.

In the experiments of Klein and Schilder the optic image was a small circle round the spot touchèd. But this limited and seemingly disconnected impression in the consciousness was an important lead to localization. It helped to determine the position of a finger in space which was otherwise unknown. It must therefore have helped to an 'optic representation' of the space round the spot touched. But no conscious optic picture of the finger and its position in space was present. We thus come to the formulation that the optic images which are in our consciousness are only a small part of what is actually going on in the psychic sphere. Whether there are images on the unconscious level or whether we deal only with somatic vestiges cannot be decided. We shall meet this problem again. But we know that whenever a touch takes place, a variety of mental processes start, which bring this touch into connection with our other experiences. Everything points to the conclusion that the 'Localzeichen' (sign of localization) is not given with the sensation itself but is added to it.

In our case the patient was unable to localize in spite of the fact that she could differentiate two neighbouring points. It is worthy of remark that the patient usually localized correctly a touch on her nipple. There are certainly points which are so distinguished in their individuality and character that they are easily brought in connection with the optic part of the postural model of the body. The lack of power of localization is not due to a lack in the sense of posture. The patient was also unable to localize on her trunk and unable to show the relative position of a point touched on her arm and leg. Head has already pointed out that there are schemata which teach us about the relation of the different parts of the body to each other. We arrive at the following preliminary formulation:

(1) The sense of posture plays a part in the building up of the knowledge of our body.

(2) There is connected with the faculty of localization the possibility of building up the knowledge of the relation of the different parts of the surface to each other.

(3) There is an optic image of the body, which is independent of the tactile images mentioned so far.

(4) Symmetrical parts of the body are physiologically and psychologically connected with each other.

(5) The optic perception and imagination emphasize the tactile similarity of symmetrical points.

(6) The conscious optic images and perceptions are only a small part of what is going on in the optic sphere.

(7) The localization of tactile images and impressions is a process independent of the simple perception of touch.

(2) Localization on the skin and the optic part of the body-image

Some remarks are necessary about the last point. There is no question that Lotze is right in so far as he says that localization is not given with perception as such. He is right when he emphasizes the qualitative difference between the sensations, and maintains that every qualitative well-characterized sensation brings with it the visual representation of its spatial relations. He is inclined to bring these qualitative differences in connection with associated sensations. But, according to our previous remarks, we believe in primary qualitative differences. He is wrong too in his belief that the different sensations provoke the soul to produce representations of space. There is no primary perception of space. Lotze follows in this respect the erroneous opinion of Kant. Localization is built up by optic and kinaesthetic impressions, by bringing the single impression into connection with the postural model of the body. But the postural model of the body is a product of the gestalt creative powers of our psyche. In order to understand this fully, we have to know what the optic part of the postural model of the body is.

Goldstein and Gelb describe a case of so-called perceptive mind-blindness. Even very simple optic perceptions were almost impossible. The patient failed to recognize a straight line. He was incapable of the perception of an optic movement. There were not only disturbances in the optic sensations; but Goldstein and Gelb mention the loss of optic images in this case and point also in a second similar case (case S.) to the serious impairment of the optic images. I have serious doubts about the correctness of this formulation. In cases of optic agnosia (mind-blindness) one sees generally that optic representations are present, though they cannot be used in the same way as before. Of course, they are present in a different way. An optic representation which cannot be used is certainly different from an optic representation which is at the disposal of the individual. Beyond that, the optic representation in these cases may show differences in structure from the normal optic representation. It would be difficult to call this agnostic optic representation, since the representations of normal persons also show characteristics which are very similar to the disturbed perception of the optic agnostic. Apparently we do not need more than parts, which may even be distorted in order to signify an object by representation. Furthermore, there is no question that the majority of the optic images of normal persons never come into the full light of consciousness. It is an unsolved problem whether these are 'unconscious' images in the psychic sense or whether we are dealing with the organic 'unconscious', which, according to the formulation given later, will have only a vague reflection in the psychic life. But in whatever direction the decision may go, I cannot believe that a complete loss of optic images can ever occur.

At any rate Goldstein and Gelb's cases acted better when they had their eyes open and could look at the limb which was supposed to act. In one case the patient was unable to start a movement, unless there was the optic perception or a muscular twitching. In the case S., where the muscular twitchings were absent, looking at the limb was absolutely necessary in order to start the movement. In both cases ataxia was absent. One may infer that disturbances of tactile and postural sensibility, in a narrow sense, were absent. In spite of that, the patient Sch. especially showed a severe disturbance in the tactile localization and in the perception of tactile configurations. He could not distinguish whether he had his finger or his whole arm in the water. His discrimination was severely impaired. He made serious mistakes in localization. He could only arrive at an adequate localization by making muscular twitchings (Tastzuckungen). He quickly moved a great number of muscles till he came near to the point touched.

Goldstein and Gelb consider that touch does not provoke a primary answer in the optic sphere, as Wundt has emphasized.

They point out the fact that blind people also localize on their body with similar methods, although the twitchings may, in the later years of the blind, disappear and be substituted by kinaes-thetic imaginations. I do not think that Goldstein and Gelb are justified in drawing such a general conclusion from an observa-tion which so far has remained isolated. It is at least probable that for the majority of normal persons optic images follow tactile perception immediately in the manner Wundt (p. 279 *l.c.*) has surmised. But it is possible that the organism has several ways by which it can arrive at a localization of tactile impression. The tactile impression may provoke the optic image directly or via kinaesthetic impressions. It is possible that kinaesthetic im-pressions follow the optic image in one case. Either one of them may be sufficient for the final task. But it is at any rate a great achievement on the part of Goldstein and Gelb to have pointed out how important optic impressions are for localization. It is also a point of great importance that even the choice of a limb for the start of a movement is only possible when the optic sphere is not too severely damaged and the body-image of the optic sphere does not show too great an impairment. We also see that the ' Localzeichen ' is indeed dependent on a process which correlates the single impression with the whole of the impressions of the body-image.

We have also gained, through Goldstein and Gelb, the addi-tional knowledge that the body-image and especially its optic parts are necessary for the beginning of a movement. There is at any rate an optic factor in the postural model of the body. With-out it, tactile localization is impossible. But kinaesthetic ex-periences may take the place of the optic factors. The patient Sch. reaches a satisfactory localization of touch by experimenting, by trying out whether the character of the muscular twitches is sufficiently similar to the character of the touch. The successive twitches serve the construction of the body-image. They are more or less voluntary. The optic stimuli as well as the kinaesthetic are connected with the high level of cortical activity. When, as in the so-called Japanese illusion, hands and fingers are doubly crossed and intertwined, the optic impression of hands and fingers be-comes so complicated that the optic gnosia is not sufficient to disentangle the picture. We are dealing then with a relative optic agnosia concerning one's own body. Tactile and kinaesthetic helps are then necessary to start the movement of a specific finger. Tactile and kinaesthetic impressions are used therefore for the orientation concerning one's own body, whenever the optic impressions become insufficient. We see how much activity is necessary to come to an orientation concerning one's own body which is basic for every localization.

(3) *Further remarks on the apparatus which serves localization*

After transection of peripheral nerves on himself Head observed serious trouble in localization when the protopathic primitive sensibility returned. But this trouble in localization never went so far that the knowledge of the side of the body was impaired. Only the full function of the peripheral nerves guarantees exact localization of stimuli. This guarantee is very closely allied to the anatomical structure. Fuchs has described contralateral paraesthesias and pain after lesion of the peripheral nerves. He called this disturbance Alloparalgia. But many observations by Oppenheim, Weygandt, Mann, and Förster prove that the transfer to the contralateral side is not the important thing. Sträussler emphasized that any irritation in any part of the body provokes pain sensations in the region of the nerve lesion. I have made similar observations myself.

We do not know how the hyper-excitability in the regions of the injured nerve occurs. It seems that every acting nerve attracts other irritations. We have to do with principles similar to those indicated by Uchtomski, to the effect that an irritation may become dominant and may attract all irritations of minor degrees. Uchtomski has studied this phenomenon in connection with more central processes like the spinal heat reflex of the frog. But it is probable that all over the nervous system we deal with the principle just described, and its occurrence, therefore, does not tell us anything about the localization. But it remains remarkable that paraesthesias may so easily become contralateral. Since Fuchs' cases probably belong to the field of causalgia (lasting pain sensations after peripheral injuries) which at the present time is considered as being connected with a sympathetic disturbance, we may adopt the theory that the relation between two symmetrical parts is partly based on sympathetic connections. Whether this connection goes over the spinal cord or not cannot be decided. But it must be remembered that vasomotor phenomena are often symmetrical. We should not consider the nervous system in isolation. After all, there are the blood-vessels, and the relation of the nervous system to structures of other kinds is certainly very close.

We stand on firmer ground when discussing the spinal mechanisms which can provoke alloaesthesia.[1] Some time ago Mott observed alloaesthesia after hemisection of the spinal cords of monkeys. Dusser de Barenne provoked a local hyperexcitability of one side of a spinal segment by the application of strychnine and cut the sensory spinal pathways above the strychninized segment on the same side.[2] A dog operated upon in this way feels continuous paraesthesias in the segment contralateral to the operation, and also feels stimuli applied to the other side on the side of the strychninization. But when there is a distance of more than three segments between the strychninization and the hemisection, the subjective phenomena are present on both sides. When the two experimental exchanges are less than three segments distant from each other, there are then only the alloaesthetic sensations present, which are on the side contralateral to the operation. In the light of these experiments, we suppose that hypersensibility and simultaneous blockade makes impulses irradiate to symmetrical parts. One might think that by the hemisection the sensory impressions coming to the postural model are insufficient and that they are transported to the side of the body which has the better tactile sensation. But against this view there is the fact that when the distance is more

[1] We use the term Alloaesthesia when a stimulus on one side of the body provokes a sensation on the other side of the body. Alloaesthetic sensations may be symmetrical or not. Jones uses the term Alloaesthesia only in connection with organic disturbances and reserves the term Allochiria, which was used by Obersteiner indiscriminately, only for psychogenic cases. But the organic and psychogenic mistakes concerning right or left have, as I shall show later, many things in common, so that we should not emphasize the difference between Allochiria (which is supposed to be strictly symmetrical) and Alloaesthesia. Generally we follow Jones's nomenclature.

[2] For the anatomical facts, cf. Appendix 2.

than three segments, the irritation is on the normal as well as on the impaired side of the body. It seems, therefore, that the two symmetrical parts of the body are connected with each other anatomically, although generally this connection does not come into action. Only if the amount of excitation is increased and the centripetal conduction is impaired will the stream flow in a direction that is not usually open. It seems that we must give up rigid ideas about anatomy in its relation to function when the general situation changes. Many passages can be used which otherwise do not function. Function is in a wide range dependent on the actual situation and independent of passages, if one considers a passage as a definite and anatomical entity.[1]

In Dusser de Barenne's dogs it is apparently a paraesthesia, which is transferred from one side to the other, and it is more than probable also that the touch to which the animal reacts has a particular quality. In human pathology we are able to study this problem more carefully. In cases of tabes dorsalis, hypaesthesia of a medium degree is often accompanied by after-sensations, which are generally localized distal from the primary irritated point. This secondary sensation is often symmetrically transferred to the other side. This sensation is not only weak, but it has an inner movement. Spontaneous paraesthesias are present in these cases too. The sensation may be transferred from right to left as well as from left to right. We are dealing with the irradiation of primitive sensations to symmetrical points. Cases of that kind in tabes are not rare.

We come to the conclusion that spinal mechanisms connect two symmetrical points of the body. We also formulate the proposition that this primitive connection is especially a connection concerning sensations of a very primitive type.[2]

---

[1] This is another aspect of the problem which is generally called 'Schaltung', switching over. Magnus and his co-workers, Goldstein and Hoff and Schilder, have repeatedly drawn attention to the importance of the Schaltung in the motor field. Förster has pointed out that in the conduction of pain different passages are available and used according to the situation. The function uses the anatomy. This is another formulation of principles which are embodied in the gestalt theory and also in behaviorism. Both theories emphasize the situation as the unity to which the mechanical anatomy is only co-ordinated.

[2] In tabes cases, after-sensations are very often moved. Simple irritations may provoke the impression of complicated to-and-fro movements. At the

Just as there are connections between symmetrical sensory points by the spinal cord there are also close connections between the spinal motor innervations of both sides. According to Axel Owre, in incomplete transverse transections of the spinal cord, when there is a paraplegia in flexion, there is often a double flexion reflex to a one-sided irritation. In complete transverse lesions one finds mass reflexes, double flexion reflex, contraction of the abdominal muscles, evacuation of the bladder, and excessive perspiration as an answer to one-sided irritation.[1]

The postural model of the body also has its basis partially in spinal mechanisms. The connection between contralateral points is of course only a small part of the spinal apparatus and the spinal impulses, which afford the possibility of correlating the different perception impulses concerning localization and motility. I have mentioned that in tabes cases one touch may be felt in two different points in different localization and that there are very often moving after-sensations. In a case of alloaesthesia after an apoplectic lesion in the medulla oblongata, examined by Kramer, temperature and pain stimuli which were perceived as touch on the affected side were transferred to the unaffected side as prick, paraesthesia, or heat. It is at least possible that, in this case of Kramer's also, spinal mechanisms were responsible for the transfer from one side to the other. We may suppose also that in Kramer's case a blockade was responsible for the symmetrical transfer.

Another of Kramer's cases gives us deeper insight into the problem. This was a case of left-sided hemiplegia, troubles in the sensibility, and left-sided hemianopsia. The patient did not feel

same time straight lines drawn on the skin are very often felt as curves. Similar observations have been made by Stein, Weizsäcker, and Stengel. There are many other important changes in the perception of gestalten on the skin under the influence of spinal or more central lesions of the sensibility. According to one of my general theories, primitive sensations are always moved in the optic sphere as well as in the tactile sphere. Phenomena which are absolutely identical with the phenomena observed in central lesions of the sensibility can be observed according to Bromberg and Schilder in normal persons, when one studies the after-effects of tactile sensations, which we generally neglect.

[1] Leibowitz has carefully studied the contralateral irritation of the sole. In about one-third of normal subjects there can be observed on the contralateral side slight plantarflexion and supination of the foot, abduction of the little toe, plantarflexion of the lateral toes. The plantar reflex is certainly not only spinal; Leibowitz rightly draws attention to its relation to the crossed extensor reflex.

that he was paralysed. He ignored the left side of his body completely. His head was continually turned to the right, and his eyes also looked continually to the right. There was a remarkable tendency to euphoria with a tendency to punning, but no confusion and no disturbances in the memory. There is no question that in this case we have to do with a cortical lesion. It is at least probable that the same mechanism which prevents the patient from appreciating his hemiplegia and the whole left side of the body is also responsible for the transfer of the sensation from the one side of the body to the other. The patient, who does not want to know about one side of his body, transposes his sensations, since he has to acknowledge them, to the other side of his body. The case proves, at any rate, that there are cortical layers which are of importance for the building up of the body-image and for the differentiation between right and left. I said that the patient did not want to perceive one side of his body. Is this a fully conscious tendency? I do not believe so, but it could be an instinctive urge to overlook a useless part of the body. It would be a process of repression. If this interpretation is correct, we could explain the phenomenon by psychological methods alone. But we should keep in mind that the so-called purely psychic processes are at the same time organic processes of a specific character and complication. There are no psychic processes in which no brain-mechanisms are involved. But it is a brain-mechanism different from the so-called organic mechanisms, which reflect only into the psychic sphere. The destruction which encephalitis causes in the undeveloped brain provokes an enormous increase in motor activities. Children subject to it not only have an increase in motility, but also an increase in motor impulses. Psychic life builds itself up in different layers, which are connected with different plans of organization in the brain. Will may also play some part in Kramer's case of body-image imperception, and again this particular psychic attitude is connected with a massive organic lesion of the brain. But in order to come to a conclusion about Kramer's case and to a more exact formulation of the important psychological problem involved, we must analyse a group of cases in which similar phenomena have been observed.

(4) *Imperception of impairment of somatic functions*[1] *and of parts of the body-image (body-image imperception)*

There is an interesting group of cases who do not realize that they are blind, deaf, or paralysed. Anton was the first to draw attention to these phenomena of non-perception of one's own defects and to show their connection with localized lesions of the brain. The localized lesion causes a group of experiences to be excluded from the general consciousness. A part of the psychic life is amputated. Redlich and Bonvicini, who have very carefully studied a case of cortical blindness, point out the fact that their patient showed a particular type of general psychic change. He was not demented, but his general attitude was similar to the attitude of the so-called Korsakoff cases, in which the retention of memory is impaired. Cases of that type are in their opinion due not to a localized brain lesion, but to a more general impairment of cortical function. Albrecht supports Anton's point of view. Pötzl tries to mediate between the different opinions.

Let us start with the study of those hemiplegics who behave as if they were not paralysed. Some of those patients assert that their paralysed arm is as good as their other and that they can walk as well as they did before. When they are ordered to raise both arms, they of course move only the healthy one, but insist that they have raised the paralysed one too. Asked to raise the paralysed arm or shake hands with the paralysed hand, they perform the movement with the other arm and are convinced that they have succeeded in the task. In some cases the patients pay no attention to the paralysed side. They also remain indifferent if their attention is directed towards it. Some of them do not consider their paralysed limbs as limbs of their own. This occurred in one of Anton's cases and also in both of Pötzl's cases.

It is remarkable that most of the cases reported are concerned with the left side. Babinski especially has called attention to this fact. In one of Pötzl's cases a left-sided hemiplegia was connected with a complete left-sided hemianaesthesia for all qualities.

---

[1] Babinski has called this anosognosia, which means agnosia for disease (nosos).

[2] Recently Gamper has tried to ascribe the Korsakoff cases to a lesion at the basis of the third ventricle, especially of the corpora mamillaria; but there is not sufficient proof for his statement.

Orientation, speech, memory, and attention were good. There was often a delirium during the night. The patient behaved as if he knew nothing about his hemiplegia, or as if he had forgotten about it. He repeatedly tried to get up, found that he could not, but tried again a quarter of an hour later. He had a vivid impression that the limbs of his paralysed side were moving correctly. Numerous experiments gave Pötzl the impression that passive movements of the limbs provoked the sensations of movement; but that they did not reach the consciousness of the patient. He refused to look at his paralysed left side. If his paralysed arm was brought before his eyes, he would declare that it was the hand of another person, "probably from the patient nearby", or would say, "I don't know where it comes from; it is so long and lifeless and as dead as a snake". When he became delirious, he very often called his hemiplegic hand a long thick snake. He would also often complain that a strange person was on his left side in the bed and was trying to push him away. Asked to move the left side of his body, he did not move at all or moved the right arm and said that he had moved the left. The autopsy showed a destruction in the capsula interna and lesions in the gyrus supramarginalis. In Pötzl's second case, the patient felt his left hand estranged and separated from himself. The movements the patient was asked to make with his left hand were often performed with the right hand. In this case there was a left hemianopsia. The autopsy showed a superficial softening in the right parietal lobe, lesions in the occipital lobe, and a large softening in the right thalamus. There were also smaller lesions in the right pedunculus.

Pötzl draws attention to the tendency of his first case to look away to the right. In a case of Kramer's the whole body, eyes, and head were continually turned to the right side. The motor impulses thus conform with the total neglect of the left side and its paralysis, and are directed only to the side which the patient acknowledges. In the majority of cases reported so far the neglected side of the body shows trouble in the sensibility. Pinéas emphasizes that the findings in the autopsies are divergent and that almost the whole region of the brain behind the central gyrus might be of importance. Pötzl believes that the phenomenon is based upon the coincidence of lesions in the thalamus opticus and the parietal lobe. The great majority of the cases observed are cases in which the left hemiplegia or the left side of the body is not appreciated. But one should not generalize too much. In one of the cases I have observed the patient showed a severe right hemiplegia with disturbances, in the sensibility, of the cortical type. The patient would often look at her hand and leg and emphasize that these limbs were not her own limbs. She would say that her hand and face were swollen. Sometimes she also said that she had a fracture of the right arm and the right leg. We are dealing here with a case in which there is a non-perception of the right hemiplegia and of the right side of the body. It is remarkable that this patient looks rather freely at her right side, and is inclined to be interested in it (cf. Appendix 1, case *b*).

What makes these patients neglect their paralyses? What makes them disown one half of their bodies? We must return to the discussion of the psychic levels I have mentioned above. We may want to forget a defectiveness. We may want to suppress the thought that we are disabled, but the tormenting consciousness of the defect will still come back again and again. We may speak of the conscious psychic level. It is clear that in the cases mentioned this mechanism does not take place. But if we continue in our efforts, we may finally forget the difficulty, and then we shall be dealing with mechanism in which the conscious attitude has found sufficient support from the 'unconscious'. But then we find also a clear-cut psychic motive, which is fully understandable. This 'unconscious' motive may also occur without the preceding conscious wish. We will speak of the unconscious psychic level. It is not probable that we are dealing with the unconscious psychic level in our cases. If we were to deal with the unconscious wish, we should be dealing with cases of superimposed hysteria. Hysteria is the disease in which the unconscious wish leads to a changed perception and function of our body. There is no question that cases of that kind exist. Later on we shall discuss Jones's observations in full.

There may be a mechanism of forgetting that is based on organic disturbances of the memory. The Korsakoff cases with their inability to remember recent events exclude especially disagreeable experiences from their consciousness. This is a defence mechanism on an organic basis. Betlheim and Hartmann were able to show that the inability to remember sexual material is especially pronounced. I may add that Korsakoff cases with a polyneuritis often even forget that they are paralysed. We are dealing then in these peripheral paralyses with a phenomenon very similar to the phenomenon of non-perception of a hemiplegic extremity. Redlich and Bonvicini are justified therefore in supposing that such a mechanism can provoke the phenomena. This mechanism would be somewhat akin to phenomena of the unconscious wish. But still it is different. The unconscious wish is much deeper rooted if it is based on an organic lesion. I speak therefore of an organic repression[1] or of the effects of the organic unconsious. But Redlich and Bonvicini are mistaken in their opinion that all the cases of body-image imperception are based upon such mechanism.

It is remarkable that the organic unconscious repression is very often combined with changes in the mood. The patients show a particular type of euphoria and there is a tendency to punning. We have to do with a psychic attitude rooted in changes in the body. It is a general disturbance in the mechanism of the brain which is reflected in the psychic attitude. This attitude is similar to, but not identical with, the 'unconscious' attitudes of the so-called purely psychic character. But in the cases discussed here we are dealing with something different. There may be a psychic attitude more or less similar to the attitude in Korsakoff cases; but it is due not to a more or less general impairment of the cortical function, but to a localized lesion. It expresses itself only in connection with a particular limb and a particular part of the body. In other words, it is a focal mechanism and a focal organic repression that we are dealing with in these cases. I attribute a great importance to this formulation. When I use the term 'organic repression', I wish to emphasize that we are concerned with a phenomenon, which, on a structural level, repeats what is going on in other repressions in the so-called purely psychic level. This focal organic repression as well as organic repression generally very often carries with it psychic attitudes which are partially identical with the psychic

[1] I have introduced this term in a study with Hartmann on head injuries.

repression. This phenomenon is based on the deep community between the psychic life and the organic function. Every change in the organic function is liable to bring forth with it psychic mechanisms which are akin to this organic function. And this reflection into the psychic sphere will help us to understand the essence of the organic function.

I want to emphasize that in the majority of cases the psychic structures connected with organic repression, whether general or focal, will be of the type of a rather blind urge which is still more primitive than the unconscious wish. The principles involved here are not limited to the problem we are dealing with, but have to be applied to the whole field of cerebral activities. We deal with similar problems in the instinctive organic urge of hyperkinesis.[1] This hyperkinesis may be a hyperkinesis of the cortical level as in sensory aphasia, or it may be a hyperkinesis of a sub-cortical level as in post-encephalitis. Here, immediately, we find new questions. There exists a hyperkinesis of still more primitive structure, as in the epileptic attack. Even spinal lesions may lead to an increase in impulses. One may even ask whether the organic urge has not levels which are even outside the nervous system, and thence we come to the question of the urge in the organism generally in its relation to growth. These deepest levels do not, however, reflect into the consciousness. But we shall not insist upon the philosophical aspect, and shall restrict ourselves to the formulation that the organic urge and the organic repression are probably built up in manifold levels, and that even the focal organic urge and repression are not the deepest levels of the psychological functions connected with organic life.

Since we deal with the same basic phenomenon in the wishes and attitudes of the different levels, we shall not expect that all these functions will be isolated from each other. The focal organic attitude carries with it, as mentioned, unconscious wishes and even conscious ones. The same is true of the general organic attitude. When there is an urge to forget one half of the body, the patient will readily develop an unconscious and conscious wish in addition to the primitive urge. The deeper levels of attitudes carry with them those of higher levels. We may even ask whether

[1] Cf. my study on organic problems in child-guidance.

the deeper organic attitudes do not likewise carry with them specific psychosexual attitudes. Not only do the hypermotility of the post-encephalitic and the hypermotility of the epileptic fit express themselves in urges to actions, but also these urges often carry a specific psychosexual colouring. The post-encephalitic child becomes destructive and sadistic, and in the post-epileptic dreamy state general and specific destructive violence comes to the surface. We have, therefore, to ask what the specific psycho-sexual attitudes are which are connected with the focal repression of one half or of parts of the body. But we cannot deny that the opposite way is also open. I have mentioned that the conscious wish very often provokes appropriate unconscious tendencies. The conscious wish brings forth similar attitudes out of the un-conscious. But there can again be no doubt that these conscious and unconscious attitudes are not in the air. They are going on in the body, carry with them organic activities, and may be con-nected with the processes of generalized and focal attitudes. The four types of attitude are therefore closely interwoven with each other, and every attitude carries traces of the other attitudes in itself. It will therefore be our particular task to study the psycho-genic non-perception of one half of the body; those cases, which, according to Jones, are true achiria and allochiria. But I desire to emphasize that we are again dealing with a general problem of wide range.

In the foregoing remarks I have emphasized the close relation between perception and action. Every perception is connected with an attitude and every perception has its motility. Pötzl has pointed out that cases of non-perception of one half of the body very often look away from their bodies. This is certainly not true in every case. In four of the Pinéas cases there is no par-ticular tendency to turn the head away from the paralysed side. Only in his first case is there a conjugate deviation to the right side. It is remarkable that in this case there is not only an allo-aesthesia for tactile impressions, but the subject also sees on the right side objects that are offered to him on the left side. In addition the tactile objects put into his left hand are felt in the right hand. Optic alloaesthesia is here connected with the tactile alloaesthesia.[1] But I am convinced that in left-sided non-perception the motor impulses to the right side play an important part, since, according to Hoff and Schilder, every conjugate deviation carries with it impulses of the whole body to turn to the side of the deviation. But in my case of right-sided non-perception the patient is absolutely free in her motor impulses to look to the right side.

Before I attempt the interpretation of these contradictory findings, I wish to draw attention to the observation of an important case (case *c* in Appendix).[1] In this case the patient had a marked tendency of the left side of the body to become transferred to the right side. The left leg was often crossed over the right leg. Accordingly, the patient, when asked for the left limbs, used the right limbs. He had somehow lost the knowledge and use of his left side. His left arm was hardly used at all in spite of the fact that there was no paresis. Touches on the left side were called by him touches on the right side, though often he would point correctly to the point touched. His alloaesthesia therefore was not based upon a real transfer of sensations, but upon the loss of the appreciation of the left side, which was turned away by motor impulses over to the right side.

This makes it clear that in alloaesthesia one may deal with a transfer of sensations as such or with the transfer of one half of the body schema. Sensation may in this latter case even remain in its proper place. The motor impulses, which try to turn the body round the longitudinal axis, have, according to Hoff and Schilder and also to Gerstmann, one of their centres in the parietal-occipital lobe; or, more accurately, the lesion of the parietal-occipital lobe (probably of Brodmann's field 19, in particular) increases the postural impulses to turn round the longitudinal axis. Whenever there is a turning impulse of this kind the postural model of the body accompanies it, or, generally, impulses to turn round the longitudinal axis carry with them the postural model of the body. Pötzl has developed similar theories. But there immediately arises the question why the motor impulses are intact in some cases of alloaesthesia and non-perception. We have

[1] Herrmann and Pötzl have carefully discussed the problem of optic alloaesthesia, based on autoptic findings. They point out that there is a close relation between optic and tactile alloaesthesia.

apparently to differentiate between a more sensory type which is represented by the first of our cases and the type in which the motor impulses turn the postural model of the body, and with it the sensations, to the other side. The non-perception of one half of the body can also be based upon a motor tendency to look away, but, instead of the motor tendency, there can be only the inner tendency to neglect the impressions coming from this side. We should not forget that alloaesthesia and non-perception of the paralysis of one half of the body are not identical phenomena; they are only allied to each other.

(5) *Alloaesthesia, non-perception, right and left, synaesthesia in the body-schema*

We have gained the following formulations:

(1) Alloaesthesia can be based upon anatomical connections between symmetrical parts of the body.

(2) This connection can be a connection in the spinal cord.

(3) The blocking of the normal pathway and the overflowing very probably play an important part.

(4) Alloaesthesia can probably also be based upon an anatomical connection in higher levels.

(5) The transfer of sensations can be a part phenomenon in the lack of acknowledgement of one side of the body.

(6) The transfer can be, but need not be, in connection with motor impulses.

(7) The neglect of impressions of one half of the body and the non-perception of one half of the body may occur without a tendency to transfer the impulses to the other side.

(8) It can be based upon mechanisms of the so-called purely psychic type (conscious or unconscious), but it can also be based on organic mechanisms (organic repressions), which are akin to the psychological mechanisms.

(9) This organic repressive mechanism can be a general one (Korsakoff), but it can also be a mechanism based upon focal lesions. This is the mechanism which is present in the cases studied.

(10) The organic repression may either lead to overlooking

the hemiplegia ; (we are then concerned with Babinski's anosognosia) ; or it may lead to the total neglect of this side of the body. It may finally lead to illusions and distortions concerning the perceptiou of this side.

(11) In the majority of those cases, disturbances of the sensibility are present, which point to a serious lesion in the sensory apparatus. But beyond that, there is a disturbance in the special parietal mechanism, the integrity of which secures the tactile postural model of the body.

This discussion would be incomplete, if we did not try to account for the reason why, in the majority of the cases, the left side of the body is affected. Hauptmann is of the opinion that the postural model of the body has its localization chiefly in the left hemisphere. In this respect, the left hemisphere would be leading over the right. But in the cases so far studied, we deal with a right-sided lesion of the brain, and these cases point on the contrary to right-sided centres for the left side of the body.   If Hauptmann's theory were correct, we should expect that the right anosognosia would be accompanied by a lesser left-sided anosognosia. But the case presented shows that this assumption is incorrect. One might assume that only centres in the right hemisphere have a sufficiently close relation to central emotional activities. Hirschl has developed the idea, which is favoured by Pötzl,[1] that the right hemisphere has a special influence on vegetative functions. But the material which could prove this contention is insufficient. Thus we have to look for a more psychological interpretation.

It seems that human beings generally make more use of the right side of their body. The right side of the body is not only stronger, but is also more 'dexterous'. Also the tonic impulses are stronger on the right side. Our whole motor impulses go more easily to the right side. When the hands are outstretched and the eyes closed, the right arm generally rises higher than the left. The neck reflexes are stronger on the right side than on the left. When the hunter in the desert or in fog loses his orientation and after describing a circle comes back to the place he started from, it will generally be a circle to the right side. When hands and fingers are doubly crossed and a movement of a specific finger is

[1] In the book on 'Worttaubheit'.

ordered, it is much simpler to move a finger of the right hand than one of the left hand. There is somehow a physiological tendency in everybody to neglect the left side of the body. This physiological tendency is certainly the expression of physiological differences in the apparatus described. It will probably not be so easy to overcome this physiological tendency to neglect the left side of the body, and most of the focal lesions will not be able to have this effect. The same focal lesion added to the physiological tendency to neglect the left side will provoke the picture of non-perception of the left side of the body. In this respect it is remarkable that according to the literature on the subject non-perception concerning the left arm is more common than non-perception of the left leg. We generally feel the superiority of the right arm much more than we feel the superiority of the right leg, if we feel it at all. The focal non-perception of the left side of the body is therefore the exaggeration of an attitude which we normally have towards the left side of the body. One sees immediately that focal lesions can help general psychic attitudes to come to a clearer expression.

We deal at any rate in those cases with an impairment of the cortical apparatus and of the tactile cortical part of the image of the body. This expression should not mislead us. Our patient with the right-sided non-perception says that her arm looks different, that it is swollen. The changed tactile impression brings with it a change in the optic field also. It is not the case that the schema of the body has two different parts, the one optic and the other tactile. It is in its essence a synaesthesia. But we should not forget that every sensation is generally synaesthetic. This means that there does not exist any primary isolation between the different senses. The isolation is secondary. We perceive and we may with some difficulty decide that one part of the perception is based upon the optic impressions. The synaesthesia, therefore, is the normal situation. The isolated sensation is the product of an analysis. In the scheme of the body tactile-kinaesthetic and optic impulses can only be separated from each other by artificial methods. What we have studied is the change in the unity of the postural model of the body by change in the sensation of the tactile and optic sphere. The nervous system acts as a unit according to the total situation. The unit of perception is the object which presents itself through the senses and through *all* the senses. Perception is synaesthetic. There is no question that the object 'body' presents itself to all senses.

(6) *Some remarks about the relation of the body schema to tactile—kinaesthetic movements*

We have not discussed as yet some of the problems connected with the tactile postural model of the body. The first case I have mentioned (Appendix 1) very often did not know whether a movement had been made on her skin or whether one of her limbs was moved. The same was true about our second case. Head and Holmes have made similar observations. It seems therefore that a given perception does not have any definite quality which characterizes it as coming from a movement on the skin or from one of a limb. Only the circumstances and the structure of the postural model of the body determine the elaboration of a stimulus in this respect. According to von Frey, there are no deep sensations coming from the joints and only the special configuration of stimuli on the skin leads us to the perception of passive movements of our limbs. But at any rate the postural model of the body-image determines the localization of the limbs in space, the relative position of two stimuli, and also the differentiation between a movement on the skin and a movement of a limb. This leads immediately to an allied problem. Our first case did not perceive movements on her skin. She felt instead a single touch or several simultaneous touches. Sometimes, as mentioned, she felt, instead of the movements on the skin, a movement in her joints. Apparently, movements get their final meaning only in connection with the postural model of the body, but it is more than probable that there also exists more primitive apparatus, the integrity of which is necessary for the perception of movement. But one could at least compare the non-perception of movement in the tactile cases with the non-perception of movement in optic cases observed by Pötzl and Redlich and Goldstein and Gelb.

(7) *Agnosia concerning the body-image (autotopagnosia)*;
fingeragnosia

Pathology shows us cases that cannot be called cases of an optic or tactile disturbance, but cases in which the postural model as such is disturbed. Patients of this kind are helpless when they are asked to show parts of their own body. When Pick saw his first case of this kind, the patient first sought her left ear on the table. Only upon the repetition of the order did she grasp her left ear. She did not succeed in finding her left eye and finally said : " I don't know, I must have lost it." When she was asked to show her hands, she tried to find them on the table and said : " nowhere, for heaven's sake ; I have lost them, but they must be somewhere." But the orientation of right and left was also lost. She did not know if there was right or left on her own body. When the patient made her movements she was able to orient herself better. The orientation on head and back, parts which are generally outside the optic perception, was extremely poor. In most of Pick's cases there was a diffuse disease of the brain.

Similarly in cases of Rosenberg's, who concentrated his attention on the difficulties these patients show in the orientation between left and right. Rosenberg emphasizes especially that the disturbance spreads also into the field of action. One of Pick's cases showed disturbances in grasping objects. He reached either behind or to the right or to the left side of the object. Pick has shown that these disturbances in localization are due to bilateral lesion of the parietal lobe, which is confirmed by observations of Anton and F. Hartmann.

Pötzl has lately observed a difficulty in the choice between right and left in connection with a lesion of the left lower parietal lobe. The patient did not know where her right and left hand were. She also made mistakes when instructed to go to the left or right side of the room. Pötzl writes: "The uncertainty between right and left could not be considered, strictly speaking, either as a motor or as a pure sensory disturbance. It appeared as a continual change of sensory deficiencies in motor ones via special disturbances in feelings which occurred only when the patient had to choose between an action with the left or right hand. In the extreme case of a more amnestic character the patient declared she could not feel which was her right hand and which her left. She said she had forgotten. In the extreme case, where the disturbance resembled a passing paralysis, she declared herself unable to move her paralysed hand. This happened in the right hand as well as in the left. But later on she performed the movements she was asked to do with the left or right hand and said, 'It came into her mind where the hand was, and that made the paralysis pass.' In between these two extreme reactions were actions where the patient declared that with the uncertainty of right and left there developed a heaviness in her hand. The whole disturbance was rather similar to the grasping paralysis of some apractics (Liepmann), but differed from it in the clear co-ordination to the uncertainty in the right and left perception, whereas the grasping paralysis of apractics occurs only when they are asked to choose a specific object out of a variety of objects".

But the clearest instance of a disturbance in the postural model of the body proper is offered in the finger agnosia described by Gerstmann. Cases of that kind are unable to recognize and name the different fingers of the hand. They are also unable to indicate specific fingers. They show the same difficulties concerning the hands and fingers of other persons. This difficulty is always connected with a difficulty in recognition of right and left on one's own body, a difficulty in writing (agraphia), and difficulties in calculating (acalculia). The syndrome is not very rare. I have myself observed three cases besides the cases in Gerstmann's first two publications. There are always difficulties in actions connected with the difficulties in a perception. It is remarkable that all these cases do not show any particular difficulties in the perception of other parts of the body. Pötzl and Herrmann localize the syndrome in the region between the gyrus angularis and the second occipital convolution. Lange's case points to a similar localization. Lesions of the left side of the hemisphere provoke the syndrome. Only in Pötzl and Herrmann's case was the syndrome caused by a tumour on the right side. But the patient was ambidextrous. We can draw the general conclusion that there exists indeed a superiority of the left hemisphere over the right, also concerning the postural model of the body or at least concerning the fingers in the postural model.

We could interpret the coincidence between finger agnosia and agraphia (inability to write irrespective of the preserved sensibility and motility of the fingers) as due to the necessity of knowing about our fingers when we write. And one could surmise that correct writing is dependent on the integrity of the postural model of the body. But there is at least the possibility that both disturbances are localized in parts of the brain which are near to each other. The coincidence between acalculia and finger agnosia could be due to the fact that primitive mathematical operations are at first performed on the fingers.[1] But I do not believe that we are dealing with actual psychological connections. It is much more probable that between finger agnosia, writing, and calculating exist some inner similarities which are responsible for the localizations in parts of the brains near to each other. We know that in the brain those functions that have some inner connection with each other are generally localized near each other. The sensory

---

[1] Every book on primitive thinking mentions the fact that counting and numbers and our whole system of numeration are in close relation with and have a close reference to parts of the body. In British New Guinea, for instance, we find the following system used in reckoning (Lévy-Bruhl, *How Natives Think*, p. 186):

(1) monou—little finger of the left hand.
(2) reere—next finger.
(3) kaupu—middle finger.
(4) moreere—index.
(5) aira—thumb.
(6) ankora—wrist.
(7) mirika mako—between wrist and elbow.
(8) na—elbow.
(9) ara—shoulder.
(10) ano—neck.
(11) ame—left breast.
(12) unkari—chest.
(13) amenekai—right breast.
(14) ano—right side of the neck, etc.

It is remarkable that in most of these systems the toes do not play any particular part. We must not forget the particular motility of the fingers. In the system of numeration mentioned here, besides the fingers only those parts of the body which can be reached easily by the hands are of importance. We shall see later that in the construction of the body-image the fingers and the hand help in the exploration of the body. The idea of multiplicity is probably closely connected with speculation about the multiplicity of the body and a continual experimentation we undertake on the body. The fingers are not only protruding parts, but are also under the special influence of our intentions. They are in some way among the first objects on which we act. But I do not think that these rather sketchy remarks exhaust the problem of systems of numeration.

area shows an organization very similar to the motor area of the cortex, and the motor and sensory points for a particular part of the body are near each other.

Lange has developed the theory that we have to do with a general disturbance in the perception of direction. But the patients have a very good perception concerning other directions and space. They have no difficulties in the perception of direction in reading. I do not believe, therefore, that these formulations of Lange's are justified by the facts. One may of course ask why disturbances in the postural model of the body are so extremely rare concerning other parts of the body. It might be that agnosia of the fingers is connected with a particular spot which can be injured in an isolated way. It is possible that the other parts of the postural model of the body have relations to other parts of the brain, the isolated lesion of which is not possible. When there is an apraxia, it is indeed almost impossible to find out whether there is an agnosia concerning these parts of the body also. The finger agnosia could be due to a particular localization of this part of the postural model of the body. The other possible interpretation is that differentiating the fingers is a particularly difficult task. Investigations by Freeman, which are not finished yet, show that children develop the complete knowledge of the fingers and their use rather late. The finger agnosia then would be the most complicated function in the recognition of the body and therefore could be more easily disturbed than any other function. But whatever the interpretation may be, it certainly is possible to speak of localization of the postural model of the body and to assert again that the postural model of the body has its specific access to the motility. We deal with true agnosias, not with those concerning a special sensory impression, but with those concerning an object of particular importance, the body-image.

(8) Interrelations of the body-image

Whenever there are disturbances in the postural model of the body, the patients also have difficulty in recognizing the different parts of the bodies of others. They cannot distinguish between their fingers; they cannot recognize the left and right side of the bodies of others. We arrive at the general formulation that the postural models of human beings are connected with each other and that where we are not able to come to a true perception of our own body, we are also unable to perceive the bodies of others. One may question if the difficulty in recognizing the different parts of the bodies of others is not primary and the difficulty in recognizing parts of our own body secondary. But there would still remain the question why the postural model of our own body cannot be built up in spite of the fact that we have more data concerning our own body. In addition to this, the disturbances concerning our own body are mostly stronger than the disturbances concerning the postural model of the bodies of others. I have to mention also that the non-perception of our own body and its defectiveness is limited to our own body. There is also convincing evidence that the difficulty in the perception of our own body precedes the difficulty in the perception of the bodies of others. But we still point to the deep community between the postural models of human beings. The disturbance may go even further, and persons with non-perception of the left side of the body may be unable to be orientated in the left side of space.

Pinéas has published an observation on this point. It concerns a patient with senile dementia (memory difficulties, disorientation in space and time). But the patient shows also a peculiar disturbance in acting, difficulties in reading of words (verbal alexia), inability to write (total agraphia) and an inability to build little figures and structures (constructive apraxia), finger agnosia and inability to calculate, total non-perception of the left side of the body and the left side of the room, and consecutive disturbances in the recognition of right and left. The patient is perfectly familiar with the connotation of the word 'left.' She knows that there exist a left and a right ear, eye, leg, and arm. She is unable to indicate the right arm or the right ear of a person sitting opposite to her. She also has alloaesthesia. I do not think that the disturbance in the perception of the left side of space follows immediately out of her difficulties in the postural model of the body. If this were so, it would be impossible to explain why the majority of alloaesthesia cases show no disturbances in the orientation in space.   Orientation in space is again an independent function, which is only allied to the left and right orientation on the body. We deal probably with a different cerebral apparatus concerning the direction on one's own body. I do not wish to deny that these functions are linked with each other and have many elements in common, but still there are independent functions. One of Herrmann's observations shows an independent disturbance concerning outside space, especially concerning the union between the left side and the right side of the space. We come to the general conclusion that there are many specific functions in the brain, which are based upon specific apparatus. That within this specific apparatus there exist connections is beyond doubt. But still the phenomena are, basically at least, partially independent of each other.

(9) *Apraxia and agnosia in their relations to the schema of the body*

When the knowledge of our own body is incomplete and faulty, all actions for which this particular knowledge is necessary will be faulty too. We need the body-image in order to start movements. We need it especially, when actions are directed towards our own body. Every trouble in gnosia and in perception generally will lead to a change in the action. We have again and again emphasized the close relation between the perceptive (afferent-impressive) side of our psychic life and the motor (afferent-expressive) activities. Consequently peripheral changes in the sensibility must lead to disturbances in actions. Central disturbances like agnosias will also be disturbances of actions.

In a case I have described with Isakower the patient suffered from an optic agnosia and had particular difficulties in differentiating her fingers. All her finger actions were accordingly clumsy, and often the wrong finger was chosen. But this disturbance in the praxia is not what we usually call apraxia. Pötzl in particular has stated that finger agnosia is in its essence a finger apraxia. I cannot endorse his point of view. The term apraxia was introduced by Liepmann into scientific literature. It is characteristic of the apractic that he knows what he ought to do. He has the complete knowledge and in some cases can express it by words, while in others he can show the theoretical knowledge of what he should do by the actions of the unaffected parts of the body. His difficulties are, at least supposedly, present in spite of an intact perceptive and agnostic faculty.

One can also speak of apraxia only when this disturbance in the movement is not due to paresis, tension, or disturbance in co-ordination. When such a patient tries to light a match, he may take the matchbox in his fingers and press it with his thumb and index finger in spite of the fact that he has full knowledge of the object. Even if helped by having the matchbox opened for him, he will not profit by this. He now touches the wrong side of the box. When he finally succeeds in taking a match, he strikes it on the broad side of the box, putting it flatly on the box. When given the lighted match, he cannot bring it near a candlestick. Given an unlighted match, he may try to light the candle in spite of the fact that he knows the match is not lit.

Disturbances of that type may occur in one half of the body. Apraxia is the inability to use the knowledge of objects in an action in spite of the fact that this knowledge can be expressed in words or with the action of unaffected limbs. Whereas even the finger agnosia is a comparatively rare occurrence, and other isolated agnosias concerning the body hardly even known,[1] the inability to use the knowledge of one's own body (body-image) in action is a rather common occurrence. Patients who can handle objects without manifest disturbances are often unable to show parts of their body. For the most part they also have difficulties in expressive movements like waving, threatening, and swearing, when they are asked to perform these actions at command. Sometimes they also have difficulties when they are asked to act on imagined objects, for instance, to catch a fly when there is no fly present. Nevertheless, the difficulty in finding their own nose and eyes is outstanding. It is a disturbance of actions towards one's own body. Liepmann has called actions of this kind reflexive actions, and I would call an apraxia of this type reflexive apraxia. Many of those cases cannot choose the right or left arm at command, in spite of the fact that they know perfectly well which is the left and which is the right side of their body. Often they act with both limbs simultaneously when they are asked to move

[1] Engerth has described cases in which autotopagnosia affecting the face was connected with finger agnosia.

either the right or the left side. They also make so-called associated movements on the other side.

There exists a particular type of contralateral associated movements, which have in many respects the characteristics of voluntary movements and are therefore different from contralateral associated movements of a different origin. These mechanisms become especially clear when isolated movements of fingers are requested. In spite of the fact that in the pronounced cases the patients are able to name their fingers, they are not able to move a specific finger according to their intention. They are apt to move another finger instead, and often they move a finger on the other hand, either simultaneously or even on the wrong side only. I have called this phenomenon 'finger apraxia'.

Finger apraxia is an almost regular occurrence in any kind of apraxia. Even in the object apraxia, when there is an apraxia for objects, there is almost invariably reflexive apraxia also present, and in this reflexive apraxia the finger apraxia and the left and right difficulty are always outstanding. When a reflexive apraxia is disappearing, the finger apraxia remains as the last sign. Finger apraxia is also present before any other signs of apraxia appear. It has, therefore, an important diagnostic significance.

Finger apraxia must be differentiated from difficulties in isolated movements of the fingers in paralysis or in extra-pyramidal disturbances. In choreics, the phenomenon may show some similarity, but generally it will be easy to make the necessary differentiations. Reflexive apraxia is, therefore, the apractic counterpart of the agnosia concerning the body-image. One may even go further and say that the not uncommon tendency of apractics to make no use of one side of the body in actions is the counterpart of the non-perception of one part of the body. There are certainly cases in which the disturbance is stronger on one side than on the other side as, for example, in case 10 of my first publication, in which the patient usually made mistakes when he was asked to move the fingers of the left, apractic side. B. Schlesinger has observed a case of constructive apraxia in which the patient was able to move a specific finger, but was unable to imitate postures of the fingers. The disturbance was more expressed on the one side than on the other.

I have not yet sufficiently stressed the difficulty shown by many patients with reflexive apraxia. They are unable to transfer from the one side of the body to the other. They incur special difficulties when they are asked to show their left ear or eye with the right hand and *vice versa*. Pick and Rosenberg have drawn attention to this disturbance.

In the postural model of the body the middle line certainly plays a specific part. There can be no question that the middle line of the head is different from that of other parts of the body. Patients, who are unable to cross the middle line in the region of the head, are quite well able to show their left knee with their right hand and *vice versa*. The psychological middle line and the geometrical middle line are certainly not identical with each other. The middle line of the body, of course, finds its continuation into external space. The disturbance in the crossed grasping is sometimes also present in external space and can, as in one of Herrmann's cases, be even limited to external space. I must repeat that external space and the body-image are certainly related to each other, but they are connected with separate functions of the brain. In Herrmann's case a parietal occipital lesion was present.

It is remarkable that all the difficulties in grasping the parts of one's own body are mostly accompanied by difficulties in grasping the parts of the bodies of others. We meet again the principle of the connections between body-images. In these apractic cases, this is very clearly expressed, since these patients very often reach for the nose, eye, or ear of the examiner, when asked to show their own. But I again think that the disturbance in one's own body is usually stronger. I have observed a case in which a patient with sensory aphasic symptoms showed severe apraxia on making movements towards her own body. She was unable to imitate crossed movements. Often she pointed to the body of the examiner, when she was supposed to show her own ear, eyes, nose, etc. The opposite was much less frequent. If she was supposed to point to her eye, she first went to the middle line and from there proceeded to her eye. Once, instead of pointing to her eye, she pointed to the bridge of the examiner's nose. She always had a tendency to deviate either to her own middle line or to that of the examiner, without differentiating well between these two middle lines. Below the head, she crossed the middle line very easily and deviated even too much to the lateral side. The patient showed very little reaction to pain in the upper part of her body. The observation shows that in parietal cases the tendency to the middle line can be increased, whereas actions lateral from the middle line meet with difficulties.

Head in his studies on aphasia has observed disturbances similar to those described here as reflexive apraxia. He used the following test. The patient has to show either with his right or left hand the right or left eye or ear. Many patients make more or less serious mistakes. According to Head, a good understanding for words is necessary for this test. But the same mistake is made also, when one sits opposite the patient and makes the same movements and orders the patient to imitate with the right hand what the examiner does with his right hand. If one is standing behind the patient and the patient sees the movements in a mirror before him, he is quite well able to imitate the movements of the examiner. According to Head, this difference is based on the fact that the patient needs a verbalization, when he is asked to imitate the movement of the examiner opposite to him. When he imitates the movements in the mirror, the patient can imitate without verbalization. It is, of course, possible that some of Head's patients had difficulties in verbalization. But there is no question that in the great majority of cases these difficulties are based on inability to use the body-image for an action. The difficulty in verbalization may be an additional factor. But we should make it clear that the greater the difficulty in the function, the more outstanding will be the difficulties in verbalization.

Pötzl has remarked that an agnostic disturbance may even appear as a circumscribed aphasia. The word certainly has a close relation to the function. And, when there are agnostic difficulties concerning colours the patient sometimes only has difficulty in naming the colours. When one observes these cases, as Pötzl has done, on successive days, the disturbance may appear one day as a difficulty in naming the colour and on another day as a difficulty in recognizing it. The difficulty in naming is therefore the expression of an actual difficulty in the function and is not merely

D

aphasic. When Goldstein and Gelb consider amnesia for the names of colours as a difficulty in thinking in clear-cut categories, they also bring the localized aphasias in connection with specific functions. But one should separate these disturbances from aphasic disturbances. The hesitation in naming is in these cases only the expression of a difficulty in a specific function. I do not think, therefore, that we have the right to bring the disturbance as described here in connection with aphasic troubles. The difficulty in verbalization is only the expression of a difficulty in the function of using the body-image in a correct way.

(10) *Remarks on human action*

We cannot deny that a deeper insight into the structure of the body-image (postural model of the body) must lead to a new conception of human actions. The greatest progress that has been made so far in the understanding of a human action is due to Liepmann's investigations. He has shown that every action is based on an anticipatory plan. This anticipatory plan has a specific structure. It not only contains the final aim, but also comprises the insight into the single actions which are necessary for the actualization of the plan. Liepmann refers to ' Teilzielvorstellungen' (images of partial aims), which have to be actualized in a final performance of the action. This general plan for the action and every detail of the plan have to be transposed into an innervation.

We deal with an apraxia when the patient is able to work out the general plan, but is unable to transform the plan into action. When a disorder in the performance of this general plan occurs, we are dealing with an ideatory apraxia. Then the order of the detail actions may be disturbed. When the detail performances are disturbed, we have an apraxia of the motor type. In a motor apraxia the disturbance can be nearer to the purely motor execution: we speak then of the innervatory type of motor apraxia.

Liepmann speaks of the plan and of images, but the term image means to him not only that which is clearly represented in the psychic sphere, but the organic trace also. But here we are less interested in the pathology of movement; we are more interested in the psychology of movement. There is no question that such a plan exists. But it would be wrong to believe that this plan exists in the full light of consciousness. The plan is not given in clear representations and images. When we want to move our arm, when we want to grasp an object, when we want to light a match, there is no question that very little of the necessary actions and innervations is in our mind. We are not clear which part of the body we want to move. We are also not clear to which particular part of the object our action will be directed. The plan for the movement is given as a germ, as undeveloped psychic knowledge, as a mere thought in the sense of the Wuertzburg school of psychology, or in Ach's terminology as a ' Bewusstheit.' We are dealing with a knowledge in which the sensual elements play little or no part (' Bewusstheiten ').

It is an important part of general psychology that our psychic life is only in small part based upon fully conscious perceptions and images. There are tendencies. We feel a psychic direction, a psychic stream, an intention going forward towards an aim. We do not know clearly, but still we have an instinctive insight where this intention may lead to.

There is no question that these intentions are inner directions, drives, and tensions in a field in which there is on one side the ego and on the other side the object, the world. In the language of the gestalt psychology, we are dealing here with tensions in a psychic field. There is no question that this germ of the plan to a movement finds its development only during the performance of the action, and the sensations provoked by the action will have a developing influence on the plan.

In this plan the knowledge of one's own body is an absolute necessity. There must always be the knowledge that I am acting with my body, that I have to start the movement with my body, that I have to use a particular part of my body. But in the plan there must also be the aim of my actions. There is always an object towards which the action is directed. This aim may be one's own body or it may be an object in the outside world. In order to act, we must know something about the quality of the object of our intention. And, finally, we must also know in what

way we want to approach the object. The formula contains therefore the image of the limb or of the part of the body which is
performing the movement. It may remain undecided whether
this image will be a clear one. An intellectual knowledge is
certainly, as pathology proves, insufficient. (The apractics know
what they should do, but still they cannot do it.) But it could be
a living thought, a Bewusstheit, in the sense mentioned above.
The patients of Goldstein and Gelb with their serious impairment
in the development of optic representations were unable to start
the movements.

It seems that either an optic perception or an optic image is
necessary for the beginning of a movement. But this formulation
would be erroneous, if by image we mean only an image of the
full consciousness. There are many people who do not have optic
images in the proper sense but are still able to begin a movement,
even with closed eyes. But normal persons without optic images
still have optic thoughts, or what I would like to call subliminal
optic representations, or living optic thinking. Martin attaches
special importance to the kinaesthetic impressions and images,
but she also considers that, at least for the beginning of the
movement, optic representations are of importance. We know
also that when an actual movement has once started it will go on
with less images. But are they really absent then? I do not believe
it. They must be present in traces, but I do not think that these
traces have no psychic representations. I think rather that they
are present in the psyche as primitive Bewusstheiten, as germs to
representations which could be developed. When an optic image
is not present, it can be at least in readiness. According to
G. E. Müller, most human beings use optic or acoustico-motor
representations, according to the circumstances.

At the beginning of any movement the optic picture seems to
be of special importance. In Goldstein and Gelb's case
kinaesthetic impressions can be partially substituted for it. In the
Japanese illusion (double crossing and intertwining of fingers)
which makes the optic picture so complicated that it cannot be
used for orientation, small movements help to the building up
of a correct postural body-image, which is necessary for the
beginning of the movement of a specific finger. Generally

speaking, the beginning of every movement is dependent on the model of the body, and it seems that the different sources of the schema of the body can be substituted for each other at least in some degree. It will also be important that the whole body gets ready for this part of the movement, and also the choice of the plans of the action will occur in this preparatory stage of the movement. According to Goldstein, this choice of the plan of the action is chiefly dependent on optic impressions and representations. But the plans of the actions will be chosen in close relation to the total model of the body.

In the plan of the movement there must be also the knowledge of the aim of the movement, at least if we deal with actions and not with purely expressive movement. Every action is directed towards something. The object can be seen, can be touched; it can be given in representations of the optic, tactile, or acoustic sphere; or it may even be given by images in readiness. According to the general principles evolved above, isolated senses do not exist. We are always directed towards objects which are given to us with their optic as well as tactile and acoustic qualities. These qualities may be given by perceptions, or by images, or by images in readiness. There arises the question whether a plan of a movement is ever given without the tendency to movement. We come again to the general formulation that whatever may go on in the sensory field will bring with it a specific motility. The germ of the plan and the plan itself will have a special tendency to be transformed into a full movement. It is not clear as yet how much of the way of the movement and of the type of the movement is given with the plan for the movement. We also do not know which part of the project is actuated after the start of the movement. But I do not think that whatever occurs in the organic field of the movement is without any reflection in the consciousness.

According to Martin, the part played by images is small when once the movement has started. When we start a movement, we must first decide which side we want to make the movement. When the body-image is disturbed, we shall not be able to make the right differentiation and we shall choose the wrong side for the start of the movement. But we may even be certain about the side with which we want to start and still not be able to use this knowledge in action. The experiences reported so far make it clear that the choice of the particular muscle or limb is also dependent on the postural model of the body. We know how often recruits are unable to make a correct choice between left and right. It is not so much that they do not know the difference between right and left as that they are not able to use their knowledge in action.

It is remarkable that in Goldstein's observations as well as my own the difficulties in choosing the correct side and the correct limb are much greater when the patients are not acting under the tension of an object in the field of vision. Many of these cases can manipulate an object quite well with both hands, but they fail when they have to show the right or the left finger. Again the recruit may fail when he is ordered to look to the left or right side, but he does not fail so easily when he is ordered to take some action in regard to an object in his right or left visual field.

Martin's normal subjects were often disturbed at the beginning of a movement by images and intentions concerning the other part of the body. When Martin ordered a left-handed subject with optic representations to move the right hand or leg at the beginning of a movement, she often felt inclined to raise the left extremities under the influence of kinaesthetic representations. The optic image corrected the sensory impulse. I must again draw attention to the Japanese illusion, in which the subjects often make a movement with the wrong side of their body, but correct it under the influence of tactile and kinaesthetic sensations. We arrive at the conclusion that the beginning of a movement is a very active process. The limb with which the movement has to start does not offer itself spontaneously; it has to be found out, and an active process of probing sets in, in which perception of any field is used according to the actual situation.[1]

[1] I have often mentioned the so-called Japanese illusion. When one crosses one elbow above the other and intertwines the fingers and thumbs around the hands again, one has before the eye another complicated picture of the fingers. If the subject is now ordered by pointing to move a specific finger, he is very often unable to do so. He moves either the next finger or the finger of the opposite hand. The subject is always able to move a specific finger, if that finger is touched. Mistakes with the left hand are more common than with the right hand. The difficulties with the third and fourth fingers are

The way in which we start a movement gives us a deep insight into the activity of the mind. The knowledge of the existence and uses of a limb is not given by a physiological process. But we have at first a vague, general knowledge. That such a knowledge exists becomes clear through the fact of the so-called absolute localization. When a finger is touched in the posture of the Japanese illusion, the clear-cut optic picture appears connected with an area of tactile sensation. We know the point in space which has been touched, but are not aware in what way this feeling and the represented space have to be brought in connection with the other part of the body. It seems to float in space. But still, there is a knowledge (Bewusstheit) that it belongs to one's own body and that one will be able to work out the exact relation. The development therefore is from a vague knowledge to concrete perception until the final sensual insight has been reached. One goes through a very active process. It might be called a method of trial and error. But we must keep in mind that we are dealing with an active choice, taking up a new piece of experience, and seeing how it fits. It is rejected if it does not fit. We are dealing with an active, psychic choice, which is only possible when new experiences are continually acquired by contact with the object, in this case the human body. The observations of Goldstein and Gelb and those of Klein and Schilder on the Japanese illusion should be sufficient to ensure the rejection of any theory which supposes that complicated units of experience, gestalten, wander into the individual's mind. They contradict the gestalt theories of the type that Wertheimer, Köhler, and Koffka have developed. Experience is an active process. Wertheimer, Köhler, and Koffka believe in the development of gestalten, but they think that these developments go on by the

greater than with the other fingers. Klein and I have found that the body-image has to be built up again, when by the double-twisting the optic and tactile sensations have lost their clear structure. By introspective methods, it is not difficult to prove that there is a continual active choosing and probing in the subject. The difficulties in starting the movement, in using the right finger, are greater, the less the motility of the finger is developed. The better the motility of a limb, the clearer is the optic picture. When there is not a clear structure in the optic and kinaesthetic sensations, the fingers do not seem to be a part of the body until the postural model of the body is reconstructed. It is remarkable that the third and fourth fingers are also those which are mostly afflicted in finger agnosia.

inner forces and by the inner laws of the gestalt. We do not deal with such an inner development in our observations. The development is only possible by continual contact with experience. Experience in itself is not a ready-made entity, but gets its shape by active probing. Our experiences likewise discard the gestalt theories developed by Meinong and his school.

Meinong is of the opinion that the gestalt is based upon impressions of a lower order. The structural process of the gestaltung adds something to it. The basic contents remain in a new unit. He speaks of 'fundierender Inhalt' (basic contents). But the experiments quoted above show that the gestalt and insight in our body undergoes a development with an active addition of new experiences. But these new experiences are not only an addition to the prior experiences. They raise a vague, general knowledge by the way of development on a level which no longer contains the more primitive experience in itself. The first experience, therefore, is not 'fundierender Inhalt', but is the first embryonic appearance of what later on is developed to its full existence. When I use this metaphor, I mean it is more than a metaphor. But here I want to emphasize only that the embryonic structure is no longer present in the structure of the developed organism. It is present only as history, as the past, as the matrix.

There is no question that Meinong and his school are right, when they refer to the production in the final shape. But they have overlooked the fact that there is not only a production, but a complete reconstruction. They have also overlooked the continual active psychic work done in this constructive and productive process. This whole process is guided by continual contacts with reality which make the final shape possible. One does not really own the postural model of the body which is necessary for the start of any movement. One has to gain it by an active process which consists in bringing new parts of the reality into the reach of the active mind. The final appearance, the gestalt, is therefore the result of an inner activity and of an action. The muscular twitchings in Goldstein and Gelb's case, the probing movement in the Japanese illusion, are the final proof that we are really dealing with an activity and that every activity has to do with innervations and motility.

This active process first determines the side that has to act, but after that the limb has to be determined and the particular part of the limb. The relation of the limb to the whole body has to be taken into consideration at the same time. Only by continuous effort are these possibilities given. It is clear that the choice of a limb for an action is the first act of the action as such. In the continuation of the action the cortical and sub-cortical apparatus of motility which later on guarantee the continuation of the movement are of importance. The principle that pictures and images mean movements clearly emerges here.

We do not know very much about the psychic processes when the movement is continued. It is probable that sensomotor regulations play the most important part here. Or, in other words, we are dealing with an organic function, which sends only vague reflections into the consciousness. But there is no question that the knowledge of the general directions of the space of the plane in which the movement takes place must be continually present. The difficulty in coming to a clear formulation about the direction of the movement is finally based upon the psychological fact that the most important factor in any movement is the inner tension between the goal and the beginning. In some way every movement is based upon the structures which extend between the beginning and the end of a movement. Martin could not find many representations as soon as the movement had started. The movement as such continually provokes new sensations of the kinaesthetic and tactile type, which go into the field of tension and change in tensions.

Psychologically, the tensions and energies at the beginning of a movement are of course completely different from those at any other point in the course of the movement. The fall of energy has a complicated structure, and every single movement has its specific melody. The aims of a movement can be very varied. The aim can be an aim in the outside world, in the outside space. It can be an aim in the region of one's own body. It can be the reaching of a particular point, or the acting on a particular object.

Experience in pathology, which I cannot discuss here in detail, leads me to the conclusion that the psychological space concerning one's own body is different from other space. Space, therefore, psychologically shows a lack of homogeneity. The outside space and the body space differ in their structure. There are cases in pathology in which it is impossible to find a point in the outside world correctly, whereas it is possible to localize points of one's own body by correct action.[1]

(11) *Summary and recapitulation on apraxia and agnosia and the representations of movement*

When a point where a movement has to go is determined, the action has to be adapted to the object towards which the movement is directed. The knowledge of this object is necessary for the handling of it. Whenever an agnosia or any difficulty as such hinders us from a clear-cut perception of an object, the action must be deficient. But apraxia is the inability to handle an object in spite of the preserved knowledge of the object. It has always been extremely difficult to differentiate between disturbances of the perception, and especially agnosias, and difficulties in actions. Heilbronner in particular has pointed out this difficulty. We are well aware, from a methodological point of view, that whenever such difficulties arise, problems of some importance will be involved. It is true that every full perception is only possible when we can handle the object felt. The whole trend of our discussion shows that knowledge and perception are not the product of a passive attitude, but acquired by a very active process, in which motility as such takes part.

This whole problem is of course incomprehensible, if we take motility as an undifferentiated unit. But motility has very different

I wrote previously: "In spite of the correct plan for the movement and correct perception of space, the correct perception of space cannot be used correctly in actions. A patient of that group would fail to grasp correctly, although he knew the correct aim. He would also make the same mistake concerning his own body, well knowing the correct localization. I have indeed observed such a case with Pötzl. There were no other apractic troubles present. We are not dealing with an optic mistake, as another case showed this disturbance in a not isolated way. The mistake was more marked in the right hand than in the left. We have reasons to believe that the perception of space needs transformation into praxia, and this praxia can be disturbed without any disturbance of the perception as such. . . . Case 6 and Balint's case prove that the mistake can be prevented only by actions directed towards the external space. In both cases there were no disturbances in pointing to a part of the patient's own body. . . . We arrive at the conclusion that the space of one's own body and the other space are not identical from the point of view of praxia".

levels. When there is apraxia present, a great part of motility of another level is preserved. Otherwise no perception of any value would be possible. Even the lack of actions in the higher level will provoke a definite impairment of our knowledge of objects. In some ways, the structure of this apractic lack of knowledge will be different from the structure of the agnostic lack of knowledge. Recently, Grünbaum has emphasized the difficulty which apractic patients have in their gnostic functions. Pick, Pötzl, and I myself have also emphasized that an erroneous action very often is not recognized as such. We believe we are correct when we have made a slip of the tongue and are often unable to understand why others laugh. Even beyond that, an erroneous action inhibits our gnostic functions. In the flow of the erroneous action, we neglect also that which we theoretically know about objects. This is only a new instance of the general principle we are concerned with, that every action carries with it a specific change in the gnostic function and that every gnostic function carries with it an action.

The action can be either an action on our own body or the body of somebody else, or it can be an action towards and on a definite object. Just as the knowledge of our own body is a gnostic function different from the gnostic functions of objects, the individual can fail in actions against his own body, whereas the actions concerning objects are preserved. In other words, the completion of a movement which has its goal on our own body is dependent on the knowledge of the postural model of the body and on the possibility of using this knowledge in the action. There is no question that movements which have their goal on our own body are psychologically and therefore also physiologically different from movements that concern objects. It is true that we do not know of cases in which the use of the knowledge of objects is disturbed while the use of the knowledge of one's own body is preserved. The using of the knowledge of the body in actions directed against one's own body is the more vulnerable function. We shall not be wrong if we attribute the greater biological importance to actions directed towards objects. It is in some ways the more vital function. Of course, it is also important for an individual to find a point on his body which is aching, but here primitive mechanisms of a lower level do help out. It is of vital importance to find the mouth on one's own body, but when the individual has failed, the final orientation is achieved with the help of an immediate tactile correction, so that one's own body offers by the manifold flow of sensations the possibility of correcting the erroneous action directed towards one's own body, when the first movement has failed. The body-image plays therefore an important part in every movement, but it has a special importance when the movement is directed towards one's own body.

It is not the purpose of this general discussion on human action to study the diverse types of apraxia. But I may mention that in Liepmann's motor apraxia we deal with the difficulties in using the knowledge of objects, and, when this difficulty has a damaging influence on the development of the further plan of the movement and of the structuralization of the single movement into a whole, we speak of ideatory apraxia. This remark is important in so far as it points again to the idea that an action develops from a germ under the guiding influence of the immediate sensations, sensory motor regulations, and their reflection into the consciousness into its definite structure. This can be seen in any psychic function. There is always a development from an embryonic state to ripeness. This whole development is not given by an inner drive but is guided by perception, sensation, sensations mediated by motility, and by the immediate contact with reality.

There is no question that in this development of the motor melody the motility as such plays an important part, especially in all those moments when the inner tension leads from the beginning of the movement to the goal. We know that in many cases we find aberrations in the motor impulses as such. These aberrations in the innervations may occur in very different motor levels. They may be due to striopallidar lesions or to lesions of cortical functions. But all this has no special importance for the problem in which we are concerned. Our aim is to show that there is no action in which the postural model of the body does not play an important part. Beyond that, we have found the continuous interaction between perception, gnosis, insight, knowledge, and motility in the broadest sense. We have reached the formulation that there is a germ for every movement, that the plan of the movement is represented at first as a general·tendency, as a drive, and that it develops actively with a decided psychic activity and ingesting new experiences into its definite shape.

The finished movement is doubtless a well-rounded shape, but again it would be erroneous to believe that this shape is given in a passive way, that it develops out of inner motives, and that it finally contains as parts its previous stages of development. The study of human action confirms us, therefore, in the idea that a gestalt has to be acquired and created and produced by inner and outward activities.

In the older literature there is a great deal about the representations of movements and the importance they may have for our actions. Our whole discussion shows clearly how utterly inadequate any attempt would be to base the psychology of action on representations of movement. Experiments by Kanner and Schilder have shown that the majority of subjects have enormous difficulties in imagining themselves in motion. I reproduce some of our protocols.

The command was: "Imagine yourself clenching your fist".

Sc. An unnatural, weightless, 'ghostly' white finger is elongated, makes queer movements in the effort of closing itself into a fist, while the real fingers are felt in their right places. In a second attempt, the patient feels his own fist disconnected from the body, a little smaller than a real one, with abnormal motility.

Bi. begins correctly. Then the arm disappears and the hand seems as though it were chopped off. The patient then brings the hand up and makes a fist in a natural way: she can feel the cords. "The fist stood out in front of me like a picture flashed on the screen, without any depth."

Ka. sees his fingers moving forward very slowly and gradually until they are at right angles with the palm and he imagines that they cannot go any further. He feels very strong kinaesthetic sensations in his knuckle-joints. Observations show that, without knowing it, he has carried out in reality about half of the movement imagined. In a second attempt he experiences a very peculiar difficulty. In whatever direction he wants to imagine his hand moving he has the feeling that one usually has when trying out the Japanese illusion for the first time.

Be. The hand comes down in spasmodic jerks, forming a small fist, while behind it the shadow of a larger hand is seen.

Next command: "Imagine yourself stretching out your arm".

Bi. There is a feeling of heaviness and extreme tension in the arm. The subject sees the arm stretching out and to the side, and has kinaesthetic sensations in the real one. The movements seem to be normal. When the arm is extended, the hand and fingers seem unusually large.

Ka. finds it impossible to imagine any action of his arm whatsoever. Bi. experiences natural motility of the image, but in the end the arm becomes unusually long.

It is remarkable that there should be such obvious difficulties in imagining self-movements, and these experiments make it absolutely clear that neither optic nor kinaesthetic representations can be the basis for the decisive human movement. The human movement is above the enormous individual differences in the imagination. It is a structure of a different order. It contains a plan, a direction, and has a meaning that brings the body either in a closer relation to the outside object, or to other parts of the body.

(12) *Expressive and reflectory movements*

So far I have dealt with volitional actions and neglected all kinds of other human activities. There is the problem of the movements which are the expression of emotions. It is remarkable that they are often preserved in apraxia, whereas the patient is unable to imitate them voluntarily. I do not doubt that movements of expression have once been directed against the world, or the body, just as there are voluntary actions now. This is also the nucleus of Darwin's theories on the expression of emotions. We understand the primitive action when we study the highly developed volitional action. In the expressive movements of wrath we are directed against the person who makes us angry. It may be a real person or it may be an imaginary one. Emotions and expressions are never present in the solitary person. It is an act in the real and imagined community. It is more difficult to understand the so-called reflectory movements. In apraxias we often observe that, in spite of the fact that the activity of the higher level is destroyed, primitive sucking and grasping reflexes are present. When patients have an apraxia in closing their eyes, they still have a normal and even increased reflectory winking. Patients who are unable to localize touches by pointing deliberately to a point touched are still able to scratch themselves when itching occurs, or to remove painful stimuli.

Henri speaks of reflectory localization and bases it on a spinal function. We are far from being able to say which part of the central nervous system acts in these reflectory movements. It is almost certain that we are not dealing with spinal mechanisms. It is impossible at present to go deeper into the psychology of these so-called reflectory actions, but general considerations, which I have discussed in my *Medical Psychology*, make it at least probable that reflectory action is very similar to the full volitional act and that reflectory action can be better understood when we take it as the simplification of a volitional act, which has in some way dropped down to a deeper level of consciousness. A volitional act is not built up from more primitive reflectory actions; but it uses the reflectory actions which are a part of a whole with many different parts. Even in reflectory localization, the individual must have some kind of conception that something is going on in his own body, that it has to be removed, that an action of his own body is necessary, and that the action has to go up to a specific point. We can see now how important the body-image is for every human action.

(13) *The phantom*

One of the clearest expressions of the existence of the postural model of the body is the so-called phantom of persons who have undergone an amputation. It seems that a sudden loss is necessary. Phantoms of arms, legs and also of breast and phallus have been observed. The phenomenon was first observed by Weir Mitchell. Most of the investigators have observed that the phantom is chiefly represented by tactile and kinaesthetic sensations. But I have noticed that optic images concerning the phantom are almost always present. The phantom in the beginning usually takes the shape of the lost extremity but in the course of years it begins to change its shape and parts of it disappear. When there is a phantom of the arm the hand comes nearer to the elbow, or in extreme cases may be immediately on the place of amputation. Also the hand may become smaller and be like the hand of a child. Similar phenomena occur on the leg. The position of the phantom is often a rigid one, and according to Katz and Riese it is often the position in which the patient has lost his limb. It is as if the phantom were trying to preserve the last moment in which the limb was still present.

The phantom follows its own laws. When the arm is moved towards a rigid object, the phantom goes into the rigid object. It may even go through the patient's own body, as I have observed in one of my cases. In one of them, the patient felt at first on the phantom leg the malleolus, toes, and heel. Later on the heel disappeared. We can be sure that we are dealing with central processes in all these processes of shaping, or disappearing of parts, in the changes of the position of the hand and feet to the stump. These facts may lead to a better insight into the structure of the postural model of the body.

Since the hand and foot of the phantom persist longer and shows a greater resistance, psychological representations of those parts must be different from the psychological representations of other parts of the body. The hand gives more sensations than any other part of the body, but it would be better to say that it is the part of the arm with the closest relation to the external world, which comes in varied relations to the objects. The other parts of the arm have comparatively little contact with the varied experience the touch of objects gives. We come to the general conclusion that the postural model of the body is especially developed by contact with the outside world, and that those parts of our body which come in a close and varied contact with reality are the most important ones. The foot gives us the most intimate touch with the earth. It seems that the contacts of the anterior part of the toe are more varied than the contacts of the heel, and we understand, therefore, why the heel disappeared first in my observation.

The part played by paraesthesias in the building up of the phantom has always been a problem. Before I enter into this discussion, I wish to mention the observation of a case who lost through amputation (after an automobile accident) the last two phalanges of the third and fourth finger of the left hand. Immediately after the operation vivid pain set in and, associated with it, the vivid tactile impression of the two fingers bent in a painful manner in the first interphalangeal joint. Paraesthesias, together with pains, played at that time a very important part. Optic images were almost regularly connected with the tactile perception. With the cessation of pain, the phantom persisted, with the fingers no longer bent, but fully outstretched and normal. The connection with paraesthesias was obvious also then. Whenever the paraesthesias were stronger, the tactile and optic postural model of the fingers became more and more vivid. Often the actual ends of the amputated fingers were felt in their place, but were felt as the normal skin of the finger tip, only smaller, and a smaller and more slender finger followed. Sometimes, on the place of amputation, finger-tips and nails were felt, and there was a vivid pain that was felt as a pain at the end of the nail. In the course of months the paraesthesias and the phantom disappeared in a parallel way. The phantom of the fingers was a vivid sensory phenomenon. But without any sensory basis the subject often forgot that the fingers were absent.

We have thus two distinct phenomena, the presence of the phantom and the forgetting of the defect. The phantom is clearly dependent on paraesthesias. No wonder, therefore, that Pitres, Souques, and Poisot have found that cocainization of the nerves makes the phantom disappear. Gallinek and Förster have also succeeded in removing the phantom by peripheral changes. Adler and Hoff diminished the perception of the phantom by applying ethylchloride to the stump. But there is no question that the peripheral phenomena are not sufficient to explain the image of the body as it appears in the phantom. It is worthy of note that in the experiments by Adler and Hoff the application of ethylchloride on the one side also influenced the postural model of the body on the other side. There is no question that phenomena of that kind can be interpreted only when we assume that the body-image and phantom are based upon a complicated cerebral mechanism. The paraesthesias, the peripheral sensations, are therefore only an activating factor. I have often drawn attention to the general principle that we should not ask whether a phenomenon is peripheral or central, but rather, "What are the peripheral and what are the central components in a phantom?" We have given up the point of view that periphery and centre are opposite to each other.

A phantom may also occur when the limb is not lost. Mayer-Gross observed a phantom after the nerves of the brachial plexus were completely torn and after a transversal lesion of the spinal cord. Zador succeeded in provoking a phantom in the left arm of a poliomyelitis case by applying the esmarch tube. But it is doubtful what the relation of these phantoms where the extremity is still present may be to the phantoms which are substitutes for an absent limb. It is very easy to provoke in normal subjects more or less vivid images of their own extremities. That many individual differences exist the protocols of Kanner and Schilder demonstrate. Such an imagined limb may also be smaller than the actual one. Any attempt on the part of a normal subject to imagine one of his own limbs moving when it is at rest may lead to phenomena that are in many respects similar to phantoms. Nevertheless, the real phantoms have another basis.

Head reports that in one case after a cerebral operation the phantom disappeared. So far as I am aware no detailed report of this case has been given.

We have to ask: What do these phenomena actually mean? Why does the phantom shrink? Katz is of the opinion that the self-experience of childhood comes back. I am convinced that in many cases this interpretation will be found correct. But in the observation mentioned above about the amputated fingers another interpretation is at least possible. The paraesthesias mark in some way the point up to which the schema of the body is going. We know that points with strong sensations will always be the marks into which the postural model of the body is drawn. The tendency to have a complete finger has therefore to be adapted to the space that is available, and we then get a smaller image of the body.

Probably, according to general psychological experiences, the postural model of the body is present in us in its original shape. This original shape is based upon continual transformations from the postural model of the child into the postural model of the adult. There is a long series of images. But one of the most important characteristics of psychic life is the tendency to multiply images and to vary them with every multiplication. It is one of the inherent characteristics of our psychic life that we continually change our images; we multiply them and make them appear differently. This general rule is true also for the postural model of the body. We let it shrink playfully and come to the idea of Lilliputians, or we transform it into giants. We have, therefore, an almost unlimited number of body-images. Probably the amputated person tries in a more or less playful manner to find which one he can use.

When the phantom is small, it can be changed by hypnosis into its normal size. If the hand is close to the body, it can be stretched to its normal place by hypnosis. (Betlheim.) We can understand the phenomena when we speak of a ready-made pattern of the postural model of the body which is activated by peripheral sensations. But when we refer to the ready-made pattern, we should not forget that psychological patterns are not something static, but a tendency and a function. The pattern of the body-image consists of processes which construct and build up with the help of sensations and perception, but emotional processes are the force and source of energy of these constructive processes, and they direct them.

We are accustomed to have a complete body. The phantom of an amputated person is therefore the reactivation of a given perceptive pattern by emotional forces. The great variety in phantoms is only to be understood when we consider the emotional reactions of individuals towards their own body. One of Betlheim's patients felt that his right arm was preserved somewhere and would be given back to him. These are phenomena very similar to the phenomena in non-perception cases. These patients may feel that their healthy limbs are somewhere else. We may mention here an interesting case of Kogerer's. It is the case of a woman, 58 years old, who, seven years before she came under observation, went through a series of operations in connection with a septic infection on the right middle finger. Finally the extremity had to be amputated. The patient now feels the hand near the shoulder. She feels some of her operation wounds in a painful way, especially those operations which took place after her first enucleation (it concerned the middle finger). The operations had been made in narcosis. Kogerer interprets this phenomenon rightly by saying that she feels the wounds of those operations in which she feared a definite mutilation.

It is clear that the final picture of a phantom is to a great extent dependent on the emotional factors and the life situation. Probably the way in which the schema of the body is built up and appears in the phantom has a general significance. It is a model of how psychic life in general is going on. Something is happening in the periphery of the body. But only the interaction between periphery and centre makes the final appearance. This interaction is based upon the playful multiplication of psychic experiences. The shaping of the experiences repeatedly uses actual sensations. But the real meaning, the real significance of an experience is due to the emotional attitudes, or, in other words, to the life situation. Our own body and the image of our own body is, of course, the object of the strongest emotions. After the amputation, the individual has to face a new situation, but since he is reluctant to do so he tries to maintain the integrity of his own body. According to Riese, the phantom is the expression of a difficulty in adaptation to a sudden defect of an important peripheral part of the body. We have spoken so far as if the phantom always remained unmoved, but many patients feel that it moves spontaneously or can be moved at will.

In a case of my own (amputation of the upper leg) every movement of the healthy leg provoked the impression in the patient that the phantom was moving in an identical way. Whenever the patient felt that the phantom was moving, movements were going on in the muscles of the stump. There was always a vivid play in the muscles of the stump, but it was easy to demonstrate that his impression of a movement in the phantom was not due to the movement in the muscles of the stump, since movements of the toes and of the foot of the healthy side were also transmitted to the phantom, and the amputation had taken place on the upper leg. Even when an innervation of the upper part of the healthy leg was transmitted to the phantom, the interplay of the muscles of the stump did not coincide with the experienced movement of the phantom. When the patient intended to move the phantom, he moved his healthy leg instead.

Associated movements on the phantom have not been seen by every observer. Katz and E. Meyer have missed them. In one of my cases, movements of the left arm always provoked a clenching of the fist on the phantom of the right side. It is known since Curschmann pointed it out that most amputated persons have associated movements in the healthy leg and arm, when they are ordered to move the phantom. Curschmann explains this phenomenon by saying that the effort provokes contralateral symmetrical associated movements. We have here new hints of the close relation of the motility of the two sides of our body. Contralateral, symmetrical associated movements are based on anatomical connections and apparatus, the centre of which is probably in the basal ganglia. Every effort to movement will provoke the symmetrical associated movement, as Curschmann again has shown. But the transfer of the movement from the intact side to the phantom can only be interpreted by the theory that the plan of the movement and the cortical kinaesthetic melody of movement is transferred symmetrically to the phantom. The movements in the stump which are never absent may help to give the vivid colouring of a sensation to these impressions. The actual movements are certainly not responsible for the final shape of the movement on the phantom, since they often go in a direction different from the direction of the phantom felt. There is no necessity to discuss 'Innervations—Empfindungen' (sensations provoked by the central impulse to innervation). This old and much-discussed problem has been decided in a negative sense.

Pathology shows clearly that we build up a plan for movements, that we develop this plan in continual contact with actual experiences, that the plan as such is already the beginning of motor activity, and that the motor activity originates from an intention of our inner direction towards a goal, which comes through in the actual movement. When the amputated patient tries to move his phantom, he has a plan for movement ('Bewegungsentwurf'). The motor activity comes out in the contralateral movement, and it depends on the whole structure of the phantom in what way the many motor and kinaesthetic experiences on the stump and on the contralateral side will give to the plan of the movement the actual vividness of the impression of the movement.

Katz has not given enough attention to the imagination of movements in limbs at rest (cf. above). The phenomena which normal subjects experience in such imagined limbs closely resemble the reports we get from amputated persons. There are many individual differences in the corresponding experience in the imagination of normal persons; but there are very often muscular tensions in the actual limb, which provoke muscular sensations that probably play a similar part in the final elaboration of the imagination as the sensations the amputated person experiences by the movement of the stump. The movements of the stump of the amputated person deserve greater attention than has so far been given to them. A number of irregular movements and muscular twitchings are always going on in the stump. They do not reach the full consciousness of the amputated person. He is unable to balance the innervatory impulses of the stump, which has no immediate contact with reality. The movements are therefore the expression of postural tendencies, which are no longer co-ordinated by direction towards a definite aim in the outside world. Only contact with the outside world provides sufficient regulating sensations.

(14) *Psychogenic body-image imperception and allochiria. Their relation to organic changes*

When there are organic changes in the self-perception of one half of the body, this organic nucleus often becomes the basis for a new, psychogenic structure. One of Ehrenwald's patients. who was unconscious of her left hemiplegia, her menstruation, and the disturbance in her bladder function, became more and more hypochondriac and stated that her whole body did not exist any longer, that it was changed and rotting. She also said that her surroundings had changed and that well-known faces appeared to her like strange ones. It is obvious that, in those cases also, the borderline between one's own body and the body of others is not clearly distinguished. In another of these cases the patient talks of his hand as if it were not his real hand; the new hand is bigger and more voluminous than the old one. He adds that he cannot show his old arm, because he does not know where he left it. He says that immediately after the attack there were several hands near his knee. He often talks about his new left hand and about his right hand. The patient had also had serious disturbances of the sensibility of the left side. There was also a very serious paresis on the left side of the body. It is remarkable that this patient talks of both the new and the old left arm. This is reminiscent of Betlheim's case in which the patient says that the phantom is not his arm and that his own arm is hidden somewhere else. It is obvious that in cases of that kind and in the phantom cases the same mechanisms are present. It is also obvious that no fundamental difference exists between the organic and the psychogenic mechanisms. We thus come immediately to the discussion of the important problem of the so-called dyschiria (Jones).

I have already mentioned Obersteiner's allochiria. A stimulus applied to the one side is felt at the symmetrical point on the other side. Obersteiner stated that the symptom is independent of a defectiveness in sensory acuity and in localization. But he still brought alloaesthesia, in which sensory disturbances are present, into a close relation with allochiria. Alloaesthesia means transposition of sensations in organic cases in which there is a difficulty in localization. Jones emphasizes the fundamental difference. According to him, this dyschiria is characterized by the fact that every sensation has peculiar qualities which he calls phrictopathic. Also, the introspective motor and sensory phenomena are, according to him, completely different from the phenomena in alloaesthesia. He distinguishes between achiria, when the patient completely forgets one side of the body, and allochiria, when one side is felt as a duplicate of the other side and when irritations from one side are transferred to the symmetrical space on the other side.

In synchiria, an irritation provokes a sensation on the side touched, but there is at the same time also a sensation on the other part of the body. In one case, which he reports in detail, there existed at first a total anaesthesia of the right side of the body. At the same time the patient had a complete amnesia for every feeling on the right side of the body, for right-handedness, and for the meaning of these terms. But he did not feel his left side as a whole, he somehow felt as if his body stopped in the middle. Fairly soon he got back the sensitivity on the right side of the body. There were abnormal perseverations; irritation of short duration provoked a sensation lasting from 50 to 60 seconds. But it lasted from 4 to 6 seconds before the sensation came into the consciousness. A perception did not take place when there was another, more normal sensation in the consciousness. When both sides were touched, the patient felt the touch on the left side only. Every irritation was connected with an immediate motor reaction. The sensation was connected with a disagreeable feeling which spread over the body. The patient did not feel as if the right side of his body belonged to him. He also felt as if the otherwise normal left side had lost its extension to the left side. The patient felt two dimensional instead of three dimensional.

In the allochiric stage, the left side was normal but the right side was felt as a second, more clever or more dead left side. The patient had also lost the knowledge that there were any other than left hands. Orders concerning the right side were effected by the left side of the body. The patient felt then that the dead left side was acting. He felt a stimulus on the right side more than on the corresponding point on the left side. Irritation on the right side could also provoke two sensations, one being of normal quality, the other one phrictopathic. In the next stage the right side was felt more personal, but more independent. This stage was disagreeable for the patient. The right side was not felt as a particular side; but when the patient moved both arms at the same time, he felt that the one was on the right side. Irritation on the right side provoked two sensations, one of which was right and the other left. The homolateral was phrictopathic.

Jones discusses the nature of dyschiria in all these states. According to his statement, we have here an amnestic disturbance with the inability to associate a given sensation with psychic processes which help us to determine the side. He states that the defectiveness is independent of any sensory disturbance. Allochiria, according to his opinion, is based on an abnormal association between the feeling of one side and the remembrance of the other side. He does not believe that a change in the sensations is of any importance. He gives the same interpretation for synchiria. He is of the opinion that one is dealing with a hysterical dissociation. It is not a simple transfer of the sensations from the one side to the other. He reaches the conclusion that dischiria is not based upon impairment of the sensory acuity, but upon a difficulty in the synthesis of the chirognostic feeling. It is a loss of remembrance concerning one side of the body.

As my previous remarks show, Jones has overrated the differences between allochiria and alloaesthesia. In alloaesthesia, especially in the more central types of cases, patients transfer their sensations from one side to the other. At the same time the left side loses its meaning for them. Pötzl was right in his opinion that the left side of the body is transferred to the right side. When we read the descriptions I have given concerning organic cases and compare them with Jones's description, we see that there exists an almost complete identity. Jones is right in emphasizing that we are not dealing only with a change in the sensations. The blockade and the transfer from one side to the other side of the body find their final meaning only when brought in connection with the image of the body.

Jones speaks of the synthesis of the feeling of the sidedness. It is of especial interest in this connection that in the psychogenic cases as well as in the organic cases paraesthesias (Jones calls them phrictopathic sensations) play such an important part. I again draw attention to the case-history of my own case, in which paraesthesias and after-sensations are so important. One can almost see that for every one of the carefully described details in Jones's hysterical cases one finds an analogy in the purely organic sphere. I am not of the opinion that the organic and psychogenic cases are identical in their structure. The psychogenic cases take place in absolutely different levels. But the same basic principles direct the psychogenic and organic disorder. The organic patterns of the body-image, the structure of which we have discussed above, are not really impaired or destroyed in the psychogenic cases, though they are not used. The organic apparatus is out of function. It could be used, if the emotions of the patient would allow this. But the psychogenic repression also always takes with it something of the organic sphere. Only in this way can we interpret the queer sensations in all those cases, which are so similar to the paraesthesias of the organic cases. I have mentioned already that the organic repression will on the other hand help those psychic processes which go in a similar direction to that of the organic repression.

The pictures occurring in the dyschiria cases are in many respects reminiscent of depersonalization cases. In depersonalization also the individual feels that his limb is not his own limb although there are sensations coming from it. Dyschiria is separated from hysterical anaesthesia by the persistence of tactile sensations. But that there is something in common between hysterical anaesthesia and dyschiria is proved by one of Jones's cases, where hemianaesthesia preceded the dyschiria. In hysterical anaesthesia the individual forgets more completely about the part of the body that he wants to forget, following the demand of the life situation. It is true that we can understand hysterical anaesthesias only if we understand the schema of the body. Janet has shown that patients who are anaesthetic on one side can move their healthy arm promptly. When they are ordered to raise the anaesthetic arm, they move both at once. Another patient obeys the command to raise the arm with a movement of the opposite side. We see again that the change in the perception of the body leads to actions which correspond to the changed perception. We have found a new instance of the general law of the close relation between sensibility and motility.

Certainly allochiria is a rare phenomenon. But other changes in the perception of the body on a hysterical basis are still more unusual, unless one counts the hysterical anaesthesias. So far as my knowledge of the literature goes, only in one case of Pick's did the patient lose topognosia concerning his own back.

(15) *Muscle tone and body-image. The persistence of tone*

So far we have studied the sensory apparatus involved in the building up of the image of the body. We have seen that every sensory process has its way out into the motility and that whatever goes on in the sensory structure of the postural model of the body has a consequence in the motility based upon it. But we have neglected so far the motor components, which are of importance for the building up of the body-image. I have to emphasize here an experiment which Hoff and I have introduced in psychology and psychopathology. Others who have examined the phenomenon have come to identical conclusions (Eidelberg, Selling).

We order a subject to stretch his hands forward, so that one arm is parallel to the other. One arm is now raised in an angle of about 45 degrees above the horizontal. (One may also bring the arm 45 degrees below the horizontal plane.) Bring the arm of the subject passively to the inclined position or let the subject take this position in an active way. Either support the resting arm (R. arm) and the raised (or lowered) mobile arm (M. arm) or let the subject keep the position actively. The subject may have his eyes open or closed. After 25 seconds, the subject is ordered to close his eyes (if they were open) and to bring his M. arm into the same position as the R. arm. When the M. arm is raised, the subject does not bring his arm into the same plane as the R. arm, but the M. arm remains several centimetres higher than the R. arm. When the M. arm is lowered, the M. arm is not brought back to the horizontal line, but remains several centimetres lower than the R. arm. The subject does not know that he has made a mistake and is of the opinion that both arms are at the same height. After a few seconds, the M. arm returns into the same position as the R. arm. The subjects generally do not know that they have changed the position. A registration with the kymograph shows that the disappearance of the difference does not decrease steadily, but by jerks which bring the arm back into the position of the R. arm.

We have called this phenomenon 'phenomenon of the persistence of tone'. It is not due to a persistence of muscular innervation, because otherwise the lowered arm would also have to go higher than the R. arm. It is a persistence of the postural impulses which try to bring back the arm to its previous position. It is a persistence of tone. The phenomenon has nothing to do with a mistake in judgment. If we order the subjects to bring their M. arm with open eyes into the same position as the R. arm and then order them to close their eyes and to keep their arms still, the previously raised M. arm starts to rise and the previously lowered M. arm starts to go down without the subject being aware of it. Therefore, we are dealing here with a muscular pull, which attempts to restore the previous posture.[1]

It is worthy of note that the individual does not learn by experience. We may repeat this experiment a dozen times with the same results, even when the subject knows that he has made a mistake before. When the arms have been brought to the same level with open eyes, the M. arm, which was previously raised, moves upward again when the eyes are closed. The subject does not realize this. He still believes his arm to be in the previous position. Or, in other words, the muscular pull which tries to restore the previous position and its effect remain unconscious. We are dealing therefore with a deception concerning the posture of our limbs in space. This can be proved by a variation in the experiment.

In this experiment the subject has nothing to do at all. After the M. arm has been in its position for about 25 seconds, the experimenter brings it passively to the same level as the R. arm. When the arm has been raised, the subject will feel that the M. arm is not at the same height as the R. arm, but several centimetres lower. When the experimenter brings the M. arm not to

---

[1] It is instructive to compare this phenomenon with one which is doubtless based upon the persistence of muscular innervation—the so-called Kohnstamm phenomenon. When one innervates one arm against an immovable resistance and the resistance is removed suddenly, the arm starts to move in the direction of the effort, although the subject has no intention of moving the arm in this way. The arm seems to rise by itself and becomes at the same time lighter, when the hand is pushed against the resistance which is upwards to the arm. When the arm was pressing downwards against a resistance below the arm, the arm continues with a movement downwards. It does not matter in which posture the arm has been. When the arm was in the lower quadrant and is pushed against an obstacle, it will rise in the same way as when the arm was pushed against an obstacle in the upper quadrant. The Kohnstamm phenomenon is indeed one that is based upon the persistence of muscular innervation. (Cf. Matthaeis' paper).

the same level as the R. arm, but a few centimetres above it, the subject will feel that both arms are now at the same height. The same phenomena occur, of course, in the opposite direction, when the M. arm has been lowered and is then brought to the same level as the R. arm or a few centimetres below it. The subject then feels the previously lowered M. arm either lower or at the same level as the R. arm. We call this 'Sensory persistence of tone'.

The theoretical meaning of this phenomenon is that the normal position of the M. arm, after the tone has influenced it, is the position into which the tone-pull would bring the arm; or the tone of the postural persistence influences the body-image in the sense that it is pulled into the direction of tone. The limb, therefore, is felt in a position which is opposite to the direction of the muscular pull. Or, in a more general formulation, the postural model of the body is dependent on the pull of the tone. This formulation has considerable general importance. The phenomenon of postural persistence is a phenomenon all over the body. It is present in every muscle of the body. It is also present for every single posture of the body. We are dealing therefore with a phenomenon of general significance.

Hoff and Schilder have shown that the phenomenon of persistence of tone belongs to the group of the postural reflexes of Magnus and de Kleyn. We know that tonic phenomena of this kind play an enormous part in the maintenance of the posture of one's own body. Every movement changes the muscular pull of other parts of the body. When the head of a normal person is turned, the arms deviate to the side to which the head is turned. At the same time, the chin arm is going higher. The subject is not aware of it. He still feels that both arms are at the same height. When one now brings the chin arm passively into the same position as the other arm, the individual feels the chin arm standing lower. It is true that the sideways deviation of the arms is partially conscious. But even so the individual has the feeling that the arms are less deviated than they actually are.

Experiences in pathological material have shown that the same principles are valid for the tones which are originated by vestibular irritation, by cerebellar lesion, and by parieto-occipital lesions. All these tones pull the limbs into a position which is unknown to the individual. The normal posture then becomes the posture into which the tone would pull the limb. From this posture every other posture is judged, and the limb is always felt in a posture opposite to the direction of the pull of the tone. Hoff and Schilder have shown that cerebellar cases have a tendency to an increased flexion in the knee, when they imitate the healthy side with the affected side. They call this the phenomenon of cerebellar hyperflexion. This hyperflexion also belongs to the group of tonic changes which influence the postural model of the body. The individual accordingly feels the leg less flexed than it actually is, and the knee (in the recumbent patient) seems to be lower than the knee of the unaffected side, when they are brought into the same position. There is no question that the cerebellar deviation tendency, which we cannot discuss here in detail, has the same influence on the postural model of the body. To sum up, there are many types of muscular tone which influence the postural model of the body. The most important ones are:

(1) Vestibular tone.

(2) Cerebellar deviation tone and cerebellar hyperflexion tone.

(3) The tone of the Magnus and de Kleyn reflexes (attitude and righting reflexes).

(4) The parieto-occipital changes in the righting reflexes.

(5) The tone of postural persistence.

I would like to emphasize that there are types of tone which do not influence the body-image. These are the tone of extrapyramidal rigidity and the tone of pyramidal lesions. It is obvious that these streams of tone, which are steadily going through our body, are continually changing our actual knowledge of the body. We are perpetually subjected to righting tendencies. It is worth while to remember the original conception of Magnus and De Kleyn concerning the reflexes of posture and the righting reflexes. The reflexes of attitude try to maintain a position which is important from the point of view of the living organism. Some of the postural reflexes have to do with the maintenance of standing. Others are concerned with bringing back the animal from an uncomfortable and unusual position to a customary and usual one. When the head is turned, the body has the tendency to follow the head until the body and the head are facing in the same direction again. When this movement is partially performed, the individual does not know that he has moved. He still believes that the head is turned away, and that the body has not followed at all. It is as if the organism would not acknowledge the correction which has taken place involuntarily. Since the body, as I have mentioned, tends to move by postural and righting reflexes into a comfortable position, we can generally say that we feel the body-image in a position which is more uncomfortable than it actually is, so that the incentive to get into a more comfortable position does not disappear.

This problem can be examined in a reaction which has been studied by Wilson, Goldstein, Hoff and Schilder. It is the reaction we have called 'Pronation tendency'. When an individual stretches his hands horizontally, so that the palmar surface is horizontal and turned upwards, and then closes his eyes, the hands do not remain in this uncomfortable, supinated (outward-turned) posture. In every normal person pronation takes place in some degree, and the thumbs are turned upward and inward to a more comfortable position. But in spite of this action towards a more comfortable position (Goldstein) the individual still has the feeling of being in a more uncomfortable position and feels his hands more supinated than they actually are.

Supination is, according to Gierlich, a new acquisition from the phylogenetic point of view. The postural tone counteracts the newly acquired function, which is exerted in maintaining an uncomfortable position. We know that the human body is continually under the influence of those impulses which try to bring back the individual into a posture and attitude which we may call the normal posture and attitude. But what the normal posture and attitude is cannot be found out in a theoretical way. It has to be determined experimentally. It has long been known that for the eyes there exists a position from which other positions can be reached without rotations. This is also the position to which the eyes come back again and again. Skramlik has made similar experiments in studying the influence of the turning of the head on the perception of the deviation of the arms.[1] The normal posture, when the arms are hanging down, is a slight flexion in the elbow. The dorsal plane of the hand faces outwards. The fingers are in semi-flexion. When the hands are stretched forward horizontally, there is always some slight rising tendency of the arms in the shoulders and a mild tendency to further pronation. But it seems that the arms in a horizontal parallel position are not in normal posture. There are motor tendencies driving the arms to divergency which escape the consciousness. Only when the arms form an angle between 45 and 60 degrees with the parallel position, no tendency to movements occurs. It seems, therefore, that this position is one of the normal positions.

There is no question that the normal position of the head to the body is when the plane of the face and of the chest are in one line. Every change from the normal position of the head provokes turning impulses in the body. But it is obvious that for every movement there exists a new normal position. After all, the normal position is not something static, but changes continually according to particular tasks which the individual has in his motility.

We have shown clearly that the postural model of the body is often different from the actual position in which the body is. It is clear that in pathological conditions the discrepancy between the postural model of the body and its actual position may become still greater. To put it briefly, we may say that many of the tonic changes in the posture of the limbs change the actual body only and not the body-image. It is necessary to examine in every single case how far this discrepancy can go and which compromises take place under particular conditions. But it cannot be emphasized enough that regulation takes place continually. We

[1] Skramlik did not give the correct interpretation to this part of his experiments. He brought them into connection with the prevalence of habitual positions in our consciousness. But he has not observed that according to this principle, which, we shall show later, has an importance, the sidewards turning of the head should provoke the feeling that the body is turned in the same direction. One would expect that the subject would then move his arms more medially than would be natural. But in reality the subjects do not know about their motor impulses which turn the body in the direction of the head. They feel their arm more medial than it actually is and make a mistake by putting their arms too much outside. We have again the general principle that the body schema is transposed opposite to the direction of the motor pull.

may generally say that it is very difficult to maintain a posture, unless we have sensory helps, which increase our orientation concerning the body. It is comparatively easy to keep the hand and fingers in any position, so long as the fingers touch each other. When the fingers do not touch and we look at our hand, there is generally some difficulty in keeping the fingers unmoved. The very moment we close our eyes we are unable to maintain the position of our fingers and abduction takes place, which is especially marked in the little finger. This phenomenon, which Hoff and I have called the phenomenon of the little finger, is increased considerably in cerebellar diseases. These movements take place outside the consciousness (even if the individual should try to perceive them) and do not influence the image of our body.

Since cerebellar lesions increase the postural reflexes, we must expect that the discrepancy between the actual position and the postural model of the body will be increased in cerebellar lesions. Goldstein mentions that the body-image becomes larger in cerebellar disease. But I would like to emphasize that the body-image changes according to the specific pull of the muscles affected, and we deal for the most part not with an enlargement, but with distortions of the body-image, which occur in the normal person, but are exaggerated in the cerebellar patient, in whom the pull of the tone is released.[1]

(16) *The influence of habitual posture on the postural model*

There are many other discrepancies between the actual position of our body and the body-image. Many active voluntary movements are neglected by the individual. Skramlik has made a careful study of the Aristotelian deception. When we touch a little object between the two crossed fingers of one hand, so that the object touches the outer side of the crossed fingers and the inner side of the other fingers, we feel two objects. Skramlik has discovered that when we change the position of the touching surface we are deceived about the connection of these two points in space as well as about their distance. The subjective position

[1] The cerebellum is an organ which inhibits certain tonic impulses. Goldstein, Hoff, and Schilder have developed this theory in detail. Cf. my paper in the archives of neurology and psychiatry.

and length of the connecting line is determined by two factors: by the relation in which the touching limbs usually are to each other, and also by the objective position, as it is represented in the mind. These two factors combined with each other, and the factor of the normal position of the limbs, have the greater influence the more they are different from the normal position. Skramlik shows that every habitual posture is so deeply engraved in our mind that postures which are actually different are experienced as similar to this habitual posture.

It is important to notice that this principle of Skramlik's is absolutely different from the principle of the distortion of the postural model of the body by muscular pull. It is in some way a sensory after-effect. These two principles act in opposite directions. When the hand is supinated, the radial side is felt higher than it is in reality when the posture is brought into correspondence with the habitual posture. Here we have an after-effect of the sensory normal position, and the hand seems nearer to the normal position than it actually is. But we know that when there is a strong pronation tendency, in cerebellar lesions for instance, the hand goes actually into pronation, but is still felt in a more supinated position. The postural model of the body is also distorted in a direction opposite to the pull. This principle works contrary to the after-effect of the habitual posture. It may be noted that even when a hand is touched when going into pronation, this point seems to be transported more towards the supinated side. But these disturbances in localization are, according to Hoff and Schilder, rare. According to Goldstein, they are the rule. We are dealing probably with a very complicated situation, where the individual tries to compromise between the absolute localization, which has been changed by the pull of the tone of the limb, and the localization on the limb, which otherwise would have remained normal. No definite decision about these problems can be given as yet.

When we try to come back to the essence of the Aristotelian deception and similar deceptions described by Skramlik, we come to the general conclusion that when we put our limbs in an unusual position we do not accept this change, and feel as if it had not taken place at all, or at least only partially. Our theoretical knowledge that we have made this change does not go into our body-image. The same principle can be applied to the Japanese illusion, in which the theoretical knowledge of the actions that have taken place does not help in the orientation of the fingers. It is just as if the actions had not taken place or had been forgotten, except that in the Japanese illusion there is the additional difficulty that the complicated optic picture is a new obstacle in the orientation. We can formulate from a general point of view that muscular pulls of an unconscious type and voluntary actions which take the limb too much out of its habitual position are not used in the postural model of the body. It is clear that there are two different factors involved. One is a factor of the motor type and the other of a more sensory type. We have taken as an instance of the first factor the persistence of tone, which is a motor phenomenon, whereas the second factor is based upon the impression concerning the habitual posture of our body. It is the persistence of a sensory impression.

(17) *The image of the face. Autoscopic experiments*

That the normal position is deeply engraved in our mind is proved by the experiments of Rupp. He found that in the Japanese illusion the hand touched is very often represented in a normal posture. The experience of the crossing, which may occur either through the subject's own decision or in a passive way, is not completely accepted. Ross has made experiments on the perception of the face when the eyes are closed. When the head is turned sideways and the subject tries to get an impression of his own face, he gets the impression that his face is looking forward but is flattened out. Also the eyes seem to be looking forward, or the individual somehow tries to maintain in a sensory way the normal relation between face and body. It seems that the individual cannot completely neglect the changed sensations; hence the feeling that the face is flattened. Besides that, the individual translates himself somehow into the rôle of the outside observer who sees the person from the front.

We see how complicated are the factors here involved. There is the tendency to the maintenance of a primary position. There is also the optic component, which plays such an important part in the perception of our body. We come here for the first time to the important principle that we not only see our own body in the same way as we see outside objects, but we also represent our own body as we represent an outside object, and the tactile impressions follow this optic representation. For this purpose, we create a mental point of observation opposite ourselves and outside ourselves and observe ourselves as if we were observing another person.

When the individual puts his head in another unusual position, for example, bending it forward to an extreme degree, he very often feels his face in the horizontal plane although it is not completely in the horizontal plane. The horizontal plane of the face affords a simple opportunity of correlating the impressions. Some subjects have the feeling that they are observing themselves from above and can somehow see through the skull. Others see their face shortened, as it might appear to an observer opposite them. We can generally say that in the perception of our own body we try to maintain normal positions and observe ourselves as if we were outside objects. This is true not only when we see, but also when we imagine.

Some years ago, when I was interested in the phenomena of autoscopy (seeing one's own self), I made some experiments with normal subjects. I gave them the order to imagine themselves with closed eyes standing or sitting in front of themselves. The second instruction was to imagine themselves, but without an optic image in addition to the body which they felt. They were to imagine themselves as they saw themselves when they looked at their body, but they were also to imagine their face. All subjects could easily imagine themselves. They saw themselves more like a picture, sometimes a little smaller. At any rate the picture is not very plastic. It is not very different from any other picture we may imagine. When one tries to imagine oneself according to the second instruction, there is very often a spiritual eye, which is in front of the subject and looks all over the body. This spiritual, inner eye need not be outside. It can be inside. It is like a psychic organ, which wanders round in the body and sees the outside of the body from the inside. It looks through the body, which is in some way empty, yet it does not see the inside of the body, but the surface. This immaterial eye wanders according to the point of the surface that has to be observed. The impression of emptiness in the body which occurs in these experiments is very queer. We are led here for the first time to the problem of the perception of the inside of our body.

(18) *How we perceive the outer surface of our body*

When we sit or stand quietly and ask ourselves what we feel (that is the way the subject puts it: it is of course, a perception of a more or less vague character) and what we know concerning our body, we feel our skin. This feeling of the skin is different in the different parts of our body. We feel it especially on the parts which are tense over the bones, for instance, on the hands we feel especially the knuckles, on the face the cheek-bone (zygoma). Then, of course, one feels all the parts which are in connection with the outside world—the parts we sit on, the parts we stand on. There are also the parts which are touched by the clothes. It is true that if we do not move all these impressions are vague and we may forget about them. It is furthermore true that when we sit, at first we generally feel the skin of the body less than the chair we sit on, then we feel also that there is something in between, and finally, when we pay special attention, we feel our skin. The same holds true for the soles. We feel the ground, the leather in between, and finally the skin of the soles.

When we let our eyes wander about our body, we get, as Mach especially has emphasized, a rather incomplete optic picture of ourselves. But we usually do not bother about ourselves, and when conducting experiments it will generally be advisable to make the subject close his eyes. A more careful analysis about what is felt on the skin immediately reveals astonishing results. There are vague feelings of temperature. It is more or less the feeling of warmth. But the outline of the skin is not felt as a smooth and straight surface. This outline is blurred. There are no sharp borderlines between the outside world and the body. The surface of the body can be compared in its indistinctness of feeling with the indistinctness of Katz's so-called space colour .[1]

Another astonishing fact is that when subjects compare what

[1] Space colours float in space without definite relations to objects.

they feel and perceive tactually on their body with the optic imagination or the optic perceptions of the body, they find that there is a discrepancy. The skin that is felt is distinctly below the surface of the optic perception of the body. It is of great interest to study the changes which occur in the feeling of our skin and of the tactile surface of our body, when an object is touching the skin or when we touch an object with our hands or with another surface of our body. At this very moment, the surface becomes smooth, clear, and distinct. The tactile and the optic outlines are now identical with each other. It is a remarkable psychological fact that though we distinctly feel the object and distinctly feel our own body and its surface, yet they do not touch each other completely. They are not fused together. There is a distinct space between. In other words, object and body are psychologically separated by a space in between.

It is an interesting experiment to diminish the pressure of the fingers against the object. We feel the object less and less and the fingers more and more. When the fingers are finally only just touching the object, the object is scarcely perceived any longer, but we have a distinct feeling in the tips of our fingers. We can now observe a paradoxical sensation. It is as if the skin were protruding over the surface and forming a slight cone, which almost reaches for the object.[1]

We may generally say that the distinct surface of our skin is perceived only when we are in touch with reality and its objects. It is true that the mere contact with an object which has no importance and is not perceived as such, already gives the strict outline to the body. There is a difference between the way in which the skin is perceived when there are no objects and the clear-cut perception of our skin when there are distinct object perceptions. This difference is analogous to the relation between space colours and surface colours. Space colours float in space without clear borderlines and without distinct relations to objects. They are

[1] Lindeman told me that he often observed phenomena of this kind in hashish intoxications. The phenomenon there is much more obvious. Beringer has seen similar things in mescaline intoxication. We come to the general formulation that intoxication and pathological changes bring to the consciousness phenomena which are present in the normal person, but are there neglected. Our tendency to live in the world of reality leads us to neglect what is going on in the field of sensations.

cloudy and vague. They may be brought in an incomplete way into connection with objects. These objects are then covered with an indistinct mass of colour. But finally they can be brought clearly into connection with the surface of the objects. We then have definite, smooth surface colours. In psychosis, one can see sometimes that the primary, vague perceptions of hallucinated colours in space get their definite distinctiveness when they are brought into connection with objects. H. Hartmann has seen a patient who at first hallucinated fire and red as space colour, but later connected these colours with her father's rage, and saw a red surface colour in the eyes of the physician. Generally speaking, impressions that are not brought into connection with definitive and distinct objects are floating without sharp borderlines in space. Only the immediate experience of objects gives them distinctiveness and clearness. We are dealing again with an important general principle, and it is worthy of note that even the tactual part of our body is indistinct so long as the body is without contact with the outside world. It does not appear that we perceive our own body differently from any other object.

There are some points which are worth discussing in greater detail. We feel, of course, that the cloudy surface of the skin, which we perceive tactually, is followed by some distinct living substance of specific character. Touching with our fingers, we have the distinct perception of the skin, which is followed by this other substance that is pressed against some resistance. There is no question that we feel the skin in some extension. This does not come out so clearly when we touch with our fingers; but when we press our back against the back of a chair, we feel first the surface of the chair, secondly the clothes in between, and thirdly the surface of our skin. But the skin has some breadth and feels almost like pasteboard which is pressed against the bones. There is no question that the physical qualities of our tissues are of great importance, and the relation of the bone-structure to the skin will give the final elaborations to all our tactile sensations and the perception of our body. We do not feel our body so much when it is at rest; but we get a clearer perception of it when it moves and when new sensations are obtained in contact with reality, that is to say, with objects.

(19) *The openings of the body*

I have mentioned that the part of the skin which is tense over bones is felt in a distinct way. But the most important parts of our body are the openings. These parts, of course, offer very particular sensations. In breathing with our mouth closed we have particular sensations in our nose. But also when we breathe with our mouth open and are not conscious that we are breathing, and even if we stop breathing, we distinctly feel the inside of our nostrils. It is important that we feel them near the opening, not at the actual point of the opening, but about one centimetre inside the body. We feel there either something specific or the coolness of the air. It seems as if the body is more sensitive about one centimetre from its opening and from its surface. The same is true about the mouth. Paradoxically, we do not feel the mouth where it opens; the sensitive zone is again about one centimetre deeper in the body from the opening. When we breathe with the mouth, we feel the air on the roof of the palate, but it seems that it is felt only in the first third of the mouth. If we breathe very deeply, we feel the air deeper in the mouth, and it even descends into the sternal region. But it does not go deeper than to the end of the sternum, and it is felt only one or two centimetres below the surface. We arrive at the general conclusion that the most sensitive zones of the body are near the openings, but one or two centimetres deeper in the body. It is true that these remarks concerning experience with our own body are very incomplete; but they give at least the outline.

The opening of the urethra again is felt deeper than it actually is. The same holds true about the anus. Both are felt about one or two centimetres inside the body. Psychologically one may formulate that the openings of our body are about two centimetres inside it. It is of course a problem of great importance where the desire to urinate is felt. There is no question that it centres round the psychological point mentioned. It is especially a feeling in the glans penis in man; and in woman, urinary tendency is also deeper than the opening of the urethra. Here there can also be a second feeling near the actual sphincter, but apparently nearer the surface than the sphincter actually is. When the bladder is very much extended, there is a feeling of pressure, but it is again near the surface of the skin and is more extended in a direction parallel to the abdominal skin. It is certainly not a feeling of a filled bag, but a queer sensation of lamella below the skin. The desire of defecating is again chiefly localized in the sensitive zone mentioned. The sensation there may have an extension of several centimetres.

Sexual desire is in the region where the opening of the urethra is felt. But it extends along the lower surface of the penis and again under the skin. In woman, sex desire is not localized in the entrance of the vulva. It seems that sex excitement in man may spread from the urethral opening into the region of the anal opening. The sensitive zone is again a little below the surface. It is probably of importance for an individual's sexual character in what part of this connecting line between the urethral and the anal opening sex excitement makes itself particularly felt.

We meet here for the first time the important principle that the individual character expresses itself in the body-image model. It is almost possible to discern from the body-image how strong the anal complexes of a person are. It appears that all our internal sensations are in this sensitive zone close below the surface. The feeling of satisfaction and well-being has some lamellar extensions in the region of the stomach. Stomach-ache originates at the same point, and this point may connect with the anal point when there is the feeling of indigestion.

It is worthy of note that pathological sensations have a tendency to be connected with the sensitive points of the openings. One of my patients, a good observer, suffered from urethritis and from time to time experienced painful sensations in the right lower part of the glans penis. When the painful burning sensation started, he always felt as if his organ was twisted so that the burning point was at the opening of the urethra (of course, about one centimetre below the actual opening) or in some way the point, which is pathologically sensitive, became the opening of the urethra. Since the correct localization was still present, a compromise had to take place and the penis was experienced as twisted. The urethroscopic examination revealed indeed a pathological change on the right side of the urethra, which disappeared after local treatment. The burning sensation and with it the feeling that the organ was twisted also disappeared after the treatment.

We perceive, then, that a strong sensation can be appointed as opening. The other sensations have to be adapted to the pathological opening. The observation is valuable, because it emphasizes again the importance of the sensitive points of the openings of the body. Of course, every part of the body has its specific psychology and its specific set of sensations connected with it. There is no question that the nipples, even when not touched, mark special points in the surface feeling of our body. There is unmistakably a close relation between these facts and Head's so-called zones.

According to Head, diseases of internal organs produce pain and hyperaesthesias in specific, spinal segments of the skin. But preliminary investigations have shown me that pain is generally not felt on the skin, but under it, and again in the sensitive zone one or two centimetres below the skin. Apparently, that is the most vital part in the perception of our body. It will be one of the tasks of the future to study the symptomatology of the subjective sensations of patients with internal diseases.

Pickler touched upon an important problem in asking where we feel our will acting on the muscles. It appears that we appreciate the weight and the shape to be moved and that we try to move it like any other heavy mass. When we raise our leg while standing, we have the impression that we are moving it about the middle of the upper leg. When we bend our head backwards, the pull seems to act on the point of the greatest circumference of the head. When we make a dorsal flexion of our foot, we seem to move and to intend to move the middle of the foot. Our will seems to be in some way directed towards the centre of gravity of a limb. The will is not directed to the moving of the muscle, and the actual location of the tendon and of the muscle-tissue has nothing to do with our intention concerning the place at which we want to move the limb. (Pickler himself came to different conclusions).

(20) *The heavy mass of the body*

In our tendencies to movement we treat our body like any other heavy mass. This leads to the important problem of the gravity and the perception of gravity of our own body. Some preliminary remarks about the perception of gravity in general are necessary. I would here recall Friedländer's researches. When we hold an object in our hands, for example, a cube of wood or metal, we may direct our attention to the object. We then feel its weight. It is worthy of remark that immediately the representation appears the object is filled with a heavy substance. Even if we know that we are dealing with a homogeneous object, the substance is not perceived as equally distributed in the object. It is as if the substance became denser towards the bottom of the object. The upper part of the object is almost empty or the substance is thinly distributed in it. The layer nearest the hand which is supporting the object is filled with a very dense substance.

Optic representations often symbolize this substance. The mass is seen sometimes like clouds of foam, sometimes like dust or powder, and sometimes like something liquid. If the object is reversed, the heavy substance goes again to the bottom and the top is relatively or completely empty. We experience the feeling that the object is kept in its place by our active effort, which props up our hand against the object. When the hand is supported, similar perceptions go on. There is not so much effort and tension in the arm, but there is the sensation of pressure on the skin. Either the sensations in the arm and hand (pressure or tension), or the perception of the heaviness of the object may be stressed. Usually there will be a sensation concerning one's own body as well as perceptions concerning the outside object, but according to the circumstances there will be a greater emphasis on the one or the other experience.

When one is standing, one feels that the heavy mass is chiefly in the legs and more especially in the feet. It diminishes from the feet upwards. Another centre of gravity is in the abdomen. When one is standing, one feels the heaviness especially in the lower part of the abdomen. Apparently the abdomen is considered as a heavy mass which is supported by the femora. Yet another centre of gravity is in the head. Most people feel a heavy mass around the base of the skull, whereas the top of the skull is lighter.

The whole picture changes when one lies down. The heavy mass immediately goes down towards the back. In the head it gathers around the occiput. The top of the abdomen seems to be more or less empty. Many persons have optic representations about these heavy masses. It is evident that the body is perceived in the same way as any other heavy mass. When one breathes in deeply and keeps the chest in a position of maximum inspiration, one immediately feels one's chest as a heavy mass. This seems paradoxical, since the specific weight of the chest is, of course, diminished in deep inspiration. But here we come to an important addition to our insight. The chest feels heavier and like an almost solid heavy substance, because a muscular effort has taken place.

When we move an outside heavy mass, we have to exert our muscles. The more force we have to use, the heavier the mass seems to be. When we keep a part of our body in its position by muscular effort, this part immediately appears heavier. We can prove this easily by making one of the arms tense by innervations of all the muscles. The arm in which we innervate our muscles immediately appears heavier and more substantial than the other one. The impression of heaviness in our body varies therefore according to the muscular strength that we apply to it. When we move something with an effort it is perceived as heavier. Paralysed limbs are therefore experienced as heavier than limbs that are not paralysed. We arrive at the general formulation that we perceive our body as a heavy mass and that the perception of our body is in no way different from the perception of any other heavy mass. Paralysed persons not only feel their own limbs heavier, but also objects put on their limbs. The same principle underlies the perception of the heaviness of external objects and of one's own body. When our limbs are supported, they will feel different from when they are not supported, because the muscular tension is different. We have to keep in mind that the perception of gravity is dependent on the degree of muscular tension and on the sensations of pressure. This is shown by the investigations of Hartmann and Schilder.

This is all that we perceive of the inside of our body. Our body is nothing more than a heavy mass, and changes in the perception of the body will often be changes in the perception of this heavy mass. I have mentioned above that when we start to observe ourselves, we have a feeling of emptiness in ourselves. Many of the neurotic and pathological changes in the perception of our own body are changes in the gravity or levity of the body and are changes concerning the substance filling the body. Sollier and Comar have reported that some persons are able to feel their inner organs and even their microscopic structure. There is no question that this opinion is erroneous. Persons who know something about the structure of inner organs may project them into their body. But there is no way of perceiving inner organs; when these organs start to ache, the sensation is again felt in the sensitive zone of the body, about two centimetres below the skin.

It is now possible to consider some experiences about the appreciation of weights. In cerebellar cases, according to Lotmar, weights are underrated on the side of the cerebellar lesion. It is true that this phenomenon is rather inconstant. Holmes found no disturbance in two cases of lesion of one side of the cerebellum. In nine other cases weights were overrated. Goldstein mentions cases of irritation in the cerebellum, where weights were overrated.

We know now that the cerebellum often provokes a rising tendency in one arm. This rising tendency means that less muscular tension is necessary to maintain the posture of the arm. The arm will therefore be lighter. A weight put on this arm will accordingly also be lighter. When there is not a rising but a sinking tendency of the arm, as also occurs in cerebellar lesions, the individual will have to put out additional strength to fight against the downwards pull, and the weight will appear heavier in the same way as the arm. Every pull of the tone will therefore be either added to or subtracted from the muscular tension and will influence the perception of gravity in the limb and in a weight put on the limb. Every extremity which rises is lighter, and every extremity which sinks is heavier. Every lighter extremity underrates and every heavier extremity overrates weight. When the rising tendency is, as in the experiments of M. H. Fischer and Wodak, provoked by vestibular irritation, we must expect the same changes. In the Kohnstamm experiment the rising arm is lighter again, and Mathaei has shown that weights are underrated with this arm. We are dealing, then, with general laws, which are of great importance for pathology as well as for the knowledge of our own body.

(21) *The vestibular influence on the perception of the weight of the body*

It is clear that vestibular irritation, which has such a strong influence on the tone, must immediately change the perception of the gravity of our own body. But, before we go into this problem, it is worth while to ascertain what happens when gravitation is changed by external forces. When we are flying upwards in an aeroplane, the body is pressed by a strong force against its support. Accordingly, when we fly upwards, or go up in an elevator, the body must feel heavier. In standing we feel this increase in heaviness especially in the legs; in sitting, especially in the buttocks. The same is true when we are in a boat and the boat has an upward motion. When the aeroplane is going down, the body immediately feels lighter. The same is true when when we go down in an elevator. In other words, we somehow perceive the addition or subtraction of the physical masses to our body. But beyond that, we have the many influences of the vestibular apparatus on the muscle tone which influences the perception of gravity of our body.

I reproduce here some of the protocols which Parker and I obtained from subjects who were in fast elevators.

1. When the elevator is going up, the legs are heavier, especially the feet. When the arms are stretched forwards, they are also heavier and sink down. This sensation is only present at the start and disappears as soon as the speed has become steady.

2. When the elevator stops, the arms go higher and are lighter. There is the sensation that the body goes further upward and sinks back in a slight curve, also forward and becomes heavier. The feeling of lightness of the body at the stopping is connected with the sensation that the body has become longer. It is as if the substance were trying to go further upward than the body and the soles.

3. After going up repeatedly, the apparent movement, especially when the eyes are closed, persists and the mass goes upward, whereas the legs remain unmoved or move upwards only a little. Something goes out of the body. A general slight swaying without predilection for a particular direction is present. It is again as if something were trying to come out of the body, especially of the head, which feels larger, and the mass goes out of the head.

4. When the elevator goes down, the arms go up and become lighter. The same is true about the body until the speed has become steady. Then the body becomes lighter and seems to elongate.

5. When the elevator is stopped, the legs become heavier, but the rest of the body continues to go down, so that below the feet there are two lighter phantom feet. At the same time the body becomes shorter. Afterwards the body goes back in a slight curve to its previous position. The arms first sink and then go into the normal position. At first they are heavier and then become lighter.

6. A further after-sensation may come. A phantom, a mass, goes down and the body shortens.

Whenever the arms go down, they are experienced as heavier. Often it feels as if they were pushed into the body. When the arms go higher, one feels as if one were being pushed backwards. The sensation of heaviness is stronger in the legs. Only the increase in speed has an influence. Also, the perception of the movement is dependent on the increase in speed. Mach and M. H. Fischer have had the same experience. As I have mentioned, body and arms are felt heavier after the start, according to the laws of the inertia of mass. It is very remarkable that when the subject is going down (protocol 4) the body not only is lighter, but also becomes longer. It is as if a part of the head were not following the movement and remains in its place. It is an after-effect of the posture of the head, and this after-sensation is stronger than the actual sensation of the posture of the head. This becomes certain, considering what happens when the elevator stops. The after-sensations are brought into relation to the phantom of the body and not to the real body. We know where the body is. It is either felt unmoved, or moved in a very small degree. It is remarkable that the tactile and kinaesthetic and also optic impressions of the body do not influence the experience of the position of the head. The sensation of our soles gives us the final impression where our feet are. Under the influence of vertical movements a dissociation occurs in the image of the body, so that a part of the substance of the body goes out of the body in the sense of the positive after-sensation.

The emanation of the substance of the head out of its frame is of special importance. This emanating substance is the carrier of the localization of the ego. Claparède has shown that we localize our ego generally in the height of the basis of the frontal bone between the eyes. We have only to add that where there is a vestibular after-sensation it becomes the carrier of the ego. It is in this respect more important than the body-image based on the other senses. We appreciate the length of our body according to the actual sensation of the sole and the localization of our ego, which depends on a vestibular after-sensation. Lengthening and shortening of the body will be experienced accordingly. This reaction, the lengthening and shortening of the body according to dissociation between vestibular head and real legs, is especially clear when, according to the protocols 3 and 6, after-sensations occur in persons with a sensitive vestibular apparatus. When the unspecific swaying occurs, which is probably due to an unspecific irritation of the vestibular apparatus, substance emanates out of the head, which appears larger.

It is a well-known phenomenon that the head appears to be larger after alcoholic intoxication. Alcohol influences the vestibular apparatus, as is well known. The dissociation in the image of our body under the influence of accelerated vertical movements has a more general significance. The vestibular irritation, which occurs under these conditions, dissociates the vestibular gravity experiences from the others. With the vestibular irritation, a part of the substance of the body wanders. This wandering part of the body is like a phantom with indistinct outlines. It contains the head portion of the body substance. The centre of the other sensations of gravity is in the legs, at least when one is standing up.

The body becomes lighter when substance emanates from it. It is as if a part of the heavy mass of the body were emptied. In other words, the body is a unit only when there are no particular irritations in the vestibular field. Unusual irritation of the vestibular nerve dissociates the postural model of the body. According to M. H. Fischer, vertical acceleration affects the otoliths. The dissociations described here are probably due to an excitation in the sphere of the otoliths. But it is more than probable that the unspecific swaying and the consequent apparent enlargement of the head is due to an irritation of the semi-circular canals.

There is no question that turning in the turning-chair or irrigation of the ear with hot or cold water provokes very similar phenomena concerning the postural model of the body, which have not yet been sufficiently studied. But when there is an apparent movement of the body or of an outstretched extremity, the substance of the body moves in the direction of this apparent movement. The apparent movement carries with it a part of the substance of the body; a phantom and the other part of the body, orientated according to the outstanding sensations of the body, especially the soles, remain. We come, then, to the conclusion that the otolith apparatus as well as the semi-circular canals have an influence on the perception of gravity of the body and that vestibular apparent movements carry a part of the heavy substance of the body with themselves.

There are also special parts of the body which are more important in orientation in relation to the body than others. These are especially the parts which are under the influence of gravity, the soles, when we are standing, the buttocks, when we are sitting, and in addition there is an important point in the head in which, according to Claparède, the ego is localized.

We shall not be wrong if we connect this particular localization partially with the eye-muscles and the position of the eye. According to the primary position of the eyes, the ego is directed forwards. The actual, kinaesthetic, and tactile sensations form a unit with the vestibular and with the optic impressions. Whenever there is abnormal irritation in the vestibular field, important dissociations are taking place. When we try to get an image of our own body, we first get some outstanding point, a frame, in which we fit the body-image. The soles give us the contact with the

G

earth and the necessary basis for orientation in the adjoining space. The head is the carrier for the distance receptors (Sherrington). The centre of the ego, accordingly, is between the eyes. Further orientation is gained by the openings of the body and the parts of the skin that are tense over bones. When the frame of the body-image is drawn, further gradual elaboration of the frame, which is marked by the important points, sets in.

For the psychology of neurasthenia and hypochondria these remarks are of great importance. According to Leidler and Loewy, we find vestibular changes in a high percentage of neurotics. This vestibular irritation will influence the feeling of the sensation of gravity of the body. It will especially change the impression about the heavy mass in the body. Neurasthenics often complain that something has become loose in their body. They talk of bubbles in their heads and in their limbs. They also speak of emptiness and changes in their heads, as if something were getting loose or as if the inner parts of the body were dissolving. It may be mentioned again that normal subjects sometimes feel the heaviness of the body not as a homogeneous, but as a foamy substance. We shall see later that we deal in neurasthenia with a particular weakness of the body schema. Wherever vestibular irritation occurs by conversion, the structure of the model of the body will be impaired. We shall discuss later which kind of tendencies lead to dissociation in the body-image.

(22) *Pain*

The problem of pain can only be solved by studying the relation of pains to the schema. There has long been an argument on this subject between Goldscheider and von Frey. Goldscheider maintains that there are no specific nerves for pain, whereas von Frey says that there are specific pain points on the skin. There are certainly points on the skin which are more susceptible to the perception of painful stimuli. Objections have been raised against speaking of pain perception. It has been said that the important thing is the reaction of the organism towards pain. But we have to consider that in every perception we must distinguish between the object we perceive, the sensation in connection with this perception, and finally the reaction of the total personality to the perception. We are dealing of course with a unified act. Such an analysis is always artificial. But still it is necessary to keep this separation in mind when we try to study psychology. This general scheme is not sufficient, since every sensation gets its sense and meaning only in connection with the whole of the body, so that the general scheme would be: (1) perception; (2) sensation; (3) the relation of the sensation to the body as a whole (image of the body); (4) the reaction of the total personality.

It is of course possible to form subdivisions, especially to point (4), but this is not our task at the present time. The description of every experience has to take into account all points mentioned, and the relation between the four sides of perception will be a fundamental characteristic of our experience. In the optic sphere perception is distant and separated from sensation. Sensation as such (the experience on the body) does not play an important part. We even need some attention to discover that optic perception is accompanied by sensation. It is not for the specific experience that we need the body for seeing. In the reaction of the total personality, the reaction of the body is accordingly less important than the reaction of the emotion and the so-called higher functions of the mind.

Almost the same is true about hearing. Of both the optic and acoustic group of experiences it may be said that sensation and perception are far distant in space from each other. In the tactile sphere sensation and perception come closer to each other. The postural model plays a much more obvious part. In almost the same category are smell and taste. Smell and taste play an objective part, but their objects are at least partially inside the body, and accordingly the reaction of the instinctive sphere of the body becomes stronger.

In pain, the object becomes comparatively unimportant. When we suffer pain, we care less for the quality of the object than for the sensation. At the same time object and subject come so close together that differentiation becomes difficult. The sensation, as such, has a tendency to irradiation. The reaction of the body is very strong. Coenaesthesia plays a very important part, and is the basis for the strong somatic answer of the total personality. The higher emotions of individuals play a less important part, at least primarily. There is no reason to deny the specific quality of the pain sensation, and, as far as sensations have their specific nerves, there is no reason to deny that pain has its specific end apparatus and nerves, as far as a specificity generally goes.

We cannot discuss here the correctness or otherwise of Head's opinion that there are two systems of sensibility in the skin, a protopathic and an epicritic. The protopathic system is, according to him, more responsible for the pain sensation than the epicritic system. It may be that there is in every peripheral apparatus and nerve the capacity to provoke pain. But there probably does not exist an absolute specificity of nervous excitation in any apparatus for perception. I do not believe that J. Müller's old formulation that there are specific energies of senses ('Specifische Sinnes—Energie') covers the facts. It is at least probable that the synaesthesia principle, which is an almost universal phenomenon, has validity not only for the central nervous system, but also for the more peripheral parts of the perceptive apparatus.

If one tends to consider pain only as a total reaction and not as a sensation, one may be reminded that the lesion of the lateral tract in the spinal cord doubtless provokes a comparatively isolated loss of pain sensation. One may also be reminded that lesion of the nerve itself also makes a field insensitive towards stimuli which otherwise would provoke pain. Therefore, there is a definite system for the sensation of pain. Achelis has emphasized the reactions towards pain. But even here we are not dealing with a specific characteristic of pain. I have often emphasized that motor answer or at least the tendency to motor answer is one of the general characteristics of any perception. The separation between sensibility and motility is after all an artificial one.

Every situation has a motor answer, and it is one of the merits of Behaviourism that it has energetically pointed out these facts. When we study human behaviour or the behaviour of any organism, we deal always with sensations, perceptions, and motor reactions at the same time, and Behaviourism is right in so far as it takes behaviour as the primary entity. But Behaviourism is also compelled to acknowledge that there are stimuli or changes in the situation, and that the answer of the organism is understood as an answer. It is a great mistake of Behaviourism to think it can define the changes in the situation otherwise than in terms of perception. Perception and motor answer are the two sides of the unit behaviour. It is true that we may think that there are some motor answers which are either incomplete or even only a tendency to an answer. But when we study a reflex, we have no right to say that there is no perception at all connected with the reflex. Reflexes are also answers, as Sherrington has shown. We have no right to say that there is no perception in the answer of an isolated spinal cord in a spinal cord preparation. We have no definite knowledge about the psychology of such reflexes. We may even go deeper and ask what is the psychology of growth, what is the psychology of a reaction of a tissue? This leads us deeply into the field of the philosophy of nature, and this is not the place to try to prove statements of such generality. These remarks are only intended to emphasize my general psychological point of view. There is no question that, in the sphere in which we are interested, perception, sensation, and motor answer form a unit. The relation between the different parts of the unit may vary, and either sensation or motor answer may sink to a very low level. But they will always be at least potentially present.

It seems that, like touch, pain also, even when superficial, is felt in a layer which is psychologically below the optic surface (perceived or imagined), of the body. Pain has to be localized and therefore brought into connection with the organization of the body-image. The phenomena of irradiation are particularly interesting. It seems that when there is any pain on the surface of the body, the postural model becomes overemphasized at this particular point. It becomes distorted. There are feelings of swelling. There exists a proof for the conception that pain has to be brought into connection with the postural model of the body. There are cases in which the perception of pain is seemingly preserved, although the individual does not take into consideration the pain he actually feels. Stengel and Schilder have described an asymbolia for pain.

The first patient we observed did not react to severe pinpricks, hitting with hard objects, or pinching. When the patient was pricked several times in her back, she did not react at first, but finally she several times touched with her right hand the point where she had been pricked. When her arm was pinched, she withdrew it completely, but without changing her attitude towards the examiner. She never withdrew her arm with force. When she was hit with a brush on the ulna, she did not show any tendency to withdraw. The patient, who was afflicted with a logorrhea in connection with a sensory aphasia, might sometimes say, "It hurts", but often readily offered the limb which had been hurt. She even hurt herself. The patient did not show any lack of attention concerning the pain, but on the contrary was very much interested in it. The autopsy showed a small lesion in the frontal lobe and a rather extended lesion, which reached from Heschl's circumvolution and the upper part of the gyrus temporalis primus to the supramarginal gyrus, which was destroyed in its lower part, and extended to the angular gyrus, in which the lesion was much less pronounced than in the supramarginal gyrus, which was decidedly in the centre of the lesion.

A series of other cases confirmed our opinion that lesions of the supramarginal gyrus are of the greatest importance in the genesis of the asymbolia for pain. It is more than probable that in asymbolia for pain patients are unable to connect the pain with the image of the body. The region of the brain which is involved in these cases is indeed very near the region which in our opinion is indispensable for the building up of the schema of the body. It is remarkable that the cases of that kind also show a very incomplete reaction to dangerous situations in general.

We have already mentioned an asymbolia for danger situations. It is important to study the motor reaction of cases of that kind. There are some local reactions, but they remain isolated; there is a squirming, but never a real defence, when there is any reaction at all. It appears that with the asymbolia an incomplete reaction on the motor side is present. In some cases the incompleteness of the motor answers is in the foreground; but in these also the incomplete utilisation of the pain perception is the paramount issue. It is remarkable that two of the patients who recovered said that they could not remember feeling any pain when they were pricked. It seems that at any rate in cases of that kind the pain is less connected with the body-image; it is dissociated from it, and, accordingly, from the personality. But there is no reason to believe that no pain is felt at all.

I have not yet mentioned two outstanding features. One is that patients often offer themselves to the pain stimulus and even inflict pain on themselves. In the first case observed by Stengel and Schilder the patient pushed objects against her eye and would have hurt herself seriously, if she had not been stopped. We may even indicate an analogy to sadomasochistic tendencies observed in those cases. We may also say that the patients are curious about the sensation which they cannot perceive completely.

Patients of that kind, as I have mentioned, are also insensitive to threatening gestures and to dangerous situations generally. Danger is, after all, a danger for the body. One could even talk of an asymbolia for danger. The patients also do not react to loud noises. But the lack or the incompleteness of the reaction to pain is still the outstanding feature in cases of this type. Pain in itself signifies a danger for the organism. The reaction movements to pain are an attempt to escape a danger situation. It is more than probable that the child's conception of pain is prior to its conception of danger, and that danger means for a child something which will sooner or later inflict pain and disrupt in this way the unity of the organism and its image. The insensitivity to loud noises which has been observed in cases of so-called pure word-deafness has probably some relation to the phenomenon described here. There are probably cases which are the counterpart of the phenomenon described here, cases in which sensitivity towards pain and danger is increased. I surmise that in cases of that kind a lesion between Broca's and Wernicke's region is present.

There is no question that not only cortical apparatus serves the sensitivity to pain. In alcoholics with deep clouding of the consciousness, Bender and Schilder have observed an increased sensitivity to pain. It seems that the somatic apparatus of consciousness has a protecting influence, and, with its impairment, reaction to pain is increased; although pain has a subcortical apparatus, it has to be brought into connection with cortical activities. Even when there is a clouding of the consciousness, cortical activity has not stopped completely. One has the impression that pain overflows the whole body when the consciousness is clouded.

The effect of pain on the body-image has not hitherto been sufficiently studied. The part of the body in which the pain is felt gets all the attention. Libido is concentrated on it (Freud) and the other parts of the body-image lose in importance; but at the same time the painful part of the body becomes isolated. There is a tendency to push it out of the body-image. When the whole body is filled with pain, we try to get rid of the whole body. We take a stand outside our body and watch ourselves. When one has toothache and is near to falling asleep, one may have the feeling that one is watching oneself and that the pain belongs to another body.

(23) *Development of the body-image*

It is remarkable that infants have very incomplete reactions to pain. The same holds true of animals (cf. postea). Are there states of ontogenetic development in which the body-image is undeveloped? And is the incomplete pain reaction a sign of the insufficient integration of the body-image? We must study the libidinous structure of the body schema before we can try to give an answer to this question.

Two factors, apparently, play a special part in the creation of the body-image. The one is pain, the other the motor control over our limbs.

Preyer has especially emphasized the rôle of pain. We have to acknowledge that pain belongs to us in a special way. Bernfeld stresses the importance of the fact that our intention acts on the body in a more immediate way, but every sensation contributes to the building-up of the body-image. There is no fundamental difference between the various sensations in this respect. Sensations are always sensations of a person. There is the central factor of the ego with its intentions and strivings and desires. This central factor uses the sensations and perceptions.

Attempts have often been made to attribute to the sensations which come from the inside of the body a decisive importance in the building-up of the body-image. French writers have talked of coenaesthesia, but there is no question that the sensations coming from the inside of the body have no inner meaning before they are brought into connection with the body-image. Not one of the numerous French writers has taken pains to study the actual experiences which we have about the inside of our body. I do not think that coenaesthesia, the so-called 'Gemeinempfindungen', has any decisive part in the construction of our bodily self. Our bodily self is built up according to the needs of the personality. It is true that pain is here an important factor. It helps us to decide what we want to have nearer to our personality, to the centre of our ego, and what we want to have further away from it. This decision and choice must be closely related to the motor activities; but what is true about pain, is also true of any other sensation. Every sensation has its motility, as I have emphasized. Sensation has in itself a motor answer. Continued activity is therefore at the basis of our bodily self. We choose and reject by action. Bernfeld's contention thus finds its proper place.

Nietzsche calls the body 'Herrschaftsgebilde' (creation of the dominating will). We may say the same about the body-image. Since optic experience plays such an enormous part in our relation to the world, it will also play a dominating rôle in the creation of the body-image. But optic experience is also experience by action. By actions and determinations we give the final shape to our bodily self. It is a process of continual active development. Under the influence of the inner drive one can only separate artificially sensory experiences from inner activities and libidinous strivings, which emanate from a central personality.

The development of the body-schema probably runs to a great extent parallel with the sensory motor development. Luquet, who has studied children's drawings, talks of the synthetic incapacity of the child. "The thing is not there as a whole. The details only are given and, owing to the lack of synthetic relations, they are simply juxtaposed. Thus an eye will be placed next to the head, an arm next to a leg etc." Of course, drawing is a rather complicated psychic activity and it may be difficult to determine whether this synthetic incapacity is based at all on sensory difficulties or whether it is merely due to motor incapacities. But the child is completely satisfied with its drawings, and I believe, therefore, that the way in which children draw human figures really reflects their knowledge and sensory experience of the body-image. They express at least the mental picture they have of the human body, and the body-image is mental picture as well as perception.

Goodenough's study contains material which is of great importance for the problem of the body-image of the child. The way in which children draw fingers deserves special interest in this respect. They may multiply the fingers, they may draw them in a straight line. It seems that there is a close parallelism between the optic development and the understanding of special relations in the body-image.

Piaget has studied the development of the left and right connotation in children. Between the ages of five and eight, left and right only have a meaning concerning their own body. Between eight and eleven, they can also apply them to others. Only after that time can they use the left and right connotation freely for others, for objects in space, and for themselves. Piaget distinguishes three stages: (1) ego-centrism, (2) socialisation, and (3) complete objectivity. He believes that one has to do merely with judgment and reasoning, but I discern in the development of the left and right connotation a development in the body-image. According to Koffka, the picture of an ear or a mouth or a finger may not be recognized by a child, although it is able to recognize these parts on the complete body. We at any rate gain the impression that, from the point of view of sensory motor development, the child brings more or less isolated and uncorrelated experiences into a complete form by continual effort. Even then the parts are not in such a close relation to the whole as they are in the adult.

(24) *Two deceptions. The influence of the optic sphere on the body-image*

Two deceptions may help us to gain a deeper insight into some of the problems discussed here. I have before me a key which I hold in a vertical position. I produce a double vision by staring into the distance. I then touch the end of the key from above with the finger of my other hand so that I have a clear double vision of the finger. I now clearly see two fingers, both of which touch the key. After a while, the impression is imperative that these two keys are not only seen, but also touched. This impression is more vivid when the finger is removed several times and put on the key again. When the tactile impression is doubled, both optic impressions are vivid, and every finger seen is a living finger. The same doubling occurs when I inflict pain by pin-pricks to the double vision of the finger. Two pin-pricks are felt. The doubling is clearer when my interest is directed towards the object and not to my sensation.

In some subjects, touch or pain is often felt, not on one or both of the fingers seen, but at a point which lies between the two fingers. The finger would be seen at this point, if one had not produced a double vision, but had fixated the finger. The optic picture of the fingers then makes a rather unreal and ghostlike impression. When I produce a double vision of one of my fingers, one picture is more substantial while the other is more like a phantom. One generally feels as the real finger that finger which one brings in connection with the other body. The finger which is connected with the body is the real and living finger. If one covers the hand so that the two fingers are seen as isolated from the other body, one feels a living but invisible finger between the two visible fingers, and the two fingers give the impression of phantoms. Phenomena of this type could be observed in the majority of subjects.

The experiment shows that the optic picture can determine the tactile sensation and the tactual model of the body. But the fact that the real finger can be felt between the untouched optic images of the fingers shows that the schema of the body is determined in some cases by the optic picture and in other cases by the tactile sensation. The final structure of the model of the body depends on the situation as a whole. The optic and the tactile material are used in the body-image according to the situation. But sometimes the optic material may determine our tactile impression and, with that, the model of the body.

It is important to compare these results with the experiment made by Stratton, Wooster, and Scholl. Stratton put on a mask, which covered the left eye; before the right eye he placed a system of lenses which turned everything upside down and from right to left and *vice versa*. When sleeping, he had both eyes covered. In one of the experiments, which lasted eight days, he looked for eighty-six hours into an upside-down world. I give the excerpt of the protocol which Scholl published.

1st day. Everything appeared upside down. All movements of the hand were wrong, since they were made as if everything was normal. But the hands reached a place different from that intended. The wrong hand was continually used for grasping objects on a particular side. The unusual tension of the attention was very fatiguing. There was a temptation to omit every uncomfortable impression and to rely upon tactile impressions, movement, and the old visual images. The completion was often made in the pre-experimental way. In regard to the limbs and other parts of the body, the pre-experimental image intruded into the actual perception. Arms and legs which were actually seen were localized in a double way. There was the localization in which they were seen; but in the background there was the previous localization closely related to muscle sensations and touch. Touches provoked a visual image of the pre-experimental type. When one side of the body approached an object the touch came from the opposite side to that expected. The same was true concerning the below and above. A nervous disturbance was present and a pressure in the upper abdominal part akin to a mild nausea.

2nd day. The nervous disturbance returned. Intentional movements were less difficult and more appropriate to the present optic experiences. Objects in the outside world which were not seen could be imagined better than on the first day in agreement with the actual vision. With some effort arms and legs could be imagined in this position, but not the rest of the body. When I moved my clasped hands over my head, the disappearance of my hands under the lower end of the visual field and a continuation of the movements made the region of my chest and my shoulders appear empty, although I had anticipated the direction of such a movement in the pre-experimental visual field. The body was experienced as upright, the outside space as upside down. When I went for a walk in the evening I was unable to recognize my surroundings. If I closed my eyes, the old way of imagining came back.

3rd day. I felt more at ease. I could observe my hands during writing without disturbance. But often I stretched out the wrong hand to grasp an object lying on one side of me. Differentiation between right and left offered special difficulties when visual localization was to be correlated to the tactile motor one. Above gave the impression which was previously connected with below. Once when I was standing before the fireplace and looking at the fire, I was overwhelmed by the queer impression that I was looking at the fire from the occipital part of my head. Touches were often correctly expected in correspondence with the new situation, though they were sometimes confused with the localization of the previous type. The unseen parts of the body could be brought in connection with optic perceptions, especially when I looked at my arms and legs. When I closed my eyes there were images in the new correlations.

4th day. No further somatic discomfort. One morning before the blind was removed from my eyes I imagined the wash-basin and its surroundings in pre-experimental manner. But my movements were opposite to those which fitted in with this image. I reacted in a new way to an old system of relations instead of reacting in the old manner to the new system of correlations. The more common type of inappropriate reaction was now the movement of one hand when the actual circumstances would have asked for a movement of the other one. So when I stretched out my right hand to pick up a book which was lying to my left on the floor, by chance I discovered a simple method by which I could select the correct hand when picking up objects from the floor, which method I used afterwards with invariable success. If I tapped with my foot once or twice near the object before I bent to pick it up, the appropriate hand came into play. Curiously enough it was then still easier to start with the appropriate foot than with the hand. The image of unseen objects harmonized with seen objects. But it was impossible to reverse them. The relation between the touch of one side and the corresponding visual image became more vivid. Competition between old and new localization occurred. Two objects of different shape, one in each hand, brought into the visual field, had a position concerning right and left opposite to my expectation. The impression of upright or reversed depended on the direction of the attention. When I looked at my arms and legs, objects were upright. When I looked away from my body and from the image of the pre-experimental optic image of the body, things were standing upside down. Objects were upright when I made quick movements of the body.

5th day. The wrong hand was used more rarely. No reflection was necessary. When hand and object were visible it was only necessary to direct the attention towards the object and it was reached correctly. The gait was for the most part undisturbed. When I made quick, complicated, but well-exercised movements, localization in space concerning visual, tactile, and kinaesthetic perception was better unified than when I was sitting and looking inactively at my surroundings. During such inactive looking I involuntarily imagined head, shoulders, and chest in the old pre-experimental relation to the present objects in the visual field. But by an effort I could form the whole shape of my body on the basis of the parts seen, though I felt this picture as forced. This spontaneous picture of the unseen parts of the body was during sitting as it was in previous experience and did not fit in with the present posture of the parts visible. These were felt where they were seen, but even they came back in the previous way of feeling if they were not looked at any longer. When I attempted to move both legs in the same direction and one was in the visual field, the other outside it, I felt as if I were moving them in opposite directions.

6th day. When I brought both index fingers into the visual field, the right one being where the left one previously was, a touch could be felt in either of them, sometimes even in both. Movement, slight flexion, or stretching made a clear difference and made it impossible to experience the touch in arbitrary relations.

7th day. More than ever at home in the new surroundings. Direction of movements good, but measurement incorrect. Finger test better with closed eyes. When I looked at a limb and let its image come up in its old position, I could feel it there, but only with an effort, and the sensation was comparatively weak. When I looked away, I felt it involuntarily in its pre-experimental position, although I was also conscious of a tendency to feel it in its new position. It was a battle between new and old localization. The hair and the skin of the head were felt persistently in the old position, doubtless because I never saw them in another position. But when I moved my hands quickly backwards and forwards before my open eyes, the movement ended every time with the touch of the top of the head. It was not difficult to create a vivid spatial imagination of the skin of my head corresponding to the new visual perception. The strangeness of the landscape disappeared.

8th day. The parts not seen were not yet incorporated into the new system. Concerning the parts seen there was uncertainty and sudden changes of correlations. When I directed my attention to the new visual presentation of the body which was to be touched, and expected the touch there, the touch was felt in the new situation, and there was no change in the correlations. Immediately afterwards, a kind of after-image of the touch occurred at the other visual side. When the original touch was unexpected, the visual picture and the tactile space could be old and new at the same time; or there was only the new picture, although without the real relation of the tactile sensation to this picture. The unseen parts (forehead) remained in the old localization. By touching the forehead with the hand the attention was directed towards the point, and the new localization could be reached. The sensations of touch on the lips could not be brought so easily out of their old localization. There were contrasting localizations for the lips. A new localization of the shoulder could be reached, but the head was settled too deep in the shoulders. As long as the new position of the body was vivid, everything stood upright. But when a pre-experimental posture of the body succeeded, the surrounding world was taken as a yardstick. I seemed to observe the world from a body which had been turned round.

After the glasses were removed my surroundings provoked a queer feeling of acquaintance. Apparent movements and nausea occurred as on the first day of the experiment. Intentional movement was performed in a direction opposite to that intended.

Stratton supposes that the local signs ('Lokalzeichen') were changed. The tactile sensations were translated into another optic world. Stratton emphasizes that right and left are more easily taken for each other than below and above. He emphasizes how much active movements help in orientation. The experiments by Scholl and Wooster took a similar direction and show similar results.

There is no doubt that the experiments by Stratton, Scholl, and Wooster offer us important material which shows the influence of optic impressions on the schema of the body. The new optic orientation has an immediate influence on the knowledge concerning one's own body. On the other hand this knowledge concerning one's own body is continually formed and influenced by the old and new optic impressions and their fight with each other. It is also clear that the body-image can be disturbed by experimental changes in vision, but that it is built up again and that a new unit is formed. The experiment I mentioned above concerning the doubling of tactile impressions when we produce a double vision and the experiments of Stratton and his successors definitely prove the influence of optic impressions on the body-image. It is hard to understand why Kaila and Bürger-Prinz doubt that the body-image can be changed from the optic sphere. They have examined the postural model of the body in Korsakoff cases. They complain about the lack of examination of normal persons. But they have overlooked important parts of the literature. They come to the conclusion that Korsakoff cases when examined for a longer time finally make mistakes concerning the model of the body. But their method is very disputable. When the Korsakoff case is tired, he loses the understanding necessary to carry out such complicated orders.

It is remarkable, as Scholl also emphasizes, that movement leads to a better orientation in relation to our own body. We do not know very much about our body unless we move it. Movement is a great uniting factor between the different parts of our body. By movement we come into a definite relation to the outside world and to objects, and only in contact with this outside world are we able to correlate the diverse impressions concerning our own body. The knowledge of our own body is to a great extent dependent upon our action. In Stratton's experiments, action helps to build up a new correlation. These experiments have a general significance in so far as they show that in the postural model of the body we do not deal with a given entity, but that we acquire it in the directed and intentional action concerning the world. I may recall here that this is also the result to which the experiments of Klein and Schilder have led. The postural model of the body has to be built up. It is a creation and a construction and not a gift. It is not a shape in Wertheimer and Köhler's sense, but the production of a shape. There is no doubt that this process of structuralization is only possible in close contact with experiences concerning the world.

In Stratton's experiment, the new optical experiences tear the unity of the body. It is worthy of note and it is to be expected that the tearing up of the body-image is connected with feelings of nausea. It is, after all, a particular type of dizziness. Dizziness occurs always when the impressions of the senses cannot be united. In all cases of dizziness practically the same occurs. It has again to be emphasized that by these changes in the optic world the purposeful motor action is impaired. We deal here with phenomena which have again analogies to what one experiences in vestibular irritation and also during sea-sickness. In sea-sickness, the impossibility of adapting movements to the ever-changing surroundings plays an important part, besides the vestibular irritations.

Another important result of these experimental studies is that we learn again that the perception of our own body is not very different from the perceptions of any other outside objects. Furthermore, it may be emphasized that, as Scholl rightly states, the phenomena of allochiria and of apraxia show great similarities to the phenomena observed in cases of this kind.

Another experience is perhaps worth reporting. When one is standing on an escalator, and especially when the escalator is crowded with people, one sees that one is moving upwards on an inclined plane. The angle of the escalator is an angle between 30 and 40 degrees. When the escalator is moving one feels clearly that the feet are not standing in a right angle to the legs but are bent upwards in an angle which corresponds to the inclination of the escalator. The impression is an absolute one, and leads even to rather disagreeable sensations in the joints. One can escape this deception only when one looks at one's feet and sees that they are standing in the normal position to the legs. In this experience it is again clear that the whole optic situation determines the feeling concerning our own body. The experience is remarkable in so far as the optic influence in this experiment does not come from an optic change concerning the perception of one's own body, but from the optic situation in the outside world. The experience shows clearly that the perception of our own body is in no way more reliable than the perception of the outside world. When one moves one's foot in this experiment the deception also disappears. We know comparatively little about our body as long as it is not in motion. Only by movement and new contacts with the outside world will the knowledge about our own body increase.

Another more general remark seems to be appropriate. Certainly the body-image in its final outcome is a unit. But this unit is not rigid: it is changeable. It is true that all senses are always collaborating in the creation of the schema of the body. But still we should not forget that, as in the experiments reported, we can change parts of these experiences in one field of the perception. The change in all experiments reported here is a change in the purely optic sphere. One should not therefore carry too far the idea of units, but should always consider that every unit has parts and sides which are comparatively independent of each other. We come also to the principle of the relative independence of parts, especially in the perception of our own body.

Another important feature is the comparative looseness with which the single parts of the body are connected with each other. It is obvious that limbs and trunk can go their separate ways; and that even under the comparatively simple conditions in these experiments, psychological dismembering can take place.

(25) *The body-image in clouded consciousness and the vestibular influence on the postural model of the body*

Optic perceptions undoubtedly have a strong influence on the body-image. I do not believe that optic imagination is less important for the postural model. In earlier experiments (cf.

Wahn und Erkenntnis) I have shown that when we deliberately produce optic images concerning our own body, changes in the actual sensations occur. When the subject is asked to imagine his hands three times their normal size, he may feel his imagined giant hands heavier, and this feeling of heaviness is an actual sensation. But imaginations, including those concerning our own bodies, follow their own laws. They change under the influence of motor impulses and motor imaginations. In the protocols I published with Kanner, I mentioned that imaginations of un-natural postures lead to far-going distortions of the optic representations of one's own body. The imagination of moving the arm elongated the mental picture of the arm, but there is in any case a continuous tendency of the optic image to change its shape. There are distortions, so-called metamorphopsias. There is also a tendency to multiply the optic imagination (polyopsia). The picture also changes its size. It may become larger or smaller (macropsia and micropsia). There is a specific tendency for every optic representation to disintegrate its shape, very often accompanied by phenomena of motion in the optic picture.

We may suppose that these changes in the optic representations concerning one's own body may have an effect on the body-image. But since there is the continual flow of the actual experiences coming from the body, the change in the optic representations will only have a limited effect on the body-image. But optic representations are only quantitatively different from optic impressions. The transition from optic images to optic perceptions is facilitated by clouding of the consciousness, and we perceive no changes in the body-image which correspond to the changes which take place in the picture of the body, which was the product of deliberate representation.

Federn has carefully described the changes in the body-image which occur when we gradually fall asleep. It often completely loses its third dimension. It is distorted in all directions. The distance of symmetrical parts can appear much larger than the length of the body. The dimensions in space lose their proportions. When two or three parts of the body are experienced correctly, the remaining part becomes a vague mass, enlarged or diminished. Sometimes the body-image reaches only to the trunk or to the knees. But parts of the middle of the body may also disappear. The borderline of the body in one direction may become blurred and it seems to be moving on this side. The body-image of the face and of the head is generally free. The parts of the body which touch the support are also stabilized. But even the shape of the head can be changed. Federn emphasizes that regions which have a greater significance from the point of view of eroticism are more resistant than other parts of the body. But we shall discuss this part of the problem more in detail later on.

I have made observations very similar to those made by Federn. In one of my cases the patient felt before falling asleep that she became smaller and smaller and finally was only a few centimetres long. Another patient felt something very similar during a nicotine intoxication. Similar changes in the schema of the body can be observed in dreams. According to Federn it consists sometimes only of the legs or of the head. There are also changes in the gravity of the body in dreams. There can be a loss of many parts of the body-image in a dream and finally parts of the dreamer's own body may appear in other persons. But only the study of the libidinous structure of the body will help here to a deeper understanding. In the first stages of hypnosis similar phenomena occur. I. H. Schultz reports the following experience of a hypnotized patient. "I am lying in water, in deep water, but I can look out. Above me lies a lean body. I know how I am lying but my body is turned round at a right angle. There is a deep hole in my chest. Out of it comes a long neck like a goose-neck with a very small head. The trunk with the head turns itself out of the body."

As my investigations with Bromberg have shown, not only optic images but also tactile imaginations undergo changes of this type. We have also referred in these investigations to the fact that tactile after-effects follow very similar principles. There is also in every perception an element which tends to distortion, spatial transposition, multiplication, and changes in the size of the object perceived. All these changes must add a new element of uncertainty in change in the construction of the body-image. Kanner, Bromberg and I have also shown that the disintegrative processes in imaginations and after-effects of sensations are increased when there is a change in the function of the vestibular apparatus.

We have studied above the influence of the otolith apparatus on the perception of the mass of the body, but there are other important changes concerning the body-image under the influence of vestibular irritations. One of the patients of Hoff and myself felt her neck swell during dizziness. The same patient felt that her extremities had become larger. In an old observation of Romberg's, the hands became larger and moved in different directions. Stein mentions a patient whose feet seem to elongate. Another patient has the sensation that her neck becomes longer and longer and that her head flies away. The legs grow and tend towards the wall. Whenever there are changes in the consciousness, the vestibular influence on the postural model may increase. I mention only the flying dreams, when vestibular irritation occurs. It is true that one then experiences especially a change in the weight of the body, but the shape of the body may also be distorted. In mescal intoxication we deal with a change in the consciousness, but probably also with a change in the vestibular apparatus. Forster reports that during mescal intoxication he felt as if his left side was very thin, while his right side was five times as thick and heavy. He felt as if the limbs did not fit each other. Zador gives an account of a patient who felt smaller under similar conditions ; his legs becoming shorter as if he was shrinking. When he closed his eyes he felt as if he could get into a mousehole. A case of schizophrenia reported by Beringer, which showed phenomena similar to those in mescal cases, felt her arms shortening and lengthening. I have reported cases of alcohol hallucinosis in which the patients felt parts of their body disappear.

A deep insight into the complications of the whole problem is afforded by cases which feel an enlargement of the whole body. R. Klein has observed such changes in encephalitis cases and in psychosis. Nemlicher and Sinegubko give an account of subcortical epilepsy in connection with macroparaesthesia. The limbs felt enlarged. They refute the theory of Bechtereff and Ratner, who maintain that the phenomenon is connected with changes in the sensory pathways and try to explain it as a change in the vegetative centres. I have been unable to avail myself of the Russian papers by Bechtereff, who has observed cases in which the patients experience a multiplicity of limbs.

But, at any rate, the vestibular apparatus plays an enormous part in the integration of our sensual experiences and consequently in the construction of the body-image. It does not surprise us, therefore, that Bonnier should have observed a case of a person who, during attacks of dizziness, felt divided into two persons. Skworrzoff mentions hallucinations of being doubled, in vestibular cases.[1]

---

[1] It seems that there is a general principle in the imagination which tends to the multiplication of pictures. This principle reveals itself in the rhythmic repetitions in the after-effects of perceptions. In the higher psychic levels, it partially takes on the character of a playful repetition. It is a characteristic of the principle of playful repetition that perceptions and images may change their place in the diverse direction of space, and that the images are tried out in different sizes. It seems that the vestibular apparatus has relations to this very universal psychic mechanism in so far as it helps to adapt the pictures due to rhythmic playfulness to the total situation. (Cf. my paper on the vestibular apparatus in the *Journal of Nervous and Mental Diseases*).

PART II

THE LIBIDINOUS STRUCTURE OF THE BODY-IMAGE

(1) *Narcissism and the love of one's own body*

Freud has shown that we are interested in the integrity of our own body. Libido is said to belong to one's own body. We call this libido narcissistic. Freud states that libido is at first given to the body as a whole. We call this the stage of narcissism and we suppose that the embryo and the new-born child have only narcissistic libido. The child is interested only in himself and not at all in the outside world. The stage of narcissism (primary narcissism) is followed by an auto-erotic stage in which the libido is concentrated in parts of the body which have a special erogenic significance. There is first the auto-erotic oral libido. The child enjoys irritation coming through the mouth. It is true that psycho-analysis calls this stage cannibalistic. The organism tries to incorporate the outside world in itself. Is there not necessarily an outside world already present? But it is judged only from the point of view of whether it can give oral satisfaction or not. But the child also enjoys its own muscular activity; it enjoys the sensation coming from the skin. There is a muscle and skin eroticism. But even at that period the genitals seem to be a source of special pleasure, though in a purely auto-erotic sense; anal and urethral sensations complete the picture.

A little later the outside world is perceived and gets its share of interest. Anal and homosexual tendencies concerning external objects may occur around the third year. Finally, with the development of the Oedipus complex (the sexual love for the parent of the other sex and the death wish against the parent of the same sex) the objects (the persons who are loved) assume a clearer shape. The conquest of the outside world has begun and the genitals take on a new significance and become the leading libidinous zone of the body. At this stage of development, when the child begins to have a clear impression of the outside world, there comes the full understanding of its own body as opposed to the outside world, the final picture of its own body is re-shaped, and we have the picture of the secondary narcissism before us. This is the present analytic theory concerning the libidinous development. Narcissism is considered as the great reservoir which sends out a part of its content to the objects. The energy which has been sent out from this reservoir may be taken back at any time. The psycho-analytic theory on this point is perfectly clear.

It is more difficult to follow the psycho-analytic theory concerning sadistic impulses. Sadistic impulses are those which try to overpower the love-object and inflict pain on it—the supreme test of power over it. The individual may identify himself with the object, may turn the sadism against himself, in which case he will become masochistic. He may invest the object with the supreme power of inflicting pain and may enjoy being completely in its power. Sadism is a partial desire, a part-step of sexuality. There is a development of sadistic tendencies. In the narcissistic stage, when there is no real outside world, sadism and masochism are meaningless. In the stage of oral libido there is an enormous aggressiveness which does not care about the existence of the object. The destruction of the object is almost an aim. The anal and homosexual stage is also endowed with rather violent aggressiveness, and the destruction of the object does not matter and may even be desired.

With the development of the Oedipus complex, the child attains a real interest in the preservation and even the well-being of the love-object. Sadism becomes a weapon for overpowering the love-object and keeping the rival away. It would blend then with the tendencies by which we try to maintain ourselves and would link the sexuality and the libidinous tendencies with the tendencies of the ego, which tend to self-preservation. Since there is always a tendency present to identify ourselves with the love-object, a masochistic tendency will always run parallel to the sadistic tendency.

This was the view of the Freudian conception and the psycho-analytic theory before the appearance of Freud's book *Beyond the*

Pleasure Principle. In this book, Freud develops the conception of a primary death instinct. He states that the individual has a tendency towards self-destruction. This is, according to him, the primary masochism. The individual would go to his death if the libidinous tendencies did not try to preserve the unity of the organism. They divert the destructive tendency from one's self to the object, and the tendency to aggression, the sadistic impulse, appears. The death instinct, the destructive instinct, is the desire of the ego which was previously called the tendency to self-preservation. The death instinct becomes destructive when not neutralized by a sufficient amount of libido.

This conception is certainly not very easy to understand. According to Freud, every individual wants to live to his own death and wants to live down the energy of life in his own way. But it is a great question whether we have the right to identify aggressiveness and death instinct. There arises also the question whether there exists a tendency, an instinct for death; but it is not the task of this book to go deeper into criticism of this late Freudian conception. Sadism in the common sense would be a mixture of libidinous tendencies and tendencies of the ego which are insufficiently neutralized by the libidinous tendencies. I will confine myself to saying that I do not endorse Freud's theory concerning the death instinct, aggressiveness, and primary masochism; I keep to his prior formulation. Sadism is the connecting link between the libidinous tendencies and the tendencies of the ego, which still try to preserve the body and need for this task the possibility of grasping, taking the objects to the mouth, which involve a certain amount of aggressiveness. But the individual knows that for his own preservation, for his own meaning and existence, the THOU is necessary. The tendency to self-preservation is therefore immediately linked with the tendency to the preservation of fellow beings. In the tendencies of the ego there is therefore not only aggressiveness.[1] The tendencies of the ego

---

[1] It cannot be denied that aggressiveness exists. It is a part of the ego. It may be a destructive impulse. The destructive impulse may be directed against one's self or against others. I will deal later with the tendency to dismember one's own body or the body of others. But these destructive tendencies never aim at the final end, they are not death tendencies. They are merely a phase from which the ego goes to new constructions.

provide food and self-defence.[1] This formulation also fits in very well with Freud's theory that the tendencies of the ego are in the full light of consciousness and that the ego is the system of conscious perception and representations and their motor answers.

In the present psycho-analytic formulation it is difficult to see the connection between the ego and the tendencies of the ego. Freud's formulation about the death instinct does not fit in with his formulations concerning the ego.

But we now return to the problem of narcissism which is so closely connected with the problems discussed in this book. What is the relation of narcissism to the image of the body? No libido or energy of the desires of the ego can be present unless there is an object with which they are connected. We are in a world, and objects are part of this world. When we live we are directed towards this world. There is always a person and the attitudes of this person. An attitude is an attitude towards something. An energy of the attitude cannot exist in an isolated way. Freud himself refers to the 'Triebrepresentanzen', the representations which are necessary for the instincts. We have therefore always to ask "What is the object towards which the instinct is directed?" The narcissistic libido has as its object the image of the body. But there is no question that our own body can exist only as a part of the world. In the first part of our discussions we have shown clearly that we do not perceive our own body differently from objects in the outside world. It is, therefore,

[1] I have often emphasized that grasping, groping, and sucking are the most primitive functions of the ego. We know that they come back in the primitive form of the so-called reflex, when higher centres in the brain are injured. We deal with very primitive reflexes. According to Mayer and Reisch, we probably have to do with a mechanism which is localized in the medulla oblongata. At any rate, in Gamper's case, in which only the brain-stem was preserved, grasping and sucking were present. Mayer and Reisch arrive at a formulation identical with that which I gave in my book on *Psycho-Analytic Psychiatry*, and find the basis of the ego in these primitive tendencies of grasping and sucking. They are right when they add that there must also be a tendency of defence concerning influences from the outside world which the individual does not want to stand. The tendency to primitive tensions of resistance belongs to this group. I have previously given a very similar interpretation to the schizophrenic negativism which is so closely related to the tensions of resistance which Kleist brings into relation with lesions of the thalamic system, but which probably have medulla and brain-stem centres.

[2] I use the terms 'instinct', 'drive', 'desire', and 'impulse' indiscriminately in this study.

senseless to say that for the newborn child only the body exists and the world does not. Body and world are experiences which are correlated with each other. One is not possible without the other. When Freud states that on a narcissistic level only the body is present, he must be mistaken. The newborn child has a world, and probably even the embryo has. It is true that on such a primitive level the borderline between world and body will not be sharply defined, and it will be easier to see a part of the body in the world and a part of the world in the body.

In other words, from the point of view of adult thinking, the body will be projected into the world, and the world will be introjected into the body. But the physiological remarks in the first part show that in the adult also body and world are continually interchanged. It may be that a great part of experiences will not be finally attributed either to body or world. I have mentioned the zone of indifference between body and world, and have stated that in a narcissistic stage the zone of indifference may play a more important part. After all, the image of the body has to be developed and built up. The narcissistic libido will be attached to the different parts of the image of the body, and in the different stages of libidinous development the model of the body will change continually.

In the whole structure of the schema of the body, the erogenic zones will play the leading part, and we have to suppose that the image of the body, in the oral stage of development, will be centred around the mouth; in the anal stage, round the anus. The libidinous flow of energy will strongly influence the image of the body. But there is no reason to believe that in eroticism concerning the surface of the body the muscle activities will be without significance. We suppose that every action of the ego in the analytic sense,[1] every grasping, groping, and sucking, will again have an enormous influence on the structure of the body-image. The senses will influence the motility, the motility will influence the senses, but the motility is also directed by strivings, tendencies, and desires. It is clear that in the building-up of the schema of the

[1] I prefer to use the term 'perception ego', when I mean the ego in the analytic sense, and the term 'ego' for the total personality, in accordance with the general use of the word.

body there will be a continual interaction between ego tendencies and libidinous tendencies or, in other words, between ego and id.

(2) *Erogenic zones of the body-image*

We may start with an important general formulation. Since both the body and the world have to be built up, and since the body in this respect is not different from the world, there must be a central function of the personality which is neither world nor body. There must be a more central sphere of the personality. The body is in this respect periphery compared with the central functions of the personality. We are now better able to under-stand Federn's dream-observations. When we fall asleep and dream, the old lability of the body-image comes back, and the body contracts and expands according to our emotional needs. It is of importance in this connection to ask again how the erogenic zones are represented in the body-image. Observation quickly shows that we feel especially the eyes, the mouth, the nipples, the genitals, the urethra, and the anus, in the way we have emphasized before.

The enormous psychological importance of all openings of the body is obvious, since it is by these openings that we come in closest contact with the world. By them we ingest air, food, sex products; by them we eject urine, sex products, faeces, and air. We have therefore distinguished points in the postural model of the body. These points are at the same time points of erotic im-portance. It is worthy of note that through the openings we also fulfil the functions of our life, and we have again to point out the close interrelation of purely sensory parts of the postural model of the body, as described in the first part of our discussions, and the libidinous structures which are in such a close relation with our strivings. Manifold investigations and experiments have shown me clearly that the difference in the libidinous structures is re-flected in the structure of the postural model of the body. Indi-viduals in whom a partial desire is increased will feel the particular point of the body, the particular erogenic zone belonging to the desire, in the centre of their body-image. It is as if energy were amassed on these particular points. There will be lines of energy connecting the different erogenic points, and we shall have a variation in the structure of the body-image according to the psychosexual tendencies of the individual. I have mentioned that the eyes are always a part of the body-image which is especially emphasized. The eyes, after all, are at least symbolically a receptive organ, and the symbolic significance of the eye, which we shall discuss later, is closely related to this function of the eye as a symbolic opening through which the world wanders into ourselves. There is some psychological truth in the old Epicurean doctrine that pictures wander into our eyes from objects.

There are some experiences concerning the erogenic zones which are relatively independent of the action of other persons and of the outside world. Urethral and anal irritations are to a great extent of an endogenous nature. When we come to the genitals the situation is still further changed. There is certainly a continual inner tension in the sex organs. They are, as Freud has emphasized, a continual source of sensations and stimulations. But there is no question that the genitals, owing to their situation near the organs of excretion, are continually irritated. Like the opening for excretion, they need continual cleaning which has to be done by the persons who nurse the child and later on by the individual himself. Whenever there is an inner tension in the organ, the organ will ask for a contact either with the hand of the person or with the outside world. The organs themselves force the individual into a continual contact with the outside world, and there is no question that we discover our body at least partially by these contacts with the outside world. It is true that what has been said about the genitals is in some ways true for the whole surface of the body. The skin is easily irritated and therefore an irritating organ. Continuous sensations are present which urge the child to touch itself or to make the persons around it touch its skin. The uncleanliness inherent in all parts of our body provokes itching sensations leading to touches which, in view of what we have already said, must themselves enrich the image of the body, which only thrives on the varied experiences of contacts with the world.

It is very important to notice that a great part of the body is discovered by the hands. The hands themselves are an outside world for the parts of the body which they touch. The possibility of moving and displacing the different parts of the body in relation to each other thus becomes a psychological problem of the utmost importance. Parts of the body which can easily be reached by the hands are therefore different in their psychological structure to parts of the body which can be reached by the hands only with difficulty.

We have mentioned above the importance of the eyes in the constructive building-up of the body-image, and the difference in the parts of the body which can be seen and those which cannot be seen. But there is no question that our own activity is insufficient to build up the image of the body. The touches of others, the interest others take in the different parts of our body, will be of an enormous importance in the development of the postural model of the body. Whenever one part obtains an overwhelming importance in the image of the body, the inner symmetry and the inner equilibrium of the body-image will be destroyed. We know that neurasthenia and hypochondria are of special importance for the understanding of the body-image. We have to do, as our later discussions will show, with disruptions in the postural model of the body.

Before we enter upon the discussion of neurasthenia and hypochondria we must return to the problem of pain which we have discussed previously more from the point of view of physiology. When we suffer from an organic pain, the model of the body changes immediately in its libidinous structure. All energies now flow to the diseased organ, as Freud and Ferenczi have emphasized. The postural model of the body is overloaded with narcissistic libido in the aching part. Paraesthesias and bodily discomfort have of course an effect very similar to that of pain. With the erotic change, a change in the perception goes on. The hand returns again and again to the aching organ. When the pain is not immediately present, pressure provokes it. There is a feeling of swelling, of dryness, of moisture in the aching part. (Of course, these changes are, like all the phenomena described here, not merely subjective; there are vegetative changes of all types present.) The aching organ becomes a centre of renewed experimentation with the body. It takes a part usually taken by the erogenic zones. There is, as we shall see later, not such a great difference between organic pain and dysaesthesia and psycho-genic pain and dysaesthesia.

Pain, dysaesthesia, erogenic zones, the actions of our hand on the body, the actions of others towards our body, the interest of others concerning our body, and the itching provoked by the functions of our body are therefore important factors in the final structuralization of the body-image.

(3) *Neurasthenia*

In neurasthenia and hypochondria we deal with neuroses in which particular parts of the body behave, as Freud, Ferenczi, and I myself have emphasized, as if they were autonomous and as if they were genitals. It seems, therefore, to be of great importance to arrive at a deeper understanding of cases of neurasthenia and hypochondria. I will first take an analyzed case.

E.M., twenty years old, complained of loss of memory, difficulties in falling asleep, in urination, and in defecation. He was unable to exercise these functions in the presence of others, or even when he knew that somebody was near. He was much worried by a tendency to masturbate in his sleep. His penis was shrinking. He had a leakage which frightened him. He was tormented by frequent erections. His memory was bad. His hands and feet were cold. He experienced sexual excitement especially when he saw feet. It made no difference whether they were the feet of a man or of a woman. His own feet also excited him.

His relations with his parents were decidedly bad. His hatred against his mother was conscious. The mother tyrannized over the home and was always talking about food; there was continual quarrelling and excitement. The father and mother had no affection for each other. He himself had no tender feeling for his sisters, the elder of whom, Martha, was four years younger, the second, Adèle, six years younger than he. There were important remembrances connected with the birth of the elder sister, but these were unconscious at the beginning of the analysis. During the birth he heard his mother crying. He imagined her lying flat on her back, naked, with her legs outspread. The physician tortured her, brushed her toe-nails, and rubbed her face with a sponge. The birth itself would probably not have affected him so strongly if it had not been preceded by an itching skin disease. He remembered that at that time he observed his father scratching his back with a brush because of an itching rash. After the birth of his elder sister he started to masturbate. He used to crawl under the bed and was afraid he might be caught.

His interest in feet was partially provoked by his father who often wiped his feet in the evening. There was another element in the development of his sexuality. He had a tumour on his genitals (apparently a varicocele or hydrocele). His mother repeatedly examined him, and he was afraid of these investigations. He also had imaginations that he was tortured by the doctor in the same way as his mother had been. He identified himself in a passive feminine way with the mother. This identification meant, of course, that a castration had taken place. He failed to recall definitely whether he thought that the child was born through the anus. But his associations and dreams made it perfectly clear. He was always afraid of dead chickens. To touch chickens, cats, and dogs provoked nausea. When he was five years old he was afraid on the toilet that a dead chicken or a dead rat would crawl into his anus.

The erotic significance of the anal zone, which was already repressed when he was five years old and appeared therefore as fear concerning the anus, is proved by another episode which took place when he was seven years old. Another boy urinated on him. They played at doctors. The patient put a pin into the other boy's anus, could not extract it and was much alarmed. When he was four and five years old he was interested in the naked feet of a girl and pretended to operate on them. His interest in the anal zone was increased by the enormous attention his family paid to defecation. Remembrances which reached far back but continued throughout his whole life showed that the boy's bowel movements were always a matter of interest to his family. He was supposed to report regularly whether he had bowel movements or not, and he was given bananas, of which he was very fond, only when he had defecated. But the mother's control was also directed towards food. She terrorized him and later on his sisters in order to make them eat more. (Later on in the neurosis, food disgusted him, and he developed a series of hypochondriac ideas about it. Heavy diet made his phallus shrink, made his hands and feet cold, and provoked itching in all those places.)

The father, dominated by the mother, also worried him and made him all sorts of promises on condition that he would eat, but did not keep his promise. The over-protection of his parents pushed him again into the passive masochistic position, which led in the birth-scene to identification with the mother. This passive attitude also meant castration, which is always partially imagined on the feet. The mother, as mentioned above, frequently inspected his genitals when he was ill. He was afraid of these examinations, which apparently started at a very early age. The father tricked him into a medical examination and finally into an operation. Analysis made it clear that his mother's interest in his genitals was present before his fourth year. The operation took place between his sixth and seventh year. He was always afraid of beatings. When he was six years old, other boys wanted to fight with him, but he ran away, pretending that he had to go to the toilet. He was afraid of burglars and thought that in the dark a cat might jump on his neck, especially a dead one. Cruel acts took place very early. He tore out the legs of bees and ants. At seven or eight years of age, he told his Aunt that her two children had just been killed. At ten years of age, he pushed a pillow into his younger sister's mouth so that it almost suffocated her.

Masturbation continually ran parallel to these events. He hid himself under the bed. In his phantasies he was tortured like his mother. Later on, other cruel phantasies came up. He was naked, bound, and soiled by faeces and urine. Flies tormented him. He himself or somebody else was quartered by horses. Breasts and bodies of women were cut away. He and a girl were naked, tied to each other back to back, so that no satisfaction was possible in spite of violent sex excitement. Stories of cruelty excited him strongly.

Between his sixth and eighth year, mutual masturbation and urinary plays with other boys often occurred. He slept in the same room as his father. The neurotic symptoms began with puberty. Characteristically, intestinal symptoms came first. A frequent urge to defecate bothered him. He was unable to

J

defecate in the presence of others. Itching sensations in the anus and the genitals also occurred. He was afraid that it would be impossible for him to marry. His hands and feet became cold and itched. Hands and feet became more and more important from a sexual point of view. His feet became more important to him than anything else. They were beautiful. He had violent erections which worried him. Finger and toe nails interested him. (He had phantasies, in the analysis, of kissing the feet of his father and mother, but also those of a passing negro.) From his twelfth year he had had many incomplete heterosexual relations—kissing, petting, etc. These relations were mostly very superficial. They did not mean very much to him. There were occasional outbursts of hatred. Many phantasies (e.g. he was lying with a girl in bed, both being naked; suddenly a corpse was in the bed) made it clear that he unconsciously identified intercourse with murder.

The hatred against the mother was obvious. He thought it would be to nobody's disadvantage if she were dead. But he often thought of his father's death also. He felt shy because of his frequent erections. He was afraid that others might get to know about them. He thought that perhaps he was inferior, though he was cleverer than others. He pretended to be dumb in order to baffle others. He had phantasies that he was wrongly accused and suffered. He was innocent but they convicted him. He had many hypochondriac complaints concerning the intestinal tract. He complained of a tendency to belch. He thought that he was too thin and that everybody saw that his face was too haggard. He had to be careful in his diet. He wanted to do everything quickly. Speed gave him the feeling that he was doing something, and he got erections. He had read all kinds of books on nervousness. He was afraid that the leakages would ruin him. He once worked with energy, but his father did not like the idea of his working. Later he became too tired and left the law school because he was unable to concentrate. He thought that nature could be improved, and that defecation and urination ought not to exist. He felt guilty and inferior. He sought compensation in the intellectual sphere. He was vain and self-complacent, especially in the intellectual sphere.

Some important parts of the analysis did not come to the

surface as remembrances. But the patient himself realized that his dreams and associations led to these conclusions. The infantile sex curiosity did not come immediately into his consciousness. But once he dreamt of an animal which was supposed to be a cow but was a horse. Urine came out of it like a fountain. (In another dream he masturbated. The semen fell on him, as from a fountain.) The horse passed gas at the same time. The association was that he had often observed the defecation of cows. In his childhood he believed that milk was the cow's urine. In another dream he saw a girl's genitals, but there was a phallus and one large testicle above. He remembered only that knowledge of sex matters came to him suddenly. Characteristically, he had no remembrances concerning the genitals of his sisters, with whom he was often bathed. Although his childhood remembrances gave more than clear hints of (probably chiefly anal) ideas of castration, the castration anxiety did not come to immediate remembrance. Once he dreamt that he had intercourse with a girl. But there was an empty space in the place of her genitals.

To sum up; it is safe to conclude that he was anally excited during the birth of his sister. That birth and sex relations had an anal significance for him (probably after genital castration) is proved by his phantasies and fears on the toilet. Memories brought to the consciousness show that in his very early childhood his mother gave him enemas, which he dreaded.

His relation to his mother was from the start passive and masochistic (anally and genitally). But he also showed a tendency to identify himself with her. The physician of the early remembrance was a substitute for the father, to whom he was also in passive sexual relation. But he had a tendency to identify himself with this physician in so far as in his phantasy he lay in bed with dead persons. According to his ideas, his father was under the yoke of his mother and passively masochistic too.

The initial difficulties in the analysis consisted of a strong negative transference to the analyst of the distrust of the parents, especially the father. The patient's strong narcissism, which led him repeatedly back to his own body, caused him also to overrate his superficial education and made the further transference difficult. When this was reached, the analyst became the carrier of all the suffering about which the patient complained; and by projection into the analyst, who in the patient's opinion mastered all his problems, and by identification with him, the final recovery took place. In a transference phantasy, the patient boxed with the analyst. The patient had learned how to box and developed the very inappropriate idea that the analyst was an experienced boxer. He thought that the analyst would be, like himself, terribly ashamed, if he were compelled to show his feet naked, and that the analyst had disturbances in defecation and was unable to sleep well. Then he developed a conviction of the analyst's health, and identified himself with him. I will not venture to decide whether this occurrence, which I would like to call Narcissistic Projection, is typical. It is at any rate of importance and emphasizes again the strong narcissism which gives significance to every part of the body. There is no question that the projection tends to depreciate the analyst by emphasizing his anal passivity. But it is the way to recovery.

I have reviewed the whole life-history of the patient. It is impossible to study the libidinous structure of the body-image in isolation. It is an integral part of the inner life-history of the individual. In order to understand it we must study the libidinous development from the earliest childhood. The family history reveals that our patient was a naughty and wild child from birth. The psycho-analysis did not protrude in this very early layer of experiences. When a child is bad, wild, and naughty in a very early stage, it points to an excess of motor impulses. Wherever there is such an excess it will necessarily be of a destructive type. Study of post-encephalitic children has shown that clearly. The motor impulses will end in sadistic activities and destruction, which will provoke retaliation from the adult. These motor drives may be based on the constitution. They may also be based upon acquired lesion of the brain, either birth trauma or infantile encephalitis. There may also be a constitutional or organic background to the life-history of our patient. The earliest actual remembrances of the patient are remembrances about an itching disease. This is also a factor of great importance.

Itching provokes restlessness. But it is also very near in its character to pain. It induces the individual to scratch. When he scratches, he may induce pain in himself. The itching will lead the hand to the whole body and especially to the genital region, which is especially apt to provoke itching sensations. The whole surface of the body will be suffused with sensations of a more or less painful type. We may suppose that the masochistic tendencies of the early stage must be increased enormously. Since itching leads to restlessness, there will be not only masochism but also increased sadism in connection with early itching diseases. Since the hand acts as a weapon against the body and experiences numerous contacts with it, there will also be a libidinous overflow to the hand, which touches all parts of the body. The searching movements of the hands along the body, the knowledge of the body, will be prematurely developed.

I have shown that the knowledge of our own body is developed on the basis of a continually renewed contact with the outside world. We expect, therefore, in our patient a prematurely developed body schema, overloaded with libidinous investment. Other experiences may have contributed to that development. The father suffered from an itching disease when the patient was about four years old, and rubbed his back with a brush. It belongs, further to his early experiences that his father wiped his feet with his hand when he came home tired from his occupation as a salesman. There is also his own search on his body and his observation of his father. In addition, his mother developed an exaggerated interest in his body. The patient suffered from an anomaly in his genitals. It is impossible now to determine whether it was an hydrocele or a varicocele. His mother was very much interested in it. She examined him carefully and touched him frequently in the genital region. Although his remembrances about this point date from a little later, it is more than probable that his mother's examination of his body reached back into a very early age. He suffered by it. The idea of genital suffering became deeply impregnated in him. Bodily pain, discomfort, and suffering thus prepared him for a masochistic attitude and for an enormous interest in his body. But his mother was interested not only in his genitals, but in all his functions, especially in his defecation. His father joined in this.

Experiences of this kind also go far back into his early childhood, but they continue through his whole infancy, childhood, and adolescence. His experiences during the birth of his elder sister (he was at that time 4½ years old) fell, therefore, on a well-prepared ground. He heard the painful cries of his mother when she was in labour with his sister. He formed the idea that his mother was being tortured by the physician, who sponged her face and brushed her toe-nails and feet with a hard brush. This phantasy, partially based on experience, now became dominating, and he masturbated with this phantasy, apparently identifying himself with his mother as well as with the doctor, who was certainly a substitute for the father. This important phantasy probably has not only the manifest meaning mentioned so far. General analytic experiences and details of the case-history not recorded here make it probable that the mother's foot was a symbolical substitute for her genitals. A fear of castration was to some extent connected with this phantasy. At the time of his elder sister's birth, his parents' interest in his defecation had already developed an over-emphasis in the anal zone. One of his earliest fears was that rats might crawl into his anus. His mother had given him enemas freely from his earliest childhood. It is probable that his ideas of suffering were connected with the fear of anal torture.

This is the history of his pre-genital development. It shows that his sadomasochistic and anal tendencies had been emphasized by his early experiences. In addition to that, he had acquired an increased interest in his body-image, and this increase was partially due to the interest taken by his parents in his body in general and in his genital and anal region. The observation of his father is an additional factor. When he entered the stage of the development of the Oedipus complex, his previous pre-genital activities and fixations[1] were liable to colour the Oedipus complex. The homosexual phases of the Oedipus complex, where the libido is concentrated on the father, would be enforced in connection with the passive masochistic and anal tendencies. All

[1] In psycho-analysis, fixation denotes an over-emphasis on early stages of sexual development, either by constitution or by an important event. Such an over-emphasis may lead to an arrest of the sexual development at this stage. But the obstacle may be overcome. There remains a tendency to go back to the point of fixation and to the earliest stage of sexual development whenever a sexual difficulty arises which hinders libidinous satisfaction.

these factors would help to an identification with the suffering mother. His latent homosexuality would therefore be increased. His relation to his mother, in the final elaboration of the Oedipus complex, would be loaded with sadistic and sadomasochistic tendencies. But there is no question that the patient had reached the stage of the heterosexual Oedipus complex, with a tendency to an identification with the father. There is no question that he had built up an ideal ego, a super ego, which forced him to attempt an adaptation to reality and especially to sexual reality.

We know that in every childhood development the period of sexual activity comes to an end with the development of the Oedipus complex, which allows the erection of a moral instance, the super-ego or ego-ideal. There follows a period of latency, in which the child appears sexless. But in many cases the latency is not an absolute one. In the case we have just mentioned, masturbatory activity, with the phantasy described above, was continued up to the time of puberty. There were playful operations on the feet and on the anus of his playmates. An actual operation performed on his genitals may be of some importance for the whole picture. It was not before the time of puberty, with its libidinous strain, that he developed his neurasthenic symptoms. The same parts of the body which were previously a source of libidinous pleasure and over-emphasis now gave him neurasthenic sufferings. He felt itching not only on the genitals and on the anus but also on hands and feet. Defecation and the fear of constipation now became the source of continual suffering. Spermatorrhoea and prostatorrhoea completed the picture. He had a tendency to watch his body in a hypochondriac way. He complained that he was unable to concentrate his thoughts.

This whole development is rather typical. Ego-ideal and ego do not want the pre-genital sexuality; they fight against the satisfaction which comes from the organs overloaded with infantile sexuality. His symptoms are the transformation of libidinous infantile tendencies; or, in other words, we are concerned not with an unhampered outbreak of infantile sexuality but with the result of the fight of ego and ego-ideal against the perversion which is the expression of the infantile drive. This is the general scheme of psychoneuroses according to Freud's formulation.

Neurasthenia, with its preserved ego system and high ego-ideal, is not a perversion but a neurosis.[1]

The symptoms of a neurosis are the result of a fight between the revived or persistent infantile sexuality (the id) and the ego system. Since the ego is not strong enough to repress the infantile drive completely, it comes back in a form which recalls the primitive drive of childhood in a more or less symbolic way. Neurasthenic symptoms occur in organs which have previously given an increased sexual pleasure. Hypochondriac symptoms have the same origin. Since in his childhood the patient did not experience an increased pleasure in single organs only but in his whole body, his whole body later became the object of hypochondriac suffering. He tried to get away from his body overloaded with libido, not only by making it a source of pain but also by transferring his love from his body to his intellect. Like the majority of neurasthenics, he was very proud of his intellectual achievements. Here is one of the reasons why neurasthenics so often acquire a half-education, especially in regard to medical knowledge. It is an attempt to transfer their libido from the body ego to the intellectual ego. Since thinking thus becomes too much an expression of personal vanity, it becomes as painful as the narcissistic body, and difficulty in concentration follows out of the attempt to sublimate narcissism in thinking.

It has often been observed that neurasthenics suffer from their disease more than organic cases do. But, as is clearly shown in the case history of our patient, they seem to get an unobtrusive satisfaction out of their exaggerated sufferings and masochism.

Alexander has justly pointed out that every neurotic symptom provides not only gratification of infantile sex desires, but also suffering. This suffering bribes the super ego to allow satisfaction through the symptoms. It is a self-punishment. We may expect that the stronger the masochistic tendencies are, the greater will be the suffering through the neurotic symptom. Since neurasthenics generally show strong masochistic trends, we understand the enormous discomfort their symptoms cause them. The

[1] This chapter may be compared with W. Reich's remarkable book, which contains excellent clinical material about the problem of neurasthenia. It also contains much material about the symbolic interchange between the diverse organs of the neurasthenic.

neurasthenic suffers in his body. His neurosis is immediately due to a fault in development in the libidinous structure of the body-image. The neurosis perpetuates the infantile structure of the body-image in a symbolic way.

The spermato-prostatorrhoea of our patient provides an impressive proof that libidinous changes are not merely psychic. Freud has often emphasized that libido means not only desire but also processes going on in the body. When libido is invested in a particular part of the body, there is a change in the physiological function of these parts. Changes in the body-image tend immediately to become changes in the body. One may consider with Abraham that prostatorrhoea is an expression of urethral eroticism. But the prostate has its anatomical position between urethra and rectum. Through its anatomical position it is suited to express anal as well as urethral tendencies. Psychogenic diseases lead from the central problems of the personality to the organs. Conflicts choose for their expressions organs which have to do with the functions involved in the conflict. But there is a specificity in the organs. Whenever such an organ is diseased it will prepare the ground for those psychic conflicts which are otherwise suited to influence this very organ. Suffering from organic disease will change not only the perceptive side of the postural model of the body but also its libidinous structure. Not only does it make the individual suffer, but it will also provoke and satisfy masochistic tendencies. The change in the libidinous flow in the body-image will then again cause a change in its perceptive side.

The building-up of the postural model of the body takes place on the physiological level by continual contact with the outside world. On the libidinous level it is built up not only by the interest we ourselves have in our body, but also by the interest other persons show in the different parts of our body. They may show their interest by actions or merely by words and attitudes. But what persons around us do with their own bodies is also of enormous importance. Here is the first hint that the body-image is built up by social contacts.

The child takes parts of the bodies of others into its own body-image. It also adopts in its own personality the attitude taken by others towards parts of their own bodies. Postural models of the body are closely connected with each other. We take the body-images of others either in parts or as a whole. In the latter case we call it identification. But we may also want to give away our body-image, and we then project it into others. The patient projects his own difficulties and his whole body-image into the analyst. I have referred to narcissistic projection. Body-images of human beings communicate with each other either in parts or as wholes. In this remark we anticipate problems which will be discussed in the third part of this book. But it is not possible to isolate problems in an actual case-history of the human being. The building-up of the body-image is based not only upon the individual history of an individual, but also on his relations to others. The inner history is also the history of our relations to other human beings.

(4) *Depersonalization*

The changes in the postural model of the body in another symptom complex, that of depersonalization, will repay study. In a case of depersonalization the individual feels completely changed from what he was previously. This change is present in the ego as well as in the outside world and the individual does not recognize himself as a personality. His actions appear to him as automatic. He observes his actions and behaviour from the point of view of a spectator. The outside world is foreign and new to him and is not as real as before. We may thus describe this state from a psychological point of view. "There is no change in the central ego. Not the ego as such is changed, not the 'I' in the sense of James, but the 'Me' and the personality and the central ego perceive the change in the 'Me' in the self. In depersonalization, therefore, many faculties are preserved. The change in the self does not follow out of the change in any group of psychic elements, i.e. the sensations, the feelings, the remembrances and thought processes (if it is permissible to employ this classification), but is based on the fact that the central ego does not live in his present and previous experiences. The self appears without soul because it does not grow undivided out of the ego. It is not sufficient that sensations, feelings, representations, thoughts, are

present in the stream of consciousness. And it is also not sufficient that the central ego perceives them. But in the living
psychic experience all tendencies of the ego must be present in a
unified and uncontradicted way" (cf. my book *Selbstbewusstsein
und Persönlichkeitsbewusstsein*, pp. 54, 55).

It has no special interest in this connection that this characteristic complex of symptoms can constitute a neurosis of its own, or
can be a part of depressive and schizophrenic psychoses. But it
is important that, according to my own observations and those of
Nunberg and others, almost every neurosis has in some phases of
its development symptoms of depersonalization. Patients with
depersonalization not only feel a change in perception concerning
the outside world, but they also have clear-cut changes concerning
their own body. I wrote in 1914 that the disturbance becomes
stronger the more the perceptions belong to the subject's own
body. The patient sees his face in the mirror changed, rigid, and
distorted. His own voice seems strange and unfamiliar to him,
and he shudders at the sound of it as if it were not himself speaking.
Gottfried feels that his movements are interrupted. His body
feels as if it were dead and he has the sensation that a dynamo is
hissing in his head. The body feels too light, just as if it could fly.
A patient of Loewy's says, "I feel the body not for me but for
itself". The patients look for their limbs in the bed. A patient of
Pick's complains that his eyes are like two holes through which
he looks. Patients complain that they do not feel the urge for
urination and defecation. They feel as if they were dead, without
life, like shadows. All the patients complain about hypochondriac sensations, noises in the ears, choking sensations, bubbles in
the head, and sensations in the heart.

The interest of these phenomena is all the greater since the
psychogenesis of depersonalization is beyond doubt. It occurs,
as I have shown, especially in organs which have previously been
of a great erotic significance. I have observed a singer who showed
depersonalization concerning speech and concerning the mouth,
an organ to which she paid special attention, in herself as well as
in others. It is in this respect especially remarkable that the
estrangement concerning the outside world is often an estrangement in the optic sphere especially. We have often emphasized

the enormous importance of the optic element in the construction of the body-image. In H. Hartmann's case the depersonalization started with jealousy and a compulsion on the part of the patient to imagine his wife in intercourse with a rival. Subsequently he experienced the impossibility of imagining this, and even of imagining anything at all. Finally also his vision lost the character of reality. The depersonalization started when the patient denied himself his voyeuristic tendency.

There is no doubt that in depersonalization the individual loses interest in the outside world and loses with it the interest in his body, which, as has been seen in our previous remarks, has such close relations with the outside world. It is true that hypochondriac sensations are remnants of an exaggerated interest in the body. But the hypochondriac sensations are not the essential part of the depersonalization, and I must firmly contradict Federn and Fenichel when they place in the centre of the depersonalization an increased interest in the body, or, in analytical terminology, an increased narcissistic libido. This view certainly betrays a complete misunderstanding of the problems involved.

Depersonalization is the characteristic picture which occurs when the individual does not dare to place his libido either in the outside world or in his own body. The change in the body-image results from the withdrawing of libido from the body-image. This disturbance is almost constantly accompanied by dizziness. It is in some way the organic projection into the organ which has, as I have noted above, the function of unifying the different perceptions which help to build up the knowledge of one's own body. In an article on the vestibular apparatus in neurosis and psychosis I emphasized this point of view. Throughout pathology one repeatedly observes the close parallel between the organism and the psychic functions. Specific psychic functions have a definite relation to specific organs. Depersonalization and organic dizziness have the same psychological nucleus, though it is expressed in different levels of organization. Dizziness due to organic causes often provokes phenomena which are akin to the psychic phenomena of depersonalization of the body. This is merely an instance of a general principle. Weizsäcker has often emphasized that every organ carries with it a specific set of emotional life, and organic disease provokes the specific set which is in connection with a particular organ. But we are especially interested here in the fact that depersonalization is a disturbance in the body-image, the psychogenesis of which is not yet known. The analytic experiments of Nunberg, Reik, Sadger and myself, failed to reveal specific points of fixation in the libidinous development.[1] This defect does not matter so much in the numerous cases in which depersonalization is only a passing symptom; for these cases can be easily explained by the supposition that every neurosis and psychosis in its beginning goes through a phase in which the individual does not dare to place his libido either in the body or in the outside world. We are dealing therefore with an unspecific result of the general shock of the psychic conflict. But this explanation can hardly hold good for those cases in which depersonalization is the leading symptom of a neurosis of long duration.

My latest observations point to the idea that self-observation, which plays such an important part in depersonalization, is derived from voyeuristic tendencies. The individual denies to himself the pleasure of optic observation, and punishes himself by not fully seeing, or substitutes seeing in a symbolic way by looking at his own self. Sadomasochism is the second important component. With the self-denial of optic observation, the body-image which has so many other components must undergo changes. But still, depersonalization is a more extensive withdrawal from world and body, or, analytically speaking, from ego and body-image. We do not know what early experiences determine this weakness in the ego and the body-image. We know less about it than about the psychogenesis of neurasthenia and hypochondria.

(5) *Hypochondria*

As I have mentioned, hypochondriac symptoms are common to neurasthenia as well as to depersonalization. The interpretation of hypochondriac symptoms from an analytic point of view is

---

[1] The latest analytic experiment in depersonalization by Searl emphasizes the fear of the child that the parent may turn into an inanimate object. But it is at least doubtful whether such cases have anything to do with depersonalization.

well established. We have to do, as Freud, Ferenczi, and I have shown, with an increase of the libido in particular parts of the body. It is an increase in narcissistic libido. This increase may be given to a structure, the function of which is impaired on a somatic basis. But it will always be of the utmost importance to know what part the particular organ plays in the whole libidinous structure and the life-plan of the individual. An important psychological quality of the hypochondriac organ has to be emphasized. It is genitalized and it very often symbolizes genitals. It continually attracts attention. Patients complain that there is something sticking in their head or in other parts of the body. It is like iron, or a piece of wood, or a bone. Symbolizations of the male genitals are prevalent. Symbolizations of the female genitals—a hole in the body, or something missing—are much rarer. This is probably connected with the fact that the increased libido for an organ is liable to provoke the sensation of a swelling of the organ and not of a diminution of it. Symbolizations of the male sex-organ are therefore in the foreground.

Transposition of organs also occur in neurasthenics. In hypochondria merely narcissistic libido is transposed to the organ. It appears under the picture of genitals, since in the narcissistic stage the whole body, according to Freud's well-founded formulations, is treated like a genital. It might also be said that the hypochondriac organ behaves like an independent body. Hypochondria is a fight against narcissistic libido; the individual defends himself against the libidinous overtension of the hypochondriac organ; he tries to isolate the diseased organ, to treat it like a foreign body in the body-image. This fight is entertained by an ego system, which is at least partially preserved and which has strength enough to fight against the libidinous organ. In depersonalization there is no attempt to expel the organ. The patient may have hypochondriac symptoms, but he has not withdrawn his libido from the particular parts. They are those which are not depersonalized. Of course, the tendency to get rid of parts of the body by expelling them is in no way peculiar to hypochondria: it has a general importance. When the effort to get rid of parts of the body becomes more efficient, we may project them into the outside world. In some paranoic cases the patients project their fæces into the outside world. They become persecutors and are then still connected with the body. It is an incomplete projection. The fæces are too valuable for the individual to give them up completely. The hypochondriac clings too much to his over-libidinized organ. His attempt to get rid of it is therefore ineffective, as it remains in the body as if it were a foreign body put into it. Since the depersonalized case withdraws from the outside world as well as from the body-image as a whole, he now merely observes his psychic functions, and considers himself as an automaton.

In hypochondria, the body and the organ remain in the centre of attention. Freud and Ferenczi have shown that an organic lesion or disease will have the same effect as the hypochondriac libido tension. The diseased organ keeps the centre of the stage. When we traumatize an organ ourselves, this organ will immediately behave like an hypochondriac organ. We may help our hypochondria by inflicting trauma and pain and mutilation on an organ. When it is considered how often traumas are followed by hypochondriac symptoms, some significance will be attached to this formulation. To become traumatized is often a method by which the individual makes it easier for himself to transfer libido to an organ which before the accident was an object of narcissistic attention. It is as if the individual felt that he was not able to concentrate libido fully on an organ which he would like to have still more in the centre of attention. He is unable to get his libidinous satisfaction in a merely autoplastic way. (Ferenczi has called the faculty of producing symptoms on one's own body autoplastic function.)

One of my patients always paid a special attention to her hands. She considered the hands as the most beautiful part of a woman's body. When working in a factory she caught both her hands in a machine and received insignificant scars on both of them. She then developed hypochondriac symptoms in her hands. Before the accident she had dreamed that her hands would be hurt. We are justified in assuming that her trauma was the result of the libidinous attention she gave to her hands and was an unconscious wish-fulfillment. The hypondriac symptom is the result of an action which facilitates the autoplastic change.

The outstanding symptom of hypochondria is the hypochondriac sensation. An organic change in the organ may form the nucleus of the hypochondriac sensation, but often the autoplastic function will be sufficient to provoke the symptom. The hypochondriac sensation is often felt inside the body. When this is the case, it is mostly in the zone of the body which we have called the sensitive zone, about two centimetres inside the body. But it may also be a sensation on the surface of the body. Often the optic perception changes then also. The skin is not only felt changed but has changed its colour and appearance.

I have not so far given enough attention to the question of how we experience optically the surface of our body, skin, and complexion. The fact that we are unable to obtain a clear conception of the colour and texture of the skin is remarkable and undoubtedly connected with the enormous libidinous value of the skin. It remains continually mysterious and changing also in its optic qualities. We may look into the mirror and still not be sure what we look like. There remains always an emotional uncertainty in the perception of our skin and of the skin of others. (It is remarkable that I do not experience the same uncertainty about the skin of coloured people.) The racial difference probably diminishes the erotic interest and makes the perception clearer and more distinct. It is therefore understandable that skin may become an almost inexhaustible source of hypochondriac sensations.

In some cases we meet peculiar disturbances in the body-image. Many years ago I observed a patient who complained that she could not think clearly. She had an intense feeling that her right and left side were interchanged. The right side was too light. Objects felt different in the left hand: they had more space there. The right hand was much smaller, especially its inner space. When she clenched her fist, the fingers did not fit her hand. It is worthy of note that in her childhood the patient had been scolded by her mother for wringing the laundry with her left hand.

The problem of hypochondria is the problem of coenesthaesiopathia and paraesthesias in general. But paraesthesia is a sign for the patient that he is ill and that he has a disease. Hypochondriac sensations are therefore inseparably connected with hypochondriac ideas. On the other hand, whenever there are hypochondriac ideas, they will lead to hypochondriac sensations. Jahrreiss defines the hypochondriac idea as the imagination of being ill, but the hypochondriac idea gets its true meaning only through the sensations on which it is based, or which originate from it.

In one of Jahrreiss' cases, in which the patient complained that her body was empty, that all nerves had disappeared out of her head and heart, and that she had no blood in her heart, it is clear that the sensations played a less important rôle than the ideas and connotations. We may suppose that in cases of that kind a higher psychic station of the body-image is affected, and we may draw the general conclusion that one part of the body-image is nearer to perception and another part nearer to ideas.

Freud, Ferenczi, and I have emphasized that the libidinous change in the hypochondriac organ is not merely psychic. Vaso-vegetative and vasomotor innervation is changed. Changes in the vasovegetative innervation on an organic basis may provoke hypochondriac attitudes. The vasovegetative field is a common ground for organic and psychic disorders. It is one of the important tasks of general medicine to describe the way in which an organ is attacked from both the psychic side and the organic side. We may be dealing with organic diseases with psychogenic consequences. In this respect, the organic symptom may be designated centripetal and the psychogenic symptom centrifugal. The psychic experience of the body is not as central as the vital and libidinous problems of the individual which form the centre of ego and personality.

(6) *Pain and libido*

Paraesthesias and pain are very closely related to each other. We start therefore now with the study of pain.[1] Pain can have a purely psychogenic origin. Psychoanalytic literature contains a number of instances of this. Mohr summarizes the matter in the following way: "It is known that abdominal pains in women are very often based on sexual dissatisfaction or a sexual defence against the unloved man. Men punish themselves by paying the

[1] Reprinted from the *Psychoanalytic Review*, vol. XVIII, 1931. I am greatly indebted to Dr White for the permission to reprint this and the following case report.

cost of masturbation or other sexual misdeeds. It is not so well known that pain in the back very often has the same cause. In many cases there are special psychic factors which produce a special pain in a special place. This can only be found out by careful analysis. A lady whom I treated complained about violent pain in her right arm after grippe with neuralgia in the right arm. She had been reminded by the death of her mother of a scene in which she had attacked her mother with her raised right arm and her mother had said to her: 'You will be punished in this limb'. In another case a patient experienced severe pains in her left breast. These pains at first were apparently of a neuralgic type, but it transpired that they also expressed a longing for her lover who had caressed her there, and at the same time her repentance for having gone too far. Reasoning from numerous observations of this kind I stated a long time ago that pain is very often felt in those parts of the body where previously an especially great pleasure has been experienced, which pleasure can no longer be procured. Pain comes especially if one wants to punish oneself for the forbidden pleasure".

E. M., thirty-seven years old, business man. He complained of impotence. This impotence was intermittent. When his potency was in order the intercourse lasted a very long time. He was sometimes able to have intercourse three times in one night. The genitals were also objectively much below the average size. His first troubles of impotency occurred after masturbation in puberty. At that time he passed urine when he masturbated. He afterwards regained his potency. After having read Havelock Ellis, he felt pain in his phallus, in his arms, and in the anus. He called these pains homosexual pains. He was compelled to think about sexual intercourse with men. He felt the pain where the phallus of another man touched him in his imagination. He thought of fellatio and on imagining that the phallus of the other man was touching his palate immediately felt the pressure and pain on his palate. He thought about an active and passive coitus per anum. These thoughts hindered him when he wished to have sex intercourse with women. When he thought of masturbation he felt pain in his arm. Pain was here experienced in those parts of the body which had to do with homosexual fantasies against which his defence was directed. At the same time the pain was perverse satisfaction and the self-defence and the punishment for the perverse fantasy.

The next case analyzed during several months gives a deeper insight:

Francis E., leading official of a big company, forty-four years old, came with the complaint that he suffered from pain in his genitals. He had then been suffering for almost ten years. The pain was either in the anterior or the posterior part of the phallus. The latter pain was especially connected with tormenting sexual excitement. At first the pain was mild, but it increased more and more, and at last developed such a terrible intensity that it absorbed his attention almost completely and made it quite impossible for him to work. There were times when he felt better, but when he had the pain it drove him to despair. During his last vacation he was on the verge of suicide. When the pain was present everything excited him sexually, even when he once read about lust murder. Reading about thefts was also connected with sexual ideas. He had pains in the back and disagreeable flushings connected with the pain in the genitals.

The patient had been married since his twenty-fourth year. He felt in complete harmony with his wife but was sexually dissatisfied. He had never had any relations with other women. For many years he had felt a deep love for a girl who worked in the same office as himself and who was subordinate to him. After having had sexual intercourse with his wife he felt restless and excited. He could not sleep and tossed about. On such nights he was compelled to take sleeping-draughts. It was difficult to excite his wife sexually; she had never been active and never took the initiative. He had to touch her first in order to excite her. He very often excited her by calling her names, such as 'swine', 'prostitute', and so on. He also sometimes beat his wife's genitals. When he went to his office the next morning the events of the previous night came into his mind against his will, and he felt a vivid disgust for himself. His pain would then increase and last about a week. At such times, if he had any other intercourse, his pain became enormous. After this there was usually a week when he felt better. The following week the sexual desire increased until the sex action occurred, and with it came a repetition of the cycle.

He met his wife when he was about fifteen years old. In both families there were disagreeable quarrels. He and his wife complained about their fate to each other. In this way they were drawn nearer to each other, and soon they began to make love, but there was no sexual intercourse. Although other girls tried to attract him, he remained faithful to his future wife. Girls were fond of him. One of his wife's sisters also tried to seduce him. As a student he also attracted homosexuals. His relations with his wife continued. They indulged in mutual masturbation. But she remained reserved. After marriage she refused intercourse. They always quarrelled before they had intercourse, but when it came to the point she enjoyed it.

Both resolved not to have any children. Life appeared so undesirable that they did not want to take the responsibility of bringing a child into the world. However, fifteen years later, pregnancy occurred. The birth was difficult; infection followed, and his wife very nearly died. Endometritis with fluor began. Sex relations were interrupted for more than a year and a half. The fluor was sometimes disgusting to him. His wife lacked sexual initiative, did not take life easily, and was very sensitive. She had a strongly individual personality. Once she had a deep interest in one of her brothers-in-law. He was jealous of her. He felt an increased tenderness for the girl in his office, who was easy-going but virtuous. When he took large doses of bromide under the influence of increased pain, he became less repressed and confessed his love to her. There were kisses, but no other caresses. Even when he was with the girl for several days no bodily approaches occurred, but he afterwards felt much quieter.

At that time the patient had already been under analysis for some time, and he was much freer in his attitude toward sexuality. He was always rather severe in his moral opinions and was called a moralist by his friends, but he was more tolerant towards others than towards himself. He believed that he was exhausted from too great indulgence in sexuality, and even worked out an anatomical theory about it. The resistance in his sex system was diminished, and through this diminution of resistance he got prostatorrhea and his pain. Indeed, the patient had excretions when he suffered from the pain. He had often been examined by the urethroscope, but no local changes were found. After the distension of the urethra the pains stopped for about two months. Massage of the prostate did not help him. He believed that his sexual nerves were inflamed and wanted to be operated on. When the pain came on and he was alone, he took measures of defence against it; he would beat himself with all his strength until he bruised the skin. He hit his head with his fists and even knocked it against the wall. He pulled and tore at his genitals and would even have liked to tear out his sex-organ. He also provoked cramps in his legs, gnashed his teeth, and pulled his lower jaw forward. There was a strong anger, irritation, and fury in him. It came back when he spoke of his experiences. At such times he could indeed provoke fear. This contrasted vividly with the rest of his behaviour. He was very amiable, polite, and adaptable in his relations with other people. He never got angry with anyone else. He was rough only when he was convinced of the dishonesty of others. At high school and college he punished himself by producing cramps and beating himself in an attempt to suppress the sexual excitement which hindered him in his studies. But the analysis showed that his whole attitude went back to a much earlier time. I propose therefore to describe the patient's childhood and development by linking together his single remarks.

All this material came out piecemeal in the analysis. He had clear and conscious remembrances of his very early life. He remembered the chair on which he sat when he was two years old. He saw with his inner eye all the details of the house in which he, his parents, and his brothers lived. The house was left when he was four years old. His earliest remembrance went back to the period immediately after his first year. He learned to walk and was admired by his mother because he did it so well. He also remembered his governesses. His father very often scolded them. He was afraid of thunderstorms and wind. He sometimes got into his mother's or his governess' bed, where he felt safe. He was very much concerned about his parents. When they went away he thought they would never come back. (Later he was very much concerned lest his wife and child should fall off their bicycles.)

As a child his mother took him with her to the sea. He enjoyed it very much. He and his mother went first. His father followed afterwards. At that time he slept in his mother's room. His mother was fonder of him than of his older brother. (Here is the association that the voice of the girl reminded him of the voice of his mother.) He clung very much to his mother. His father was very strict, especially at the dining table. When he was four years old his father sold his business. His mother protested, and there were violent scenes between his father and mother. During the analysis the following scene came to the patient's mind. The mother was lying on the floor after a violent quarrel with his father. Shouting and crying, she hit her skull against the floor. (In this scene the patient recognized the origin of his own attacks of fury.) The moving of the family from the house and from the business was in some way the fatal point in the family history. Relations between his parents after that became worse and worse. He took his mother's part without speaking about it. (Apparently so many remembrances of his first years were preserved because the time before the moving was in his mind like the lost paradise. Whether the remembrance of his walking did not cover something else cannot be decided. At any rate, the scene is characteristic of his relation to his mother. I am inclined to believe that we have here a real remembrance. The fear of wind and thunderstorms may be interpreted as fear of the strict father. His anxiety was the expression of aggressive tendencies which came out very early in him.)

Between his fourth and fifth years he had a Catholic governess. She gave him an illustrated Bible for children. The crucifixion and the bearing of the cross by Christ made a deep impression upon him. He came from a cultivated and emancipated Jewish family. He developed a hatred against the Jews who had crucified Christ. From the same time he remembered a picture of the War of Independence where a general and some officers were shot.

He had no recollections of the birth of two younger brothers. They were four to six years younger than he was, but he spent the time before their birth and the days following in the house of his grandparents. The elder brother, two years his senior, was not a good student and was beaten by his parents because of it. Sometimes both parents hit him savagely. Such scenes were painful to the patient and he pitied his brother, whom he loved. Later on, between his tenth and twelfth year, he masturbated with the older brother in the latter's bed. When doing so they talked about beating and killing. Only late in the analysis, under great resistance, did he admit that they said, "Kill the Jews". Very often they spoke about the "crown of thorns".

In the same hour it developed that between his fourth and fifth year he believed that all men were Jews and all women were Christians. He also applied this to his father and mother. (His hostility against his father is here clearly portrayed. He identified himself not only with his mother, who beat and was beaten, but also with his father. His brother beaten by his father and mother represented the father and mother at the same time. The sexual act with his wife repeated the maltreatment and depreciation of women. The beating of his wife's genitals shows that the sexual act for him meant maltreatment.) His brother's private tutor took him into his bed when he was ten years old and masturbated with him. He felt very disgusted. It is remarkable that the patient's elder brother also suffered from violent pain in his genitals, though it disappeared quickly after treatment with testicular extract.

The patient suffered from constipation at a very early age. On one occasion when he was constipated at a children's party he pressed his hands deeply into his abdomen, pushing his hands in his loins. He made use of the same trick whenever he suffered from constipation. He was given enemas. They were painful, especially when made with water which was too hot. He had a hernia of both sides, and had to wear a truss. He often went to a neighbouring town to have the truss adjusted. When he was in his fifth year of elementary school he was operated on. It was said that up to that time his urine went into the testicles. The patient never had trouble in urinating, but he got sexually excited when wetted either by his or another person's urine. He also had day dreams about urinating on somebody's abdomen. This operation did not play any considerable part in his life. He was inactive for a year after the operation.

He had trouble in bowel movements throughout his whole life, and was apt to become constipated whenever anything worried him. He suffered from achylia for many years. He had spastic difficulties in defecating. There was sometimes blood in his faeces; sometimes slime also. When he suffered from pain in his genitals the pain went towards the anus. He also once suffered from gastric ulcer. When he had pain from the ulcer, the other pain stopped. When he became excited there was a feeling of pressure and pain in his stomach. When he attended the university he pushed his stomach against the back of a chair and sometimes induced a friend to sit on his stomach. (There is no question that the anal component is as important in the psychic life of our patient as the genital. Also, his anal experiences are connected with pain, and constipation provokes the same fury as the genital pain.)

He had his first emission when he was about twelve years old. It was connected with burning. He reproached himself, but he often masturbated afterwards without pain. The quarrels between his parents continued when he was about twelve or thirteen years old. His mother became very intimate with one of her relatives, who was in the habit of coming when his father was out. The patient heard him coming and going. He felt sexually excited and suffered. He began to understand his father better. His father was strict but honest, and could not show his feelings. He felt bitter and thought that Fate was against him. His financial speculations did not succeed. Finally he shot himself after the patient had graduated from college.

The whole family was always under pressure. At school he believed in an evil fate, and continued in this belief. He felt bewitched when he could not find something and hit himself. When he got excited he was often unable to find notes he had made, and thought that an evil spirit had taken them away. He then said to himself, "It not." This meant, "It, Fate, does not want me to go on the right way." He also sometimes said that things were bewitched by the devil. He believed in a demonic power, and thought that this demonic power prevented him from becoming wealthy. He also had serious financial losses through no fault of his own. He always saw himself as a beggar and feared that he might lose his job. (It is clear that he identified himself with his father. On the other hand, the father was the demonic power and provoked fear by wind and thunderstorm. His feelings went back to a very primitive, archaic layer. The shortened expression reported above recalls features of a similar type in the case-history of the schizophrenic Senats-President Schreber). He felt possessed of the devil. During a short relapse in the course of the treatment he said that a cure of this nature was only for human beings; he himself was not a human being. States of excitement and self-punishment occurred only when there were pains in the genitals, not when there were other pains. For instance, he was able to tolerate pain from a tooth-fistula very patiently.

The patient had complete control over himself. He not only fulfilled his responsible job but hid his outbreaks of fury from everybody. He had these outbreaks of fury only when he was alone. His whole attitude was a little stiff and reserved. During the analysis he lay on his right side, with his left arm often stiffly stretched in the air. He could sleep only on the right side; other positions excited him sexually.

In the incomplete analysis positive transference was prevalent. Only at times of great pain was his fury sometimes directed against the psycho-analyst. It was but rarely that this clever and witty man associated freely. His dreams were infrequent. There were dreams, especially at times of sexual excitement, in which he had to pack his luggage continuously. In another dream he rubbed his erected phallus against another. The same night he dreamed that an operation was to take place on his genitals, but the operation was postponed. The surgeon looked like a cousin of his mother's. In another emission-dream he got into the bed of a sister of his mother's. Afterwards he dreamed that his wife asked for intercourse, but there were three men who wanted her, including his elder brother. (This aunt of his who interested him sexually is a substitute for his mother. The three men who wanted intercourse with his wife are connected with the jealousy he felt concerning his mother and his wife.)

He was very fond of his youngest brother. The younger one was morally inferior. He did not care for him at all. (The analysis was incomplete concerning the question of latent homosexuality.) He loved music but was very conservative in his taste. He hated jazz. He was also conservative in his political opinions. Although he did not conceal the fact that he was a Jew, Jews were repulsive to him. In college he had an open conflict with his rabbi and was afterwards converted to Catholicism.

The history of this case is as important for the problems of sadism and masochism as for the psychology of pain. In the early history of the patient there are many hints of real pain experienced by him. He had a direct memory only of anal pain (enema and constipation), but there was also an anomaly in voiding about which the patient did not know very much. At any rate, he was compelled to wear a truss. It is at least probable that in his childhood there were genito-anal sensations of pain. Probably they would have passed without leaving any trace had not the severity of his father and the revolt of his mother been added to the pain experience. That his father and mother beat his brother in a rather cruel way makes it probable that sadomasochistic components also played a part in their life. It was for this reason that the passion of Christ impressed him. In view of such a history, the sadistic attitude of the patient is almost a matter of course. It breaks through in the homosexual experiences with his brother and in the manner in which he had sexual relations with his wife. His hatred against his father is proved by his infantile theory that all men are Jews and all women Christians. There was sometimes an identification with his father, and then his sadistic tendencies were directed against his mother (wife). In this connection the jealousy concerning his mother also plays an important rôle.

At a very early age the patient started to act against himself. It is worthy of note that his pressing against his abdomen was at first considered by him as a curative procedure. Later on he found an outlet for his aggressiveness by hitting his head if his studies did not proceed as he wished. But his technique in inflicting pain on himself did not develop before he started to fight against his sexuality. He produced muscle cramps and struck himself. It is difficult to believe that achylia, ulcer, and colitis are independent of this psychic background. Spontaneous pain in the genitals now comes into the foreground. He was conscious of its sexual colouring and tried to counter it by a furious defence and self-maltreatment which was partly directed against the genitals themselves. That the pains were psychogenic is proved by the fact that they were based on the inner life history of the patient, but that does not prove that they were nervous in the common sense. Prostatorrhea is proof that something is going on in the organ itself. It is apparently an organic change which grows out of psychogenesis. The borderlines between organic and functional changes become more and more blurred. In physiology, we no longer believe in the absolute contrast between the periphery and the centre. What we call functional changes are certainly closely related to the central brain apparatus, but the periphery is doubtless always affected also. On the other hand, what goes on in an organic way in the periphery will also influence the central attitudes and functions. We now begin to get an insight into psychic laws to which Weizsäcker was the first to draw attention.

Disease of any organ is connected with a special psychic attitude. It may be said in a schematic way that the difference between psychogenic and organic is, among other things, a difference in the direction in which the process moves. In organic disease the periphery is affected first, and the affection goes from the periphery to the centre; in psychogenic cases the change goes from the centre to the periphery.

I should like to emphasize the fact that the connotation of the prevalence of centrifugal tendencies in functional diseases and centripetal tendencies in organic diseases means not only physiological but psychological processes as well. When there is an organic disease we feel that there is something changed which belongs to the periphery of the circle of the Ego (*Ichkreis*).

Organic disease and organic change have less to do with the personality than functional disease. A functional disease is connected with the innermost problems of the individual—with the centre of his Ego. It is certain that centrifugal and centripetal currents often make a complete circle. In the case under discussion the organic phenomenon of pain played a part which was prepared by the constipation and hernia. A very careful examination of the genitals did not show any organic changes in the common sense. Whether the burning the patient felt during his first emission had an organic basis cannot be decided. That he was impressed by the fact is connected with his attitude towards pain.

Pain appears as a phenomenon closely connected with sado-masochistic attitudes. The many intertwinings of the pain motive are remarkable. Constipation, hernia, the mother's outbreaks of fury, the father's severity, the parents' hostility towards the elder brother, were the basis of the sadomasochistic tendencies which broke through in the sexual play with his brother. Severity against himself prevented him from deriving full satisfaction from heterosexuality. His heterosexuality was mixed with sadistic features. His severity also led to hostile actions against his own personality. His pain in the genitals, mixed with strongly repressed lust feelings, appeared as the expression of sadomasochism and again led to his self-tormenting and self-punishing activities.

Federn justly points out the close connection between pain phenomena in the genitals and sadism. He refers, for instance, to awakening dreams of patients who suffered from gonorrhea and pains in the genitals. The abnormal irritation led to sadistic dreams.

I observed a case of prostatitis and urethritis following a gonorrhea which had been cured many years ago. Burning pain near the end of the urethra was the first symptom. Soon obsessions with sadistic and anal content followed, but disappeared with the disappearance of the genito-anal sensations. Sadistic fantasies in puberty and very early sadistic childhood remembrances completed the picture. When the urethral troubles appeared, the patient developed an obsession that his phallus was detached from him and being immersed in a glass of water; also an obsession that it was crushed in the street by a car. When a tormenting feeling of pressure in the bladder region occurred, there was also an exteriorization in this part of the body which in obsessions took an anal content that is less interesting to us. The patient was free from any obsession during the period after puberty and also at the time of his acute gonorrhea. This case, which was purely organic in the beginning, is the counterpart of the case under discussion to which we now return.

In this case the anal components played an important part, and the self-massage first occurred in connection with outbursts of irritability because of constipation. It must be remembered that, according to Roheim's opinion, which is based on ethnological material, sadistic and anal elements are of importance for the origin of medical art. We should not forget that massage very often substitutes and overcompensates one pain for another. It is homeopathic from the point of view of the man who suffers. There is no question that under the influence of the massage something else goes on in the deeper organic layers. When there is any pain in an organ, the individual is induced to touch, rub, or massage. It is remarkable that often where touch is painful there exists a psychic constraint to touch the painful organ. It is as though there were a psychic derivation of pain. Is there something similar to what is called derivation in the somatic field? There is certainly some analogy, but no final proof. While there is pain, magic thinking will come to the surface. Pain, therefore, provokes not only anal and sadistic regression, but also a regression to the narcissistic sphere. We know that in the anal sadistic obsessional neurosis also the step to magic thinking is often made (Freud). Obsessional neurosis cases, as well as our patient, still retain criticism against magic thought. Even if the patient in an almost schizophrenic abbreviation says, "It not," he still does not live entirely in a magic world.

I have already stated that pain contains a narcissistic element. It is a real sensation. When feeling pain, we are less concerned about the object which provokes the pain than about our own sensations. The object and subject are not well differentiated from each other, but the patient's lack of differentiation is one of the conditions determined by magic archaic experiences. As Freud also points out (1914), our own body becomes the centre of attention.

One of the important problems not touched so far is the existence of enormous differences in the individual sensitivity towards pain. We do not know how far these differences are based upon anatomical differences (Förster and Jahrreiss) or whether they are based upon a different attitude acquired by early experiences. Förster suggests some difference in the inhibitory mechanism for pain which is corticofugal and striothalamic. He is of the opinion that emotion acts on the periphery but probably also on the thalamus and the cortical region. But one should not neglect the fact that psychogenic pain occurs, as our instances have shown, in parts of the body which have a special erotic significance for the individual. A short time ago I had an opportunity of observing a case of obsession neurosis with special fear of touching dirty objects with the hands or feet. In this case pain always occurred in the parts of the body which came in active contact with the dirty object or were in danger of doing so. There is no question that psychogenic pain has an organic basis, but beyond all else it has a meaning which uses a particular part of the body-image for the expression of the libidinous tendencies. These remarks may be considered as a contribution to the question of sado-masochistic impulses in connection with psychogenic pain and organic diseases. Whatever goes on in the body has its specific psychological meaning and importance.

(7) *A case of loss of unity in the body-image*[1]

Helen Hoffman, born in 1866, has been for several years under my observation. Her family history is of no importance. A daughter of her sister has a chronic psychosis. The patient, who looks about forty-five years old, complains that she has terrible states of anxiety, especially when walking in the street.

[1] Reprinted from *The Psychoanalytic Review*, Vol. XVII, 1930.

" When I get this anxiety state I cannot walk further. I run into myself. It breaks me into pieces. I am like a spray. I lose my centre of gravity. I have no weight. I am quite mechanical. I have gone to pieces. I am like a marionette. I lack something to hold me together. I am not on the earth ; I am somewhere else ; I am in between. I am rigid, I cannot cry. Once I had an uncanny dream : I floated without any feeling of belonging anywhere. In the morning when I awakened all was flown away. I have no time before me. I don't know how it will go on. I am turned upside down and wrong side up, I am only half a human being. I felt already as a child that I am not a whole being. I was kept back in school. I was never as happy as other children even when I was eight or nine years old. I could have been happier." She knew already when nine years old that two girls were going to die. " Indeed they died afterwards. That is a terrible feeling. They suddenly looked blue and yellow." She cannot bear to hear talk of natural death. " If I hear about it I melt away and remain so for weeks. I am completely in pieces, there is no ground under the feet when you are not on the earth. I feel the ground very rarely." She also knew beforehand about the death of her mother and sister. " When I am melting I have no hands, I go into a doorway in order not to be trampled on. Everything is flying away from me. In the doorway I can gather together the pieces of my body." When she passes wooden fences the boards tear her head. " It is as if something is thrown in me, bursts me asunder. Why do I divide myself in different pieces ? I feel that I am without poise, that my personality is melting and that my ego disappears and that I do not exist anymore. Everything pulls me apart, therefore I do not like the saying " to jump out of one's skin." The skin is the only possible means of keeping the different pieces together. There is no connection between the different parts of my body. Sometimes the roof of my skull flies away. When it does not come back, I stand on my head immediately and it tears me to pieces. When the anxiety in the street catches me I do not feel anything, then I hurt myself with my nails in order to feel myself. Then I do not see human beings but only uncanny beasts such as kangaroos, rhinoceri and prehistoric animals."

At school her teacher had told her about the kangaroo bearing its young in its pouch; she was very much impressed by that. Once her skull fell from her body; it lay before her feet. She was in danger of stepping on it. She feels some pulling in her body, then the upper and lower parts of her body are separated from each other. Then the roof of the skull remained on a tree(?). "I felt it there on the tree." She feels light, her body flies up and down. "Is it possible that the head is growing and then becomes smaller again? When I am lying in bed the bed flies with me." She cannot pass over bridges and open places. She has the feeling that she has to float with the water. She has dreams of a similar type, e.g., she saw many big lions in her dreams. One of the lions opened its jaws and she put her head in it; then it closed its mouth. The whole yard was full of lions. "I would take the risk." Once she dreamed that her head was battered against a wooden chest. During the last months she has seen five big heads before her; they come nearer like bells. "They go through me. They become bigger and bigger until they are $1\frac{1}{2}$ metres in diameter. They are of a vivid blue colour. Then I have no self. I am not in the world. I am beside myself." She is always afraid that somebody will step on her limbs.

She hears voices behind her right ear. There is an evil voice which orders her to pull off other people's clothing. She feels a desire to strangle people in the street and says to herself, "My God, give me strength to stand what the voice is saying." "No, that's the devil in me. I have to fight against my own self and I have none."

In the evening she sees in her fantasy wonderful things, landscapes, foreign cities, boats, garlands. In her dreams she does not walk, she flies.

When the roof of her skull goes higher she feels a devil in it. He speaks to her very clearly. He is her second self. "You cannot go before you have pulled this hook three or five times." She cannot resist this voice.

This report describes the present stage of the patient (1929).

Her descriptions do not vary very much. She has a kind and amiable personality. She often comes alone to the clinic, but feeling anxiety. She is very easily hypnotized, sinks quickly into a very deep hypnosis with extreme suggestibility, and gets considerable relief from hypnosis. She wears gloves from fear of dirt. She is a virgin and extremely shocked when sexual problems are discussed. "Those feelings do not have to exist." She would like to eliminate sexuality. In spite of her being over sixty she behaves like a shy coquettish girl. She gives the following history of her life. She had spasms at the age of two. When three or four years old she became frightened for fear she could not find her way home. At this same period she was afraid of ghosts and cried for weeks. At the age of four a pea got into her nose. In her second year at school the teacher told her that the parents usually die before the children, which frightened her. At fifteen she had her first menstruation and thought she was going to die. Her father died when she was about eighteen. She then began to feel anxiety when alone. She would go in the street only in the company of two persons. She could not do anything with knives and scissors because she was afraid she would do something wrong.

After three years she felt better, though she did not feel strong enough for marriage. She often went to cemeteries and still goes. "When I go there the corpses come out, it is a noise as if of silk and something is floating around me, it is transparent. The dead talk to me." When she was thirty years old an uncle of hers died. She said the dead man lay beside her during the night and grasped her with his arms until she felt as if screwed into them. She also felt the corpse on her genitals. She saw skulls of the dead. Subsequently she felt well for some years, and there were only a few obsessions, although she did not like to be left alone by her sister. When she was forty-two years old the mother of a friend died. When she was ill she felt the compulsion to drill a hole in her skull and to suck her brain out. She felt also a compulsion to bite the forehead of the dead woman : "That's also the voice." She wanted to enter the body in order to get its brain. She had

L

been always very fond of this person. After the death of her friend the head always came back and drilled itself in between the upper and lower part of the patient's body. At that time she could not eat any meat. She felt a disgust and at the same time the impulse to put everything into her mouth. She cannot bear to hear anything about operations ; she feels as if she wanted to put the operated part (the genitals, the leg, and so on) into her mouth. " Are you not afraid of me ? " the patient now says to me.

Once she told her mother she should be ashamed of having borne her. At that time she began to feel as if she were falling to pieces. She was very fond of her sister, but sometimes she swore at her and felt the impulse to throw her against the wall, to stretch out her arms, and finally to tear them out. After the death of this sister she started to pick up useless things. She felt not only that the dead woman was between the two parts of her body, but also that the uncle was with her. She picked up all kinds of dirty objects in the street. She dug holes in order to find something. She picked up dirty papers and stones, brought them into the entrance hall, and wanted to put them in her mouth.

Meanwhile the dead began to fasten on her. The obsession increased. She could not go into the first street-car that came along but had to wait until five had passed. She had to clean the sewer gates. She had to count the number of buttons on men's suits. She was interested as to whether others had the eyes of murderers. In the church she tore the altar-covers and wanted to see what was in the statues of the saints. She was obsessed with the question of how one gets children (she was told in her childhood that children were fished out of the Danube). She had to touch everything. She forced a friend of hers to allow her to touch her tongue. She felt a compulsion to tear it out, in order to have some part of her friend. She was completely perverted. She felt compelled to touch everything in her friend's shop. She touched the statues of saints, also that of Christ. She felt compelled to touch his genitals. She connected everything with the mouth. She was compelled to stare at shops and to look at ties, dolls, and linen.

There is no doubt that in the history of this case sadistic features prevail. It is a neurosis. The patient sometimes touches the borderline of psychosis but never crosses it. Her voices are not real voices, they are like the voice of conscience. All her delusions about her body never produce a full conviction in her mind. Believing one moment, she disbelieves the next. Her superstition does not gain a real influence on her life; she always remains sociable, even amiable. It is doubtful whether it is an anxiety neurosis or an obsession neurosis. But the anxiety, at least in the years when I was seeing the patient, was always accidental to the queer delusions concerning her body. Nevertheless, I would not classify the patient as a case of pure obsession neurosis; her hatred does not reach the height it reaches in classical obsession neuroses. The extent of her love is greater than in those cases. In connection with that there is also the fact that she is so easy to hypnotize. Her strong repression in all genital matters fits into this scheme. She certainly has a fixation in the region of the Oedipus complex in addition to her fixation (which is the more important one) in oral and sadistic spheres. We understand now that the anxiety is a part of an hysteria. Her fixation to the father must have been a strong one. It is worthy of note that the first attack of the neurosis followed the death of her father. Since every relapse in her neurosis follows the death of someone she is fond of, we have the right to suppose that she has a special relation to death. If she believes that she is able to know beforehand who will die and when, she must have wishes concerning the death of other persons, especially those whom she loves. Her superstition deals with the death of other persons as well. Her interest in cemeteries belongs to this group of phenomena. But it is not necessary in this case to make use of interpretations. The sadistic tendencies are the overt content of her compulsions. She feels compelled to bite the skin of the forehead of her friend's mother, to cut a hole in her skull, and to suck out her brain. Against the sister she loves so much, sadistic impulses come out in her wish to tear out her arms; against the friend, in her wish to tear out her tongue. We can see quite clearly that the compulsion to touch things has the same basis. The primary impulse is that of tearing and breaking to pieces; but her still strong ideal of ego prevents her from doing it and even from wishing it too openly. It is remarkable that these cruel instincts are not only instincts of tearing, but also of biting and sucking. It is an oral sadism. One of the patient's remarks deserves special attention. She says, " Whatever happens I feel it in my mouth." She feels a compelling desire to put in her mouth parts of the body cut up by operations. We see that always; whenever a partial libido prevails it attracts all events in life; every interest, every emotion becomes connected with that partial desire and with the special organ of it. One of my patients suffering from impotence told me, " Whatever emotion may go on I feel it in my genitals; they shrink in." It is as if there were one deepened canal attracting all the water. We know this principle in physiology too. Uchtomsky has called it the " Dominante." Her sadism is especially directed against the genitals; she wants to tear out Christ's genitals. Her friend's tongue is a substitute for genitals. Behind that lies the childish belief that girls have a penis. Her childish curiosity is also destructive; she wants to tear open the images of saints in order to find out what is in them. Of course, in such a picture the anal feature must be present. That is so in her case. When she picks up dirty objects and brings them in through the doorway, the dirty things represent the anal penis, the doorway, the vagina as well as the anus. Poking with scissors in holes of sewer-gates adds again a cruel note to the anal tendencies. But I would not have reported the case for that. These are well-known things in psychoanalysis, though perhaps this case shows them more clearly than usual.

It is, however, remarkable that this sadism directed against others also affects her own body. She does not feel a tendency to hurt herself, but she feels her body falling to pieces, or, in other words, there is a mechanism of conversion instead of a mechanism of compulsion. Once again we see that sadism, as I have already pointed out, is a borderline phenomenon. When there is a sadistic tendency it is likely to be directed against the object as well as against the subject (masochism). Psychoanalytic opinion as to what is primary sadism or masochism has changed in the course of years. Freud now states that there is in every individual a primary death-wish, a primary masochism, or a tendency to self-destruction. He believes that sadism is secondary to these self-destructive tendencies. The self-love (narcissism) turns the destructive tendencies from the self against others. I personally do not think that masochism and sadism are either primary or secondary. *They are both*. They are primary as well as secondary. They are borderline phenomena. Sadism and masochism are not the only borderline phenomena. The same is true of reproaches; they are self-reproaches as well as reproaches against others. Another borderline phenomenon to be mentioned is dizziness, which lies in between subject and object and wanders from one to the other. We shall presently discuss the importance of this fact that sadism as well as dizziness is a borderline phenomenon. As I have often emphasized, there are some points in the world where subject and object are closer to each other.

In pain, for instance, the hurting object is not so important as the feeling in the body. In agnosias concerning their own bodies, patients are usually also disorientated in relation to the bodies of other persons. Right and left are concepts concerning the outside world but in a specific relation to one's own body. Many psychic phenomena lie in between subject and object, and, according to the situation and the psychic need, they are either " appersonated " or " projected." It is important to note that one's own body is often treated like an outside object. The patient's feeling that she is going to fall to pieces is also a sadistic attitude against her own body. There is another important point. Her feeling that her limbs are separated from her and that there is danger that somebody may step on them might be called a projection of her own body; it is probable that she does not want to have her limbs.

It seems, however, that from a general psychological point of view, we overrate the cohesion of our body. In spite of her tactile and kinaesthetic perceptions my patient not only imagines, but also feels her body outside. A patient of mine, who in the course of a gonorrheal infection felt pain in his glans while eating at table, experienced the sensation that his burning penis was immersed in his glass. The same patient had the feeling that his bladder was lying in the street and a street car was crushing it. Sometimes he felt as if dogs in the street might carry away his phallus like a sausage. Afterwards the picture changed and he had a similar feeling about his faeces. They were not hallucinations, but vivid optic imaginations accompanied by a queer exteriorization of feeling which made him feel that parts of his own body were lying in the street. It was an obsession. Obsessions very often have this queer vividness which makes the content of the obsession almost a hallucination. The important conclusion we may draw is that feeling our body intact is not a matter of course. It is the effect of self-love. When destructive tendencies go on, the body is spread over the world. The correctness of this conclusion may be doubted. One would like to say that we lose the unity of our body only under special pathological conditions ; but we also have to remember how much the feeling of our body varies under normal conditions. When we touch an object with a stick we feel with the end of the stick. We feel that clothes eventually become a part of ourselves. We build the picture of our body again and again. I have shown this with Klein, by studying the mistakes one makes in moving one's fingers when the hands are doubly twisted. There are forces of hatred scattering the picture of our own body and forces of love putting it together. I have shown with H. Hartmann that we perceive our body as we would perceive any other heavy substance. If we perceive that heavy substance as our body we have to build up the knowledge of our body again. Neither the optic nor the kinaesthetic or tactile impressions give us a ready-made impression of our body. We have, in fact, built it up so as to give a shape to the vague material. The shaping takes place according to biological needs.

This cutting to pieces of one's own body is accompanied by some interesting sensations in the case of our patient. She feels her body lighter, as if she were flying. She also has some flying dreams. We know that when dizzy we cannot maintain the unity of our body ; the parts of the body seem dislocated. When flying in an aeroplane, as it goes down, one often feels suddenly lighter as if the substance of gravity were leaving the body eddying upwards. The destruction tendencies concerning one's own body are aroused by excitation of the nervus vestibularis. In this respect the multiple hallucinations of the patient are very remarkable. She sees five large heads. Hoff and I have shown that polyopia is not uncommon in vestibular lesions. Eisinger and I have shown that in the dreams of patients with vestibular troubles, multiplication of figures is the rule. We have the right to suppose that the conversion in this case affects the vestibular apparatus. It is impossible to say what parts of the vestibular apparatus are affected. It is possible that there is a diencephalic station of the vestibular apparatus too; the connection with anxiety would point in this direction, though we have no definite proof of it.

In my book on *Selbstbewusstsein and Persönlichkeitsbewusstsein* (1914), I first pointed out that there are very close relations between the vestibular apparatus and depersonalization, and since then I have always emphasized this connection (cf. Stern and Stengel). It is worthy of note that our patient complains about herself in exactly the same way as do cases of depersonalization. On the other hand, many cases of depersonalization complain that the poise of their body is changed. I may mention that our patient, like all patients with depersonalization, complains that she does not know how it will be possible for time to continue. The relation of vestibular sensations to time should be studied morecare fully than has hitherto been done. On the other hand, we know that every negation of one's self is connected with troubles in the perception of time. (Cf. E. Straus and E. Minkowsky). But the important thing is that here depersonalization is a sadomasochistic negation of the patient's own body—and is connected with vestibular mechanisms. And here we come to the last point of importance. Goldstein, and especially Hoff and I, have shown that the perception of one's own body is dependent on muscle tone. The tone also changes the perception of the heavy mass of our body and its limbs. The vestibular irritation changing the tone has in many ways a similar effect.

Certainly there are many primitive tonus tendencies which

drive the limbs away from the body. Goldstein refers to an outward tendency of the body. The cerebellum restrains this outward tendency. After cerebellar lesion this outward tendency comes out again. Goldstein ascribes to the cerebellum the function of keeping the body together. There must be some truth in this statement; the centripetal and centrifugal tendencies which Goldstein discusses in motility and tonus are present in the postural model of the body as well. The centrifugal and destructive tendencies are connected with sadistic tendencies, the centripetal with narcissistic ones. We consider it important that these centrifugal destructive tendencies concerning the postural model of the body exert a conversion influence on the vestibular apparatus which has to do, from the organic point of view, with a tonus in the medulla oblongata which is at least partly centrifugal.

The far-going disrupture in the postural model of our patient occurs in anxiety states. We are certainly not dealing with a typical case of an anxiety neurosis. But it seems that every anxiety impairs the experience of our body-image. This point has not yet been sufficiently studied; my own material does not contain decisive facts, nor have I been able to find them in such literature as is available on the subject.

(8) *Hysteria*

There is no question that in hysteria also there are changes in the postural model of the body. Freud, Ferenczi, and many others have shown that hysterical disturbance symbolizes the sex-organ, but we have seen that the same is true about hypochondria. In my psychoanalytic psychiatry I have already tried to give a clear account of the different parts of the body in hypochondria and in hysteria. In hypochondria and in the hypochondriac neurasthenic, the hypochondriac sensation is transferred from the sex-organ to other parts. The object relation in this symbolization is either completely absent or at least not clearly given. In hysteria the symptom is more or less a symptom connected with the genital relations to others.

It may be worth while to review the hysterical symptom from this point of view. According to analytic theory, hysterical blindness is the expression of the wish of seeing the sex-partner naked and its repression. I may add that the frequent absence of the conjunctival reflexes in hysteria is probably in a very similar category. In hypnotic experiments I suggested complete blindness. This suggestion was often followed by the absence of the conjunctival reflex (the corneal reflex is never absent in hysteria and never disappears by suggestion). The hysterical globus, the choking sensations in the throat, the feeling that a nail is driven into the head (Clavus) are the expressions of a wish concerning the male sex-organ, though not any male sex-organ but that of a particular and individual person. Hysterical anaesthesia is the expression of a repression against any sex feeling. Hyper-sensitivity towards pain, especially in the erogenic zone of the mamilla, the hysterical point over the ovaries, is a clear-cut negation of the sex tendencies of these particular parts in close relation with genital activities. It is true that it may be the patient's own genital which is transposed from one part of the body to others, but it may also be the sex-organs of another person brought symbolically into connection with different parts of the body. Even if, in all these sensations and changes in the body-image, fantasies of a more primitive and pregenital type are present, and even if homosexual, anal, oral tendencies, etc., are involved, the hysterical conversion symptoms are always more or less closely related to the genital desires. But the genital desires of hysteria are closely related to the Oedipus complex.

The symptomatology of hysteria is to a great extent a change in the image of the body. We can distinguish between two groups of phenomena ; one connected with the surface and the outward appearance of the body, the other with the inner part of the body. It is remarkable how many object relations and situations may be condensed in a hysterical change in one organ of the body. The classical instance is Freud's case, Dora, in which hysterical coughing, hysterical catarrh, is the expression of genital wishes to be infected and to take the place of the mother. At the same time it points to an infantile enuresis which is again the expression of a sex-wish concerning the father. But the whole symptom is provoked by the actual wish for sex relations with the man who is the husband of her father's mistress.

It is not the purpose of this discussion to go into the principles of psychoanalysis. I only desire to emphasize that the hysterical symptom in the body is not only the product of transposition, but that there are also innumerable condensations which lead to this transposition. It seems that in the purely hypochondriac case there are less condensations than in the hysterical change in the postural model of the body. We have not mentioned so far that the change in the postural model of the body is not only due to transposition in the subject's own body-image, but also that parts of the body-image of others are constantly taken into the subject's own body-image.

In Dora's case the coughing of the patient is the expression of an identification with the mother who has catarrh in the genitals. But we shall deal more in detail later on with this mechanism of identification, which is, after all, the expression of the close relation between the different postural models of different persons.

An hysterical symptom may be the expression of an identification with any diseased person if the patient desires for conscious or unconscious reasons to be in the place of this other person.

(9) *Some principles concerning the libidinous structure of the body-image*

The few observations we have discussed so far allow us to formulate some important principles concerning the emotional influence on the postural model of the body.

1. Emotional influence will change the relative value and clearness of the different parts of the body-image according to the libidinous tendencies.

2. This change can be a change on the surface of the body but can also be a change in the inner parts of the body.

3. There may be a change in the subjective appearance of the skin, a very common symptom in hypochondria. There may be a loss of sensation concerning any part of the body. There may be a forgetting of one limb of the body or of one

side of the body. (Cf. the chapter on Achiria and Dyschiria).

4. There may be changes in the perception of the gravity of the body. But the heavy substance of the body may contain holes or there may be consolidation in the inner parts of the body. The formation of holes, the formation of solid parts, are the only possibilities concerning the change of the body. It is an important analogy that organic growth can use only two principles : growth makes either protrusions or folds. By irregular growths holes are created. The psychological change in the solid substance of the body can be compared with the changes which take place in a solid mass of cells by irregular growth.

5. What goes on in one part of the body may be transposed to another part of the body. The hole of the female genital organs may appear as a cavity in another part of the body, the penis as a stiffness or as a piece of wood somewhere else. There is said to be a transposition of one part of the body to another part of the body. One part may be symbolic of the other. There must be some foundation for this symbolic substitution. The nose may take the significance of the phallus. The protruding parts of the body may become symbols of the male sex organ. Cavities and entrances of the body are largely interchangeable. Vagina, anus, mouth, ears, and even the entrances of the nose and ears belong to the same group. It appears as if the general connotation of opening or protrusion is basic for our attitude towards the body and the body-image. The symbolic interchange of organs by transposition may occur in the so-called purely psychic sphere ; it may be only a change in the mental attitude. But there is no psychic experience which is not reflected in the motility and in the vasomotor functions of the body. A thought about the body influences it as well as an image. This influence may not be measurable at the time, but it still exists, and a change in the body will not be very different from libidinous changes in the body-image which are connected with organ symptoms of paraesthesia or pain, or even with changes in the organic function and structure. There may be psychic or organic reasons why the organ as such is affected by the transposition in one case and not affected

in another. As the cases I have presented show, the early history of the patient will very often determine how far the body-image in its libidinous structure can influence the actual function and structure of the body.

6. The attitude towards the different parts of the body can be determined by the interest the persons around us give to our body. We elaborate our body-image according to the experiences we obtain through the actions and attitudes of others. The actions of others may provoke sensations when they touch and handle us. But they may influence us also by words and actions which direct our attention to particular parts of their body and our own body.

7. The interest others have in their body and the actions of others with their body will influence the interest in the respective parts of the subject's own body.

8. Diseases which provoke particular action towards the body will also change the postural model of the body.

9. Early infantile experiences are of special importance in this connection, but we never cease gathering experiences and exploring our own body.

10. We may take parts of the bodies of others and incorporate them in our own body-image. (This phenomenon is called " Appersonization " in general psychopathology). We may take in parts of the body of others by identifying ourselves with them. This identification may again either lead to sensations and perceptions in the body or to psychic attitudes towards parts of the body, which may either come out in the consciousness or may remain unconscious.

11. It seems that the emotional unity of the body is dependent on the development of full object relations in the Oedipus complex. The prevalence of sado-masochistic tendencies leads to a disruption of the postural model of the body.

12. Psychogenic pain is one of the expressions of sado-masochistic tendencies which causes shifts of attention in relation to the organ in the centre of the sado-masochistic attitude.

13. In hypochondria we have to do with a transposition of the genitals and their libidinous investments to other parts of

the body. This transposition can be on the surface or in the inner parts of the body. The genitals are in some way experienced as isolated and not in connection with persons.

14. In neurasthenia we find an important anal sadistic attitude towards other persons and accordingly a disruption of the postural model of the body. The relation to other persons and the individual life experiences accordingly play a very important part.

15. In connection with sadistic object relations, anxiety may lead to a far-going dismembering of the whole body.

16. In depersonalization the individual withdraws from his body-image.

17. In hysteria the fight against genitality and object relation leads to the elimination of parts of the postural model. The elimination mostly symbolizes the elimination of sex organs. But identification and object relation play an enormous part in the building-up of the body-image. When the changes in the body-image symbolize the sex organ, the sex organs are closely connected with actual sex relations to persons as a whole. The disruption of the postural model of the body seems to be less violent in cases of hysteria.

It cannot be denied that our discussion of the body-image in the various neuroses is a contribution to one of the general principles of psychoanalysis, namely that the development of genital sexuality is necessary for a full appreciation of other persons and our appreciation of their somatic integrity. According to Abraham, there is then a development from the interest in parts of the body of another person to the interest in the integrity of his whole body as an expression of his person. But the development from pregenitality to genitality is also of fundamental importance for our attitude towards our own body. We experience our body as united, as a whole, only when the genital level is harmoniously reached. Fully developed genital sexuality is indispensable for the full appreciation of our own body-image.

The analogy of our investigations on the libidinous structure of the body-image to our findings concerning the physiological structure of the body-image is very striking. The image of the body is not a static phenomenon from the physiological point of view. It is acquired, built-up, and gets its structure by a continual contact with the world. It is not a structure but a structuralization in which continual changes take place, and all these changes have relations to motility and to actions in the outside world. Difficulties arise in the building-up of the postural model of the body, and the various senses cannot be used and co-ordinated. All senses participate in this constructive process, and undoubtedly the vestibular apparatus has here a particular function. Our relation to the earth, to gravity, is an outstanding factor for the mechanics of movement and for the perception of the body-image.

The processes which construct the body-image not only go on in the field of perception but also have their parallels in the building-up in the libidinous and emotional field. External love-objects, our relations to them, and their attitudes towards us are here of enormous importance. But in this process of structuralization the concomitant of sexuality is of an outstanding importance and especially the development of the sadistic attitudes and our attitudes towards the existence of fellow human beings.

The body-image in the sphere of perception is dependent on the inanimate world or rather on the world under the aspect of the inanimate. The body-image in the libidinous sphere is to a great extent dependent upon our attitudes towards the love-object, or, in a broader sense, the animate world, or still better, the world under the aspect of animation and life. It is therefore clear that a full understanding of the problems involved is only possible if we consider the inter-relations of the body-images of various persons, or, in other words, the sociology of body-images. This discussion, however, must be postponed till later.

(10) *Conversion*

There is no question that a cortical activity is necessary for the production of the body-image. The discussions in the first part of this book demonstrate this. Of course, the postural model of the body is not in any way deposited in the cortical region ; this is only a part of the brain which is necessary for the final integration of the various processes which lead to the building-up of the structure of the body. Cortical activity in its various levels brings the perceptive process to its final end and takes it out of the vague indistinctness and generality of the primitive perception ; it makes a whole of it with distinctive parts, and simplifies the waste amount of closely interwoven impressions and impulses which are the characteristic of the lower level of perception and mentality. There is no reason to doubt that image and perception are bound up with cortical activity. The same is true about memory, thought, and judgment.

Perceptive and mental images (we shall here use the term " picture ") are connected with motor impulses of various levels. I have emphasized that these various impulses make the final elaborated perception possible. The pictures undergo a process of development from a vague and interwoven generality to clear units with distinctive parts. The process goes from the general to the individual and from complication to simplicity. The thinking of the child and of the primitive person is fuller of meaning than the thinking of the adult. They see more relations ; everything is connected with everything else. Their thinking is full of symbolizations and condensations. An object means much more than the adult mind sees in it ; it is not only animated but connected with all activities in the universe. Freud calls this type of thinking the action of the system of the unconscious ; Lévy Bruhl and the French School call it primitive or pre-logic thinking. I prefer to speak of the sphere, and mean by this term the processes which go on in the background of our minds, bringing the single parts repeatedly into all types of varied relations and proceeding under the direction of the various instinctive tendencies from the general to the individual. Pictures (representations and perceptions) have, therefore, an important development in which the psychic tendencies play an enormous part. We have the right to assume that every phase in this development is connected with a particular motility[1], and is on the other hand directed by the instinctive

[1] Allers and Scheminsky have shown that the representation of movement provokes muscular innervation and the characteristic action-currents.

tendencies. When, therefore, we speak of pictures, we simplify the actual facts. The picture is already the product of varied activities and interactions of tendencies directed towards the external situation. It has to be emphasized that isolation of single parts in the psyche is in some degree arbitrary. There is no picture which is not will, action, and emotion at the same time. When we talk of pictures and contrast them with desires, it should not be forgotten that in the final analysis they form an inseparable unit and are only the two sides of the total human activity.

But let us take this artificial unit of pictures. Whenever a picture is present it leads to a tendency to an action. This tendency comes out in the system of the muscles. I mean, of course, the system of the striped muscles. This is not the place to discuss the complications of the system, which, as has often been pointed out, has various levels. We may recall that one level is especially connected with attitudes, and is also known as tonic, while there is another level which is especially connected with activities in the proper sense. We also have phasic activities, which can be of various kinds. They may be rhythmic but they may also be arhythmic; they may be frankly directed towards the outside world or they may be chiefly imitations of what is going on in the outside world. This latter distinction can also be made concerning the tonic activities. In simpler language, when we see or imagine something, we change our attitude, imitating the object, or preparing ourselves for an action concerning the object. But we may also perform a distinct action which can be either rhythmic or arhythmic. Only the latter will have the chance of being successful; it will generally be less successful if it is not an action in the proper sense but an imitation. But when there is a picture created by an emotional drive, it will have an influence on the vegetative system of our body.

There must be a connection between the cortical activities associated with the pictures and the vegetative apparatus which has its most important stations in the gray substances around the third and fourth ventricles (inner caves of the brain). Here lie centres for all vasovegetative innervations, sympathetic and parasympathetic centres. There is no necessity to go into details ; I need only refer to the work of Hess, Aschner, Leschke, Cannon, and others. It is well known that temperature, secretion of saliva, urination, and all vegetative functions can be influenced from this part of the brain. It is of special importance that there are sex centres and metabolic centres in this region too. Possibly these centres will influence growth.

The sympathetic and parasympathetic apparatus of this region influences the whole body, but the fact that it influences the glands with internal secretion deserves special attention. The sympathetic and parasympathetic apparatus and the central regulation of the vegetative functions have at least two stations ; the one around the fourth ventricle is of a more primitive type, while the centres around the third ventricle probably serve the higher regulations. It is a question which is not completely solved whether the influence of the pictures calls directly to the sub-cortical apparatus or whether the sympathetic and parasympathetic apparatus also has its representations in the cortical region. At any rate with every picture are connected two streams of impulses, the one 'animalisch' (motor) and the other vegetative. Both streams go back after they have reached their peripheral goal, so that we deal with a closed circle of vegetative and animalic impulses—from the pictures and to the pictures. The body-image follows the same important principles. We now understand better why every change in the body-image is at the same time a change in the vegetative functions of the body and why changes in the libidinous structure of the postural image of the body are changes in the organism.

The experiments in which attempts have been made to influence the function of the inner part of the body lead to very interesting conclusions. It is very difficult to suggest to an individual that the pupil of the eye should become larger, but we are immediately successful when we make the suggestion that the subject sees something terrible going on in the outside world. Similarly when we want to produce a change in the body we can do it only when we change the pictures of the outside world or when we change something which, like the image of the body, belongs more to the outside world.

M

But in the majority of cases we do not have a body-image concerning the inner part of our body. Therefore we reach the body only by pictures of the outside world. We cannot directly suggest changes in metabolism, but we can suggest to a naked person that he feels warm, and the basal metabolism will react not in the sense of a decrease but even in the sense of an increase.[1] When we want to change the output of urine in a person by suggestion, we have to suggest to him that he is drinking a large amount of water.[2] It is true that we may get similar results by suggesting pleasure or displeasure, but, when a suggestion of pleasure or displeasure is given, the individual certainly reacts with pictures which deal with pleasure or displeasure. These pictures may be pictures of the body-image or concerning the outside world. We come to the important general conclusion that the body-image and the picture of the world lead to the vegetative changes, and it follows that our body is dominated by the image of the body which is in such close relation to the world. (For literature concerning these experiments I refer my readers to the paper by Heilig and Hoff and the book by Schilder and Kauders on Hypnosis).

There is no question that only these experiences lead to the understanding of the problems of conversion. We can understand conversion only as something which is happening in the postural model of the body.[3] According to the definition, conversion is the expression of psychic conflict in the sphere of the body, and a psychic energy, which is prevented from expressing itself, goes into the somatic field. It goes from the psychic sphere into the somatic sphere.

The term " conversion " is used rather loosely in psycho-analytic literature. An hysterical fit, an 'animalisch' (motor) phenomenon, is considered as conversion as well as anxiety, which is a vegetative phenomenon. (According to Freud's newer formulations, anxiety is a danger signal concerning the

[1] Experiments by Hansen.
[2] Experiments by Heilig and Hoff.
[3] J. H. Schultz believes that somatic changes may be produced by the mere concentration on the organ by autosuggestive training. Even if his assertion were true, it would be necessary to know what stages the auto-suggestion has passed and what kind of representations are used in order to come to the perception of the organ.

ego, but he leaves it open whether it occurs by conversion of sex energy into anxiety). Conversion may therefore be connected with the 'animalisch' as well as with the vegetative stream of impulses. It is so far an unsolved problem why in some cases the symptom remains chiefly in the psychic sphere of images, thoughts, and character changes, while in others it expresses itself in cramps or in obviously material changes of the blood circulation of the vasovegetative innervation such as gastric secretion, constipation, or, in a general way, as an organ neurosis.

Since we are chiefly interested in the psychological problem we need only allude briefly to the existence of the general change in the vasovegetative system, which is connected with every picture and especially one which is loaded with psychic energy. Every organ which is predisposed from an organic point of view (Adler speaks rather vaguely about organ inferiority) will especially attract the stream of impulses. It is as if the bed of the stream were wider in those places. It may be that the predisposition of the organ may be purely organic and is not reflected in any way in the psychic sphere. But it is more than probable that the organ which is in any way different will provide sensations different from and probably more numerous than those of the average organ; and that somehow the anatomical and physiological difference in the organ will therefore be reflected in a postural model of the body, usually not where the organ actually is but where it is felt in the zone which I have called the sensitive zone of the body. The different organic functioning will have its reflection in this part of the body, and this point will then be the point which attracts and reflects conversion.

But we must not forget that the different functions of the organ and the sensation which it provokes will change the attitude towards the objects connected with the functioning of this organ. When a particular kind of food provokes indigestion, the attitude towards the food will be changed, and the picture of the food as such will again provoke a change in the postural model of the body. Every change in the attitude towards an object in the outside world has the greater chance to lead to conversion, the more the organ system which reacts to this particular part of the outside world is psychologically and physiologically predisposed. But it is an unsolved problem how much of the predisposition of the organ and its reflection into the psychic sphere is caused by constitutional elements. Predisposition may be created by temporary or lasting organic disease in childhood or even later. In scientific terminology, we have to reckon not only with constitution but also with constellation. But we are not justified in assuming that conversion takes place only in organs which are different by constitution and constellation. What does determine the flow of energy into a so-called normal organ? Freud has indicated that the childhood experiences concerning this organ may be responsible; a real or imagined pain or any discomfort connected with a passing function (the normal function) or organic discomfort may be the cause.

In the case of psychogenic pain described above, pain experiences concerning sex organs and the anal sphere were present in childhood. In the neurasthenia case an itching disease seems to have been the basis for the later itching sensation. But I have shown in both cases that the psychic problems of the child gave the final significance to the passing sensations, and it is a question whether an actual discomfort experienced in childhood is really indispensable for the conversion. The intensity of the attention directed towards the organ of later conversion may be, and probably is, sufficient for the genesis of a conversion symptom. In psychoanalytic literature there are frequent references to the jump from the psychic into the organic and the riddle of conversion in connection with it. This formulation is misleading; it overlooks the general organic character of the psychic function. The conversion is only an accentuation of what goes on in every " Psychic Process." F. Deutsch has drawn attention to another important factor in the psychogenesis of conversion symptoms. We know that some muscles which are generally out of the reach of voluntary innervation can be exercised; e.g. a movement of the ears. We can also exercise vegetative functions to some extent by stressing the pictures connected with the particular vegetative functions. There are persons who are able to effect marked changes in their pulse-rate. I may mention J. H. Schultz's studies on auto-suggestive training and the Yoga practice. One can also exercise vegetative organs. There is no question that many of the vegetative functions, for instance bowel movements, are closely intertwined with voluntary functions and can be trained to a considerable extent. Watson has clearly demonstrated that we can influence the intestines. The exercise and the training of the vegetative organ will, of course, depend on the psychogenic structure and experiences of the individual.

(11) *Organic disease*

There arises the problem of organic disease in connection with the postural model of the body. Organic disease provokes abnormal sensations ; it immediately changes the image of the body, partly the picture side of it and partly the libidinous investment. These sensations immediately become a part of the general attitude and experience of the individual, and underlie the transformation and transposition, the condensations and symbolizations we have studied in neurotic cases. Symptoms in organic diseases as well as in psychogenic diseases take place in the postural model of the body. They can only be understood in connection with the general problem. Of course, there are symptoms which do not change the psychological sphere. A growing cancer may not make any immediate changes in the postural model of the body ; but it may lead to fatigue, weakness, and lack of appetite, which are definitely connected with the body-image.

There are, of course, purely objective phenomena which may be very valuable for the physician and may help him in a diagnosis, for instance, the absence of patellar reflexes or a nystagmus. But we are not justified in talking of symptoms unless some change in the postural model has taken place. A change in the X-ray picture of the lungs is not a symptom in this sense, but coughing, pain in the shoulder, or fever, are symptoms. We come to the preliminary differentiation between objective phenomena of a disease and symptoms ; the latter are connected with the postural model of the body. A few instances given show that symptoms are merely changes in the picture or in the sensations and representations, but they may consist also of a reflectory answer as in vomiting and coughing.

The reflectory action may lead again to a change in the sensations. The symptom may also lead to a different motor attitude and action. When an individual has a sore foot he uses his foot in a different way, or he may not use it at all. These changes in attitude may be voluntary and conscious, but they may be and often are to a great extent instinctive. When an individual has lost one leg not only is there a change in the postural model of the body concerning the leg, but also a different function which is necessary owing to the absence of the leg changes the whole motility of the individual and with it the whole postural model of the body. Every difference in the function, has therefore an immediate influence on the body-image. It is as if the change in the function were transmuted into a static difference and difference in the image. It is a fascinating psychological problem to follow these changes from function and movement into the relatively static image of the body. We shall meet this problem again later on. Generally we can appreciate movement, function-change, only concerning a relatively stabilized background. The body-image is this stable background on which changes in the functions are engraved. Ross's experiments and Skramlik's studies show clearly the tendency of the body-image to relative stability; or, in other words, psychologically the function is contrasted with the relatively stabilized form.

There is no question that the body-image is fundamentally changed by organic disease, and that this change undergoes the various transformations we have already studied. The transformation goes along typical lines. The following laws can be formulated :—

Every protrusion can take the place of another. We have possibilities of transformation between phallus, nose, ear, hands, feet, fingers, toes, nipples and breasts ; every round part can represent another—head, breasts, buttocks ; every hole can be interchanged with another—mouth, ears (in some respects, eyes and pupils), openings of the nose and anus. Each zone has typical lines of extension. The anal zone extends over the back. The mouth will generally extend in the interior plane. The details are not yet very well known. Actions may create artificial caves in the body ; the inside of the hand and the inside of the mouth and the inside of the genital region may be substituted for each other. We know still less which motility phenomena can be substituted for each other. In some tics the masturbatory reaction may wander from one part to another, from below to above, etc.

The so-called organ neurosis mediates between the organic and the psychogenic disturbances. According to Hansen an organic symptom can only provoke a psychic reaction if it is a part of a so-called unconditioned reflex (an unconditioned reflex is the production of saliva when hydrochloric acid is put into the mouth). The frequency and readiness with which organic symptoms are provoked by psychic experience are determined by their readiness to react in unconditioned reflexes. The external experience becomes the signal which provokes the unconditioned reflex. But we know very little about which part of the body is able to give such unconditioned reflexes. When we ingest food we also immediately provoke with the change in the outside world a particular attitude of the individual which expresses itself in the body-image of the mouth. Not only is the function of the whole intestinal tract changed, but also its reflection in the body-image.

Organic change is therefore always connected with a change in the body-image. When we study an organ neurosis, we are able from a psychological point of view to determine why the individual became ill at a given moment, or at least we should be able to show why he was unable to bear the stress of the situation at a particular moment and why he changed his postural model of the body and with it the function of the inner part of the body. We should also be able to determine why a particular organ was chosen for the conversion. After all, the organ neurosis in its proper sense is the clearest instance of a conversion.

We have mentioned what determines the stream of energy to

a particular part of the body-image and its dependent inner organs. We must, of course, not forget that every individual during his life gathers experiences about symptoms in connections with organs. The individual who produces a gastric neurosis has seen people with stomach-disease vomiting; he himself has experiences about symptoms later when he eats indigestible food, and perhaps he has gathered in previous experiments with himself, experiences that special representations concerning food and concerning the taste in the mouth have provoked symptoms similar to those produced by indigestible food.

I would venture to say that everybody uses the small experiences of everyday life in organic diseases for subsequent experimenting on the body-image and for the acquisition of the key representation for a particular organ which is not immediately represented in the postural model of the body. By the term 'key representation' I mean that we are able by specially arbitrarily chosen representations to change the function of intestines which are otherwise beyond our reach. We cannot decide to increase our pulse-rate, but we can imagine ourselves in a frightening situation and can thereby provoke a change in the pulse-rate. The representation of a frightening experience is the key representation to the heart and also to the dilation of the pupil. The representation of disgusting foods is the key representation for some types of salivation, nausea, and vomiting, and probably also for a change in the gastric juice.

In every individual a continual process of experimenting with key representations goes on, thus gaining indirect influence on the inner parts of the body. This experimentation with the organs probably begins in very early childhood, and every organ neurosis is, as Deutsch rightly emphasizes, prepared by such experimentations. Here we also gain a deeper insight into the influence of organic diseases in early childhood. Organic disease facilitates the handling of the key representation. We understand also why it is comparatively simple to retain a neurotic symptom after the organic disease is over. It is not the purpose of these remarks to give the psychological theory of the disease ; we are interested in those problems only so far as the body-image is concerned, and try to find the way in which inner organs can be influenced by psychic attitudes. Primarily, the psychic attitude acts on the body-image.

A change in the function of an inner organ may sooner or later change its anatomy. When asthma is provoked by psychogenesis, sooner or later the structure of the organ will be changed. When there is innervation of the stomach, sooner or later organic changes may follow. In what way the psyche changes the function, how far the disturbance in the function can go, and whether, and if so in what degree, disturbance in the function may lead to a change in the anatomy of the organ, are problems for future investigation.

I have already referred to the fact that the constitution and the constellation concerning a particular organ are important factors in the choice of the organ for a neurosis, and especially for an organ neurosis. It is a question whether for the choice of a particular organ, for an organ neurosis, a particular somatic constitution or somatic change is not indispensible. We may even go further, and ask whether, for a conversion neurosis, this particular somatic change with its expression in the body-image is not necessary. From this point of view we may justify an organic theory of the neurosis, and consider especially the individuality of the organ in which the neurosis expresses itself. I think that these remarks give a clearer meaning to what Freud in his Psychoanalysis called *Somatisches Entgegenkommen* (somatic predisposition and readiness) and Adler summarized in the rather vague connotation, ' organ inferiority.' I may mention in this connection the purely somatic theories of neurosis, especially those of Fr. Kraus. But we have, of course, to consider not only the state of the organ (cf. also Curschmann), but also the differences in the flow of the psychic energies to the organ. The psychological factors may single out the organ ; we may psychologically be able to determine especially the intensity of desires connected with a particular organ and with a particular part of the body-image, but we may even here meet the remainder which cannot be solved by present psychological methods and which we have to ascribe to different somatic factors in the flow of psychic energy. Even if we consider neurosis and organ neurosis, we come to underlying organic differences and factors which are beyond psychological reach. If we wished to express this in psychological terms we should have to say that the psychic attitude of the individual, so far as it is in the consciousness, is based upon an archaic system of strivings and tendencies which has found its expression in the structure of the body. This is one of the reasons why we have given so much attention to the organic side of the body-image.

It is not very probable that the problem of organic disease can be solved if we consider only psychogenesis. It is true that we do not know much about why an organic disease occurs at a particular moment. A fracture of the skull and its serious consequences can be caused by an accident independent of the conscious or unconscious psychic activities, and in such a case we know why the organic change occurred at that very moment. But we do not know why diabetes, heart disease, and carcinoma occur at a particular time. We also do not know why a bacterial infection becomes efficient in certain individuals only at a particular moment. But we cannot overlook the fact that even in these obscure cases the factor of outside influences and merely somatic occurrences is probably of an outstanding importance. There are, however, many organic diseases in which the psychogenic factor can apparently play a greater part, as, for instance, gastric ulcer, angina pectoris, some colds, etc. We often wonder why organic diseases occur at times when the life situation of the individual has come to a crisis, and why they so often occur where the individual seems to need them out of his innermost strivings. Even then we have to be careful. How many normal individuals do we meet who are not at a given time more or less in serious stress ? We have no statistical data for purposes of comparison.

The best formulation of this problem can be found in the book by Thornton Wilder, *The Bridge of San Luis Rey*. At noon on Friday, July 20th, 1714, the finest bridge in all Peru broke and precipitated five travellers into the gulf below. Why did it happen to those particular five ? The author shows clearly that all of them died at a crucial point of their lives. Is there a plan, a meaning, in the accident which killed them ? That is the ironic question set by the novel. We may raise the same ironic question if an organic disease occurs when the life of an individual tends to an inner crisis.

The investigations made by Groddeck, Jelliffe, and F. Deutsch have certainly furnished interesting material, and have shown the possibility of the influence of psychogenic factors on the body. But we have to be extremely careful in every case to distinguish whether we are dealing with a coincidence or with the expression of inner tendencies. Part I of *The Bridge of San Luis Rey*, has the title, " Perhaps an Accident," and the last chapter, " Perhaps an Intention." A preliminary study shows that there are some cases of organic disease which certainly are nearly an accident. Some cases are chiefly due to the inner intention of the individual. In the majority of cases disease is accidental as well as intentional. In organic disease, the accident, in the neurosis, the intention prevails.

The sign of organic disease is pain and discomfort. Disease is suffering. In disease the individual is passive. Even in a neurosis the individual finally succeeds in suffering, in being passive and masochistic. But whenever we have pain, when we are suffering, we experience a change in the postural model of the body. We arrive now at a deeper understanding of the reasons why masochism has so much to do with disease and why the sado-masochistic part in instinctive life is of such an enormous importance for the structure of the postural model of the body.[1]

[1] The psychological side of medicine should be emphasized, but not over-emphasized. The mortality of infants has decreased as well as the mortality of tuberculosis ; the fight against infectious diseases has been extremely successful ; the average duration of life has been considerably increased. These are triumphs of somatic medicine. There have been unquestionable and far-reaching results in surgery. I need mention here only tumours of the central nervous system. Psychological medicine will have to strive hard to equal these achievements. It will probably achieve more in making the physically healthy person happy and adapted to reality than in curing the physically ill person ; or, in other words, psychological medicine is a gigantic attempt to solve the moral problem of humanity. But physical disease is certainly not always merely a moral problem, though the moral element is invariably present. There is no doubt that some somatic illnesses are merely the expression of moral difficulties. But I do not think that the number of those serious moral somatic diseases is very great, and, in addition, there is considerable doubt whether a disease which has originated in the psychic sphere can always be cured by psychological methods.

(12) *Further remarks on expansion and destruction of*
the body-image

So far we have studied the schema of the body as a unit which is built up from various sources ; we have not yet considered the fact that this unit not only appersonates parts but also frequently gives them away. The unit is also in a continual danger of losing some of its parts. There are also parts in this unit which are not continually there, which are expelled. There exists not only a tendency to build up the postural model of the body but also a tendency to destroy this image, as will be observed from some of the cases I have reported. Before we start a full discussion of this problem, we must consider the relation of the body-image to the excretions. When we eat food or when we drink, something from the outside world is added to the image of the body. But as long as it has not passed the sensitive zone it remains external. This is also true about air. When the food has passed the sensitive zone it disappears as an object, but somehow it has not added to the body-image ; it is, psychologically speaking, digested immediately after it passes the sensitive zone. When we urinate we attribute the urine still in some degree to our body. It is true that this relation is, as Freud has shown, a specifically psychological one ; it·is a psychological part of the postural model of the body. What has once been part of the body does not lose this quality completely. The bowel movement also separates the faeces only physically from the body, psychologically they remain a part of ourselves. We are dealing with a spreading of the body-image into the world. More complicated is the problem of voice and language. The sound produced by me is not completely independent of me. It still remains a part of myself, and we are again dealing with the spreading of the body into the world. Finger-nails, everything which comes out of the mouth and nose, hair which has been cut off, always remain in some psychological relation to the body. The organization of the body-image is a very flexible one.[1]

On the other hand, some of the parts of our body can become

[1] Magic practices with faeces, urine, blood, nails, etc., are based on the fact that they still belong to the body-image.

loose in their connection with the body. Single parts of the body are personified. Children and nurses of children personify fingers.[1] It seems that all protruding parts can gain this relative independence in the postural model of the body. In this category belongs the fact that the male genitals especially are often personified and made into independent persons. It is true that the same happens to the female genitals too, though in my opinion less frequently. One talks of the little man, the little etc., and calls the female genitals the little woman, etc. In dreams children very often symbolize the genitals. The coherence in the postural model of the body is different in different parts. Anatomical configuration here plays an important part. A protrusion belongs less to the body. But besides this, there is the libidinous function which is of the utmost importance for the structure of the body. It seems that whenever a part of the body is less closely connected with the other parts of the image of the body, a fear arises of losing it. It is the fear for the integrity of the body which is based upon the inner qualities of the postural model of the body.

Psychoanalysis first drew attention to the existence of fear concerning the male genitals, especially the penis, and to the fear of castration. It soon came to the surface that there are many symbolizations for the castration complex, and that almost any parts of the body, especially the protruding ones, may serve as a basis for the castration complex.

[1] This little pig went to market   (thumb)
This little pig stayed at home   (index)
This little pig had bread and butter   (middle)
This little pig had none   (ring)
This little pig pee-wee-weed all the way home.   (little)

    *   *   *   *   *   *   *

Der Daumen schüttelt die Pflaumen   (Daumen)
Der klaubt sie auf   (Zeigefinger)
Der tragt sie hinein   (Mittelfinger)
Der misst sie   (Ringfinger)
und Der frisst sie   (Kleiner Finger)

    *   *   *   *   *   *   *

Das ist der Vater
Das ist die Mutter
Das ist die Schwester   (selbe Reihenfolge)
Das ist der Bruder
und Das ist das Wutzerl in der Wiagn.

In psychoanalysis these parts of the body have been considered as symbols for the sex organs. But it soon became clear that there was not only a fear of losing the penis but that there are pregenital analogies to the castration complex. There is the fear of losing the inner parts of the body, and we find in these cases a phenomenon which we may call anal castration complex. There is also a general fear about the integrity of the body, or, as I have called it, a general dismembering motive and fear. In psychosis especially this dismembering motive plays an important part. In the last analysis it is based upon the structural qualities of the body-image. The fear of operation belongs to the same category. When we build up a persistent and coherent image of the body, we build it up out of our emotional mood, which is based upon biological tendencies. The unity of the body-image thus reflects the life tendency of the biological unit. The change in the biological unit reflects itself in the more plastic image of the body ; the tendency of the organism to self-defence reflects itself in the fear of castration and pregenital castration in the fear of being dismembered. We understand why, in the psychosis in which the unit of the instincts is so much endangered, the motives of castration (Stärcke), dismembering plays such a great part. In one of the observations discussed here the patient is dismembered under the influence of her own sadistic tendencies against the outside world and against herself. At the same time there are parts of her in the outside world, and she projects herself into the outside world. In response to the emotional need, parts of the body are projected into the outside world. We again obtain an insight into the enormous lability of the postural model of the body. The lability of the postural model of the body, on the merely perceptive and imaginative side, corresponds closely to the changes of the body-image under the influence of emotion. In Federn's dream experiences and hypnogogic experiences the image of the body is changed not only from the point of view of perception, but also from the point of view of the libidinous structure. In the alcohol hallucinosis cases, one finds not only vestibular changes and optic disturbances, which disrupt inside and outside the body-image, but also far-going libidinous disruption of the body-image.   The castration complex and dismembering motives are, as Bromberg and I have shown, in the foreground of the picture in a great number of cases.

The postural model of the body is stable only for a short time and changes immediately afterwards.   Stability of pictures in psychic life probably only connotes a passing phase to which the next phase can be contrasted.   But there is no question that in our psychic life there are always tendencies to form units, gestalten, or, to use a comparison from physics, quantums. But whenever a gestalt is created the gestalt tends immediately to change and to destruction.

To discuss the part the castration motive and the dismembering motive play in psychosis would almost mean a discussion on the whole field of psychiatry.   Stärcke has postulated that in psychosis the castration complex plays the same part as the Oedipus complex plays in neurosis.   This would not be true if we considered only the genital part of the castration complex ; but there is some truth in his statement if we consider the fear concerning the integrity of the body as a whole, which comprises the pre-genital activities as well as the genital ones.   Fear of mutilation of any kind is based upon the narcissistic love of our whole body.   The dismembering motive is the expression of the castration complex on the level of narcissistic self-love ; in melancholia especially, where the sadistic tendencies are so cruel and strong, disruption of the postural model of the body is common.   The melancholic subject denies the existence of almost any part of the body. He complains that his intestines have gone, that he can no longer urinate and defecate, that he has no limbs ; or he may complain that his limbs have become enormous.   One of my patients said, " I am perforated and distorted.   I have tentacles as large as the coral animals.   There are, of course, people destroyed alive.   I think of myself as an empty barrel.   I am solely air and powder."   The patient also maintains that her head is turned to wood, and her brain has been long ago cooked in the soup.   She cut it out and ate it ; not only her own brain but perhaps also those from other heads.   (Psychoanalytic

Psych., p. 123). Other patients complain that they have been turned to stone.

It is easy to recognize that in these delusions we are dealing basically with the same phenomena as in the cases of hypochondria and the cases of neurosis in which sadistic impulses prevail, except that, according to the far-going dissociation in the emotional life and the primitivity in the instincts, the disruption of the postural model of the body is much more extensive. It is, of course, very difficult to get from patients descriptions of a kind which would allow a differentiation between what is an actual change in the senses and in the perceptions and representations concerning the postural model of the body and what is a delusion concerning the image of the body. We know that image and perceptions are based on the same basic somatic processes. But we have to consider that there are also intellectual processes, thinking processes, illusional elements concerning the body. There is a line connecting perception, imagination, and thought. Thought processes concerning the body also have their basis in the whole attitude, the libidinous strivings, and the perceptions, so that the careful study of thoughts concerning one's own body or the purely intellectual part of the body-image will lead us to a deeper understanding of the structure of the body-image.

In schizophrenia, all kinds of bizarre perceptions, imaginations, and thoughts concerning the body may occur. Case 14 in my book, *Seele und Leben*, complained that she had been made homosexual. At the same time she said that her heart had been taken away from her and that she had been made empty. In the later phases of her psychosis the patient complained that her whole body was destroyed and that her nose had been taken away from her. Schizophrenic patients often complain of being changed into something else. It is not difficult to show that we are dealing again with phenomena based upon the inherent qualities of the body-image under the influence of a dissociated libidinous structure. But these cases afford new proof of how labile the postural model of the body is, and show that the immediate experiences of the body can be easily distorted and changed by psychic influence. This change can be in the perceptive field, in the field of imagination, and in the field of the thought processes. Whenever we meet a far-going change in the libidinous structure, the postural model of the body will undergo considerable changes. These changes will be especially strong when sadistic tendencies are in the foreground.

This leads us again to the problem of destructive tendencies, especially of self-destructive tendencies. Federn sees in melancholia the clearest expression of the death instinct. But death and life are actually in no way real opposites; they are not opposites from a biological point of view. Biology does not point to an inherent instinct for death. But there is a real drive to life. It is true that there are destructive tendencies which are also self-destructive. But the depressive patient does not desire the end; he rather perpetuates self-inflicted suffering and the suffering of others. Melancholia means eternity of suffering and not the end and not rest. The melancholic patient kills and dismembers either himself or others, but the dismembered self is resurrected. Even here we find the process of destruction and construction. It is true that we disrupt the body-image as soon as we have created it. But the construction processes are always the *basso continuo* even when the disruption of the body-image takes place. That is why I chose the sub-title : " A study in the constructive forces of the psyche." Destruction is, in other words, a partial phase of construction, which is a planning and the general characteristic of life. We destroy in order to plan anew. I do not intend here to go deeply into the theory of ego instinct or sex instinct, or into the theory of the ego and the id. But I do think that the differences between them should not be exaggerated. We find in ego and in id the same fundamental tendencies and emphasize especially that construction, which is only possible on the basis of always renewed destruction, is such a general characteristic of instincts—and one that is beyond the division of instincts in ego or sex instincts. There are everywhere constructive forces.

It is clear that the problem of the body-image is basic for the understanding of psychotic cases. In many psychoses, changes

concerning the consciousness of the body are in the foreground
of the clinical picture. Wernicke has referred to somato-
psychosis, in which the orientation in relation to the body is
disturbed. (Cf. also Pick). He has given in this connection
a classical description of depersonalization. He was the first
to see clearly that this whole psychological sphere can also be
understood from the point of view of brain physiology. His
attempt to separate the psychosis into allo—somato- and auto-
psychosis is not only fundamental for a rational classification
in psychiatry but also a psychological discovery of great importance. I have tried to elaborate this point of view in a
short article, *Über Probleme der klinischen Psychiatrie*. But this
article has not attracted much attention. A short time ago
Gurewitch reported some interesting observations on what he
calls " The parietal syndrome in psychosis." These dealt with
cases of somato-psychosis. But he has neither appreciated the
historic development of the problems involved nor perceived
the many angles and complications of the problem.

(13) *Libidinous development of the body-image*

Bernfeld has collected material about the attitude of the
child concerning his body. According to Preyer's observations
(*Die Seele des Kindes*) the child has in the beginning the same
attitude towards the parts of its body as towards strange objects.
It watches its arms and legs in motion as it would follow a
candle-flame. It looks at the grasping hand as attentively as
at any other foreign action. It observes itself and touches
itself in the bath, especially the feet (39th week). It bites its
fingers, arms, and toes, so that it screams with pain (409th day).
It bangs its own head with violence (41st week). It presses
one of its hands firmly with the other on the table like a toy.
This interest in observing one's self diminishes with the second
year. It is as if the child now knew its body and had no further
interest in it. Preyer and Bernfeld draw the conclusion that
a child has practically no knowledge of its body, and has to
distinguish it from other objects by kinaesthetic motor and
visceral data. Bernfeld says correctly that it is a question of
the co-ordination of optic, tactile, and other experiences with the

motor body ego. Preyer and Dix have emphasized the importance of the pain experience in this development. But, on the
other hand, Dix reports that even in the 10th month the child's
actions against its own body do not provoke the pain reaction
one would expect. Thus a ten months old child bangs its head
against the wall as if it were a foreign object; with others, in the
earliest months, a bleeding wound provokes no pain reaction. It
seems that pain reactions towards the internal organs are stronger
at this age. Preyer and Bernfeld emphasize also the importance
of the obedience of the organ for the creation of the body-image.
It seems that some parts of the body can be dissociated from the
body even late in the development. Bernfeld says correctly
that the body ego is present from the beginning, because
from the beginning some organs obey the needs of the
body.

A nucleus of the body-image is present in the oral zone from
the beginning; head, arms, hands, trunk, legs, and feet grow
in single relays to this nucleus. Bernfeld comes to the conclusion that there is a primary development starting with the
oral zone, and that a secondary refinement differentiates the
body ego from the outside world. This process acts in two
directions. The child finds the body ego too big, the mother
has to be eliminated. In other cases it is too small, and the toes
have to be added. According to Bernfeld, obedience of the
organ or disappointment by the organ are the main factors in
this development. Bernfeld's formulations are based upon
analytic material and are very similar to our own views. It is
true that the actual empirical material about the child is very
limited. Bernfeld's summary is based upon his study of
adults.

In any case, the problem of a development of the body-image
arises. We do not know in detail how this development takes
place. We have reason to believe that there is an inner development, maturation, in all fields of psychic life, and there are inner
factors, which are given in the organism and comparatively
independent of experiences which determine this development.
But we always see that the process of maturation gets its final

shape through individual experiences, and we should not neglect this influence of individual experience.

The general principle may be explained by Arnold Gesell's well-known experiment. In a pair of identical twins, Twin T, beginning at 46 weeks, was trained 20 minutes daily for six weeks in stair-climbing. Twin C was not. At 48 weeks T scaled the stairs for the first time without assistance. At 52 weeks he was an expert, while C could not climb even with assistance. But at 53 weeks C without assistance or training climbed the stairs. Similar experiments have been made by J. R. Shepard and F. S. Breed concerning the pecking of young chicks. It is obvious that, even in functions in which maturation of a central nervous system is undoubtedly of great importance, training plays a part at least in some phases of the development. At any rate T was superior to C between the 48th and 52nd weeks. We see that even the way in which maturation develops is dependent upon the factors of experience. But we do not know what will be the later development of these two twins trained in this way. According to the experience of psycho-analysis, we have at least to reckon with the possibility that their psychic attitude towards walking and climbing stairs will be different throughout their whole life.

Concerning the image of the body, we have to suppose that there is a factor of maturation which is responsible for the primary outlines of the postural model of the body. But the way in which these outlines develop, the tempo of development, will be largely dependent on experience and activity; and we may suppose that the finer trends of the body-image will be still more dependent on the life experiences, the training, and the emotional attitudes. There is no reason why one should join either of the extremist groups, for one of which experience, learning, and conditioning are in the foreground (Watson), while for the other experience means little or nothing (Köhler, Koffka, Wertheimer, and Wheeler). Freud himself has always emphasized that besides the factor of anatomy and structuralized function there is the factor of experience and attitude. There will be functions which are merely determined by anatomy and physiology. But even in those the psychic influence and the influence of experience will, according to our latest observations, play some part. In other experiences, especially in those concerning the libidinous structure of the postural model, experience will play an outstanding part, but even so experience will be connected with anatomy and physiology. I have emphasized in earlier parts of this book that the central factor of the organism and the personality very often determines which part of the anatomy shall be used.

One has to suppose that the body-image not only has an ontogenetic development but that there is also a phylogenetic development. It will of course be difficult to determine this phylogenetic development.

Preyer and Bernfeld emphasize the important part pain plays in the development of the body-image. We know very little about pain sensations in animals. Hempelmann has collected the material on this point. The pain reactions of the lower vertebrates are rather limited. This is so even with birds. According to Ziegler human beings reach the highest level of pain-sensitivity. Can we consider pain-sensitivity as one of the important factors in the building-up of the body-image? Uexküll considers pain as a biological necessity. It is a sign of one's own body and serves to prevent self-mutilation. This is especially necessary in carnivorous animals. Rats devour their own legs when the sensory nerves are cut. It seems at any rate that pain is one of the important factors in the organization of the otherwise labile structure of the body-image.

We are still more uncertain about the invertebrates. We can never know whether the violent defence reactions of earthworms are an expression of pain or only an expression of strong irritation of the nervous system. When an earthworm is cut in two, the part of the body which does not contain the higher centres makes more violent movements. In the arthropods, especially insects, lesions and mutilations, which according to our experiences would be apt to provoke pain, do not have any particular external effect. If the antennae and the whole abdomen of an ant are cut off, it may continue quietly sucking honey. A caterpillar, the rear end of which is injured, may gnaw itself when the anterior end is turned towards the wound. A cross-spider devours its legs when they are broken off. A male spider gnawed at by the female during copulation may continue in the act. According to Uexküll a dragon-fly starts to eat up its own body when its rear end is pushed between its jaws.

We are justified in believing that we are dealing in all those instances with an incomplete organization of the postural model of the body, and we may come to the general conclusion that psychological integration of the postural model of the body is characteristic for higher levels of phylogenetic development. It is remarkable that in the instance of the rats the cutting of the sensible nerves disintegrates the postural model of the body so that actions occur which in their structure are similar to the actions of the invertebrates. Apparently the rat which devours its own leg has a body-image in which the optic part plays a less important rôle. One is reminded also of the cases of non-perception of one side of the body by lesion of the tactile sphere in which the optic impression is not sufficient to preserve the unity of the body-image. Experiences of that kind are a warning against the over-evaluation of optic factors in the building up of the postural model of the body.

It is necessary to mention here another remarkable phenomenon, the so-called autotomy. This defence reaction is to be found not only in some invertebrates but also in lizards. By a special reflex, which has its centre in the lumbar region of the spinal cord, the lizard is able to throw off its tail when caught by it. Its vertebral column breaks at the preformed weak point in the middle of the vertebra. Decapitated lizards also show this reflex.

It is clear, also, that we have mechanisms which change the body-image at a very deep organic level. It is a diminution of the body-image, which goes into the body as such. But we see, on the other hand, that there may be organic differences in the coherence of the structure of the body so that a psychological and organic dissociation of parts of the body may become simpler. The mechanism of expansion and contraction of the body-image has therefore a deep organic level, but we find the same mechanism again in the psychological structures as emphasized before.[1]

When dealing with genetic psychology, we should not forget that objects in primitive thought and objects in fully developed thought are not the same thing. Just as the body is a construction which takes place according to the total situation, objects have their meaning only in the specific set of circumstances. We are too much inclined to believe that the circumstances in our thought are the only ones which matter. In my medical psychology I have mentioned Volkelt's well-known experiments on spiders. When a fly is put directly into the mouth of the spider, it is not accepted. It is only accepted when it flies into the web and the spider has the opportunity of seizing the fly actively. The spider's object is not actually the fly, but the concussion of the web with its subsequent activity, leading to the fly and the connected series of impressions. It is well known that similar instances can be found all over the field of animal behaviour. The following well-known instance, taken from Köhler, belongs to the same category. Regarding cleanliness, Köhler tells us he has observed only one chimpanzee in captivity that was not coprophagous (faeces-eating). Yet whenever an animal stepped into faeces and lost its footing, just as a human being would in a similar predicament, it would hobble away until an opportunity was found to clean the foot. The hand was never used in the process of cleaning, although but a moment ago the same substance was being conveyed to the mouth, the animal refusing to let it go even when threatened with severe punishment. In cleaning his foot, however, the ape would make use of a stick, a piece of paper, or a rag, and his gestures showed unmistakably that the task was a disagreeable one. This was also the case whenever any part of the body was

[1] Ferenczi regards autotomy as a tendency to throwing away an overloaded organ. He considers it as a basic reaction of life and compares it with the withdrawing of psychic energy from an unpleasurable experience. He considers ejaculation from this point of view. He finds a similar tendency to push out the genitals, which are loaded with displeasure. He mentions worms which are liable to push out their whole intestines. Others burst as a whole into single parts. I do not want to go deeper into these interesting analogies. Although I doubt the validity of Ferenczi's explanation in detail, I do consider that the general principle of trying to find analogies to psychological processes in the organization of animals is absolutely justified.

dirty; the filth was removed as quickly as possible—and never by the naked hand. Faeces are viewed differently according to the total situation. I have chosen this particular instance because it pertains, at least indirectly, to the body-image. We may suppose that the lack of coherence in the body-image of animals will vary according to the situation.

When a child draws a hand with an enormous number of fingers, it does not follow that it has the same perception of this part of the body in any other situation. When it disregards spatial relations in drawings, it does not mean that it would disregard them in other circumstances.

The same problem can be met with in the whole realm of primitive thought To us the number 2 is a pretty well defined connotation, but in primitive thought the " 2 " in ' 2 apples ' and ' 2 men ' are certainly very different things. According to Lévy-Bruhl, the numerals (in the Kuki Chin group of the Tebeto-Burman family) are restricted in their sphere so as to apply to some special kind of objects. We may come to the general conclusion that connotations and objects are constructions which fit in with particular situations. It seems that primitive thought and primitive levels of development are more prone to create object and connotation according to the actual situation, and that they do not feel the necessity of co-ordinating the various situations. It is a sign of a higher level of psychic development when objects are seen and connotations are created which satisfy the needs of a multiplicity of situations.

In primitive thought there is a greater esteem for the enormous variety of situations, and no attempt, or only an insufficient attempt, is made to find a method which is fitted to all those situations. I do not believe that the thought of the adult person ever gets completely away from creating new connotations and new object perceptions according to the urgent need of a single situation. Our body-image is certainly not always the same thing. The body-image is a different object according to the use we make of it. The logical thought of the clear consciousness tries, of course, to construct the body-image so that it fits into at least the majority of situations. The development of the body-image runs in some way parallel to the development of perceptions, thought, and object relations. The undeveloped body-image therefore shows deep characteristics. It shows a greater tendency to transformations ; the single parts are less coherent with each other ; it is easier to expel them and to take other parts in. But even this incomplete and incoherent body-image is used differently according to the various aspects of the situation.

(14) *Changing the body-image by clothing, and the psychology of clothes*

The discussion of the postural model of the body has brought forward fundamental problems of psychoanalysis. This is based upon the fact that the somatic reaction and the body are the main topics of psychoanalysis. The scientific method of psychoanalysis considers especially what the individual experiences in his own body, and considers less the purpose and the aim in the outside world and still less what is going on in the central sphere of the personality. Psychoanalysis is the science of the reflexion of the world and of life in the body of the individual. Yet psychoanalysis has so far neglected the structure of the schema of the body. But every desire and libidinous tendency immediately changes the structure of the image of the body and gets its real meaning out of this change in the postural model of the body. In every action we are not only acting as personalities but we are also acting with our bodies. We live constantly with the knowledge of our body. The body-image is one of the basic experiences in everybody's life. It is one of the fundamental points of life experience. Whatever we may do, either we want to change the spatial relation of the postural model of the body or we want a change in the schema of the body itself. When we see something, muscular actions start immediately, and at once bring about a change in the perception of our body. Every striving and desire changes the substance of the body, its gravity, and its mass.

There are also immediate changes in the shape of the body. When an action takes place, it can be said that it brings the body-image from one place to another and from one shape to another. We may even go further and say that in every action and in every desire we intend a change in the body-image. It may be an immediate wish in the foreground of the consciousness, but it may also be more or less in the background. Our body, and with it our body-image, is a necessary part in every life experience. One sees immediately that the psycho-analytical method of considering life from the point of view of the body thus has real justification.

I have many times emphasized how labile and changeable the body-image is. The body-image can shrink or expand ; it can give parts to the outside world and can take other parts into itself. When we take a stick in our hands and touch an object with the end of it, we feel a sensation at the end of the stick. The stick, has, in fact, become a part of the body-image. In order to get the full sensation at the end of the stick, the stick has to be in a more or less rigid connection with the body. It then becomes a part of the bony system of the body, and we may suppose that the rigidity of the bony system is an important part in every body-image.

It is a new proof of the lability of the body-image that whatever comes into connection with the surface of our body is more or less incorporated in the body. We know that many attempts are made to change the body-image. Pictures may be drawn on the skin. Tattooing changes the optic part of ourselves. When we paint our body we change the body-image in an objective way. Tattooing, painting the lips, painting the face, bleaching or dyeing the hair, dressing the hair, are in the same category. Moreover, washing and cleanliness are also in this category. It is true that when we clean ourselves we not only change the image but also remove actual sensations of itching.

There is no question that the meaning of all these changes in the appearance is not always in the consciousness, there is also a symbolic meaning. Psychoanalysis has shown that cleanliness is a tendency to overcome anal tendencies. But cleanliness may also satisfy narcissistic tendencies, and cleaning may be a transformed masturbatory act. The crippling of the feet of Chinese girls apparently emphasizes that they are woman, *i.e.* castrated. It is, however, unnecessary to change the actual appearance of the body when one wants to change the postural model. Head has already stated that the postural model of the body reaches to the tip of the feather in a woman's hat. We must consider the psychology of clothes from this point of view. Clothes have, according to Flügel, many functions. There is the function of protection but there is also the function of decoration. Clothes become a part of the body-image. The head-dress, for instance, enlarges the body and spreads it out. The principle certainly goes very far back. The curious practice of the crab " Maja verrucosa " in masking itself and covering its back with algae, leaves, little stones, and pieces of coral is probably a primitive example of similar principles. Is that an enlargement of the body-image ?[1]

Whatever article of clothing we put on immediately becomes a part of the body-image and is filled with narcissistic libido. This is especially shown in the attitude of women towards their clothes. It may even be said that the clothes we have taken off are still a part of our body. But there is certainly a difference between the clothes which are closely connected with the body and those whose connection is more or less loose. It is true that clothes also serve the purpose of modesty. But even when we cover primary and secondary sex parts we change our postural model. With a change in clothes we change our attitude. When we take off our clothes in the evening,[2] we change our set of attitudes, partly because the body-image as such is in the closest relation to our libidinous strivings and tendencies.

Since clothes are a part of the body schema, they gain the same significance as parts of the body and can have the same symbolic significance as parts of the body. Flügel has emphasized that the phallus is often symbolized in clothes. The best known symbol is the hat, which usually has male significance, especially when it is pointed or has horn-like decorations. The shoe

[1] Concerning adornment, Köhler found his animals (chimpanzees) pre-possessed of a tendency to hang all kinds of things upon their bodies, after which the objects hanging about the body served the function of adornment in the widest sense. Köhler believes that primitive adornment does not depend upon its possible effect on others but upon a curious heightening of the animal's body feeling, self-consciousness, and pride.

[2] Freud points out the regressions which take place when we remove the enshrouding of the " body ego."

is sometimes a female symbol, since it encloses the foot (penis), but it may also be a masculine symbol, especially when it is pointed. The pointed shoe was, indeed, sometimes shaped like a phallus. The tie may symbolize the penis. Even the cloak may become a symbol for the phallus. But some ritual clothes may symbolize the universe and accordingly, the maternal womb. It is not necessary to give further examples : full details may be found in Flügel's papers which also contain the literature. But from our point of view we have to emphasize that clothes become a part of the body-image, that they are loaded with libido, and that all the transformations which we have found in the body-image as such occur also in regard to the clothes.

A full understanding of the psychology of clothes is of course not possible when we only consider the postural model of the body of one individual; we must consider also the interrelations between the diverse schemas of the body. We identify ourselves with others by means of clothes. We become like them. By imitating their clothes we change our postural image of the body by taking over the postural image of others. Clothes can thus become a means of changing our body-image completely.

When people wear enormous masks at the carnival in Nice, they are not merely changing the physiological basis of their body-image but are actually becoming giants themselves. One of the pleasures to be derived from this pageant is the possibility of playing with the enlargement of our body-image and thus increasing our own importance. Our body-image is in a continuous process of enlargement and shrinking and we enjoy these changes in it. The body-image changes continually and we triumph over the limitations of the body by adding masks and clothes to the body-image.[1] This is the explanation of the animal masks of primitive peoples which actually identify the wearer with the animal. But by changing, the magic power is increased and with the enlargement of the body-image the narcissistic power also increases. Clothes are thus only a method of transforming the body-image. The possibility of

[1] We like to have our body in a hundred sizes and a thousand variations. So long as the psychic structure of the ego is preserved we are not able to satisfy this urge of playful multiplication.

transforming the body-image is the basis of the widespread belief of primitive peoples in transformation. It appears that their power of rebuilding the body-image is greater. According to Preuss, every animal and every object can transform itself into innumerable shapes. A human being turns into a wolf. The transformation of one thing into another is the speciality of all so-called demons ; the War Gods of the Zunis possessed as a specific faculty the power of transformation and the spirit and breath of destruction.

In the fairy tales and myths of all peoples transformations of human beings into animals and of animals into human beings are common. In the primitive fairy tales most of the characters are animals and human beings at the same time. K. von den Steinen reports a case where a fugitive negro slave was pursued by Bakarai. They failed to catch him but found a turtle among the bushes. The Bakaraic people ceased their pursuit in the firm conviction that the boy had transformed himself into the turtle.

In the later development of fairy tales transformation, which hitherto had been a matter of course, became possible only by special magic. Whatever the psychic motives for the transformation myths may be, they are based on the plasticity of the body-image. We know that in psychotics the patients often have the sensation of being transformed into an animal such as a dog or a wolf. Myths concerning were-wolves belong to the same category. Primitive people and psychotics sometimes succeed in changing their body-image by mere libidinous imagination. It may be a change in the perceptual-imaginative or even the intellectual part of the body-image. So-called normal people generally only succeed in a minor degree in this " autoplastic " change in the body-image. We have then to use alloplastic methods, masks, and clothes, when we insist on far-going changes in the body-image.

In all our discussions we have not so far distinguished between belief in the transformations of others and the transformation of ourselves. Both are closely connected with each other. As we shall see later, body-images are not isolated and the community of body-images is at the basis of every social function, though on methodical principles we have here dealt only with the body-image of the isolated individual.

(15) *Gymnastics, dance and expressive movements*

Human beings are bound and tied down by their body-images. One of the motives of transformation and of clothing is the desire to overcome the rigidity of the body-image. It may be transformed by clothes, by decoration, or by jewellery, but it is also possible, as we have seen, to change the body itself as such; holes may be drilled in the body, ears, nose, lips, the genitals may be perforated, parts may be cut away, metal and wood may be inserted into the different parts of the body as among primitive peoples. One mutilates oneself. It is a continuous play with the body and with the body-image.

One may also try to change the body-image in a less violent way by gymnastics of all kinds. The contortionist pushes to extremes this play with his own body, and the pleasure we get out of watching his performance is based upon our wish to break through the borderlines of our own body. It is mixed with awe and disgust. We desire the integrity and the totality of our own body; we are afraid of every change which may take away a part of this body (castration and dismembering motive); but we are still continually experimenting with it. Our delight in imagining beings with an increased number of limbs is an example of this experimentation. I remember the strong impression made on me by a scene on the vaudeville stage when the body of a performer was so well concealed behind the body of another that only his arms and legs protruded and one saw an individual moving with four arms. This is the playful multiplication of limbs. It is the same motive which comes out in the innumerable limbs of Indian Gods and Goddesses. Very similar motives are to be found in the drawings of children.

There is another way of dissolving or weakening the rigid form of the postural model of the body, and that is movement and dance. I have mentioned above that, whenever we move, the postural model of the body changes. The previous scheme of the postural model remains in the background and upon this previous scheme the new scheme is built up. When we move, we depart from the comparatively rigid primary picture ; it seems in some way loosened and partially dissolved till the body returns into one of the primary attitudes. As Goldstein has mentioned, movement and especially dancing often use postural reflexes which are not fully in our consciousness. It is a fascinating problem to ask which movements express themselves in the body-image and which do not. It is also a problem whether during a movement the body-image does not undergo distortions connected with the postural reflexes we have previously studied.

Dancing must be considered from a similar point of view. It is perhaps worth while to mention that the optical picture during every quick movement tends in itself to multiplication. When one sees dancers on the stage turning rapidly around their longitudinal axis, provided the movements are rapid enough, one sees (also monocular) two heads instead of one.[1] During rapid movement, the optic impression tends already to multiplication and loosening of the postural model. But I have already mentioned that these movements also have an influence from the kinaesthetic side on the perception of the body. Every rapid movement, especially when it is circular, also changes the vestibular reaction and with it the lightness and heaviness of the body. This is partially due to the muscular action, but also to the vestibular irritation. Tension and relaxation of muscles, moving the body with and against gravity, with and against centrifugal impulses, may have an enormous influence on the body-image. The phenomenon of the dance is therefore a loosening and changing in the body-image. That so many dances are connected with circular movement has a deep meaning connected with the vestibular irritation, which gives a greater freedom concerning the heavy mass and substance of the body. It is remarkable that in cult-dances drugs are often taken which affect the central equilibrium via

[1] One can easily make the following experiment. When one takes a fountain pen, looks at the clip, and turns the fountain pen around its longi. tudinal axis quickly enough, to and fro, one sees two clips instead of one-During every rapid movement, as Kanner and I have shown, there exists a tendency to see several objects in the path of the movement.

the vestibular apparatus. Dancing is therefore a method of changing the body-image and loosening its rigid shape. One may add that in dancing also the connection of clothes with the body, especially with women in stage-dancing, will be changed considerably, and so will give an increased feeling of freedom concerning gravity and the cohesion of the postural model of the body. There is no question that the loosening of the body-image will bring with it a particular psychic attitude. Motion thus influences the body-image and leads from a change in the body-image to a change in the psychic attitude.

We now come to the problem of expressive movements and their relation to the postural model of the body. According to Flach, every change in the psychic attitude provokes a change in the dynamic situation as a whole, which is experienced as a change in the muscular tension as pull, striving, or loosening. Single elements of muscle-tension are not experienced, but there are specific sequences which form a whole when an expressive movement like entreaty, defiance, or sadness takes place. We have here a specific sequence of muscular states which are experienced. With the tension is connected the feeling of a display of energy ; loosening of the tension and relaxation of muscles are connected with a loss of energy and with the sensation of heaviness in different parts of the body. Tension and relaxation are the elementary components in the dynamic sequence. There is so close an interrelation between the muscular sequence and the psychic attitude that not only does the psychic attitude connect up with the muscular states, but also every sequence of tensions and relaxations provokes a specific attitude. When there is a specific motor sequence it changes the inner situation and attitudes and even provokes a phantasy situation which fits the muscular sequence.

Two protocols may be reproduced. The subject was instructed to make a gesture of entreaty. She knelt down with her hands interlocked before her chest and then changed this position by the following movement. The hands interlocked before her chest were pushed towards her body which moved forwards above the hands. The head went backwards, whereas the neck stretched itself towards the imagined person opposite her. The subject said : " It was an ardent entreaty. It was a strong pull to some imagined person opposite me, which started in the trunk and pulled the body towards the person opposite, keeping the stretched body in this tension. At the same time the intertwined hands were pressed together by this pull and pushed towards the body. The head was felt as the last extension of the body ; the fact that it fell back was due to the intensity with which the body stretched itself forward. This occurred by tension which started strongly but still developed in intensity, which was kept back as it tended towards the other person until the climax where the stretched body remained in the same tension."

In the expressive movements for defiance there is a resistance and a turning away which is connected with a sudden jerky tension. This tension is directed against the resistance and has therefore a specific direction. The tension immediately reaches a great intensity and then decreases as quickly, so that the tense parts of the body go back into their previous position. When the subjects take the attitude of sadness the limbs of the body become heavier in consequence of the relaxation of the muscles.[1] This relaxation is diffuse in the whole body and connected with a pull backward.

It is clear that every emotion expresses itself in the postural model of the body, and that every expressive attitude is connected with characteristic changes in the postural model of the body. Flach rightly emphasizes that we are dealing with total figures, with wholes, with shapes, with characteristic sequences. But these characteristic sequences are sequences of changes in the body-image, are characteristic changes in the heaviness and lightness of the diverse parts of the body. Thus the postural model of the body is changing continually, and goes back to the typical primary images of the body which are dissolved and then crystallized again. The image of the body thus shows characteristic features of our whole life. There is a continual change from crystallized rather closed entities to states of dissolution and to a stream of less stabilized experiences, and

---

[1] In I. H. Schultz's important experiments on auto-suggestive training, the relation of the muscles leads to changes in the experience of weight.

from there a return to better form and changed entity. It is therefore the continuous building up of a shape which is immediately dissolved and built up again.

There is nothing automatic in this continual process. There are the emotions which influence it; there are the active tendencies of play; there are instinctive motives and voluntary motives to reconstruct and destroy always under the guidance of the final aims of the personality and of the organism as a whole; there is an inner need of escaping every final crystallization and restriction. Flach's experiments are experiments concerning expressive movements. But every emotion is either connected with expressive movements or at least with impulses towards them. Every emotion therefore changes the body-image. The body contracts when we hate, it becomes firmer, and its outlines towards the world are more strongly marked. This is connected with the beginning of actions in the voluntary muscles, but there may also be sympathetic and parasympathetic elements in it. We expand the body when we feel friendly and loving. We open our arms, we would like to enclose humanity in them. We expand, and the borderlines of the body-image lose their distinct character. It is a task for the future to determine specific changes in the body-image in the manifold emotions.[1] In I. H. Schultz's experiments on auto-suggestive training it is important again to note that the impression of heaviness and lightness are outstanding.

We expand and we contract the postural model of the body; we take parts away and we add parts; we rebuild it; we melt the details in; we create new details; we do this with our body and with the expression of the body itself. We experiment continually with it. When the experimentation with the movement is not sufficient, then we add the influence of the vestibular apparatus and of intoxicants to the picture. When even so the body is not sufficient for the expression of the playful changes and the destructive changes in the body, then we add clothes, masks, jewellery, which again expand, contract,

[1] Kauders studied the psycho-motor disturbances of psychotics by ordering them to repeat their motor actions after they had recovered. The emotional state and the content of the psychosis came back in those circumstances. These experiments prove again the unity of picture emotion and motility.

disfigure, or emphasize the body-image and its particular parts.

One should not speak so much about growth and evolution, when one means by it something passive and automatic. One should emphasize the continual activity, the trying out. One may speak of growth and passing of shapes, ' gestalten.' But here again one should be aware that one is not dealing with automatic development but with a tendency of the constructive life energy. It is a construction and destruction connected with the needs, strivings, and energies of the total personality. It is clear that we are far removed from the classical gestalt psychology in which there is no room for spontaneity guided by experience and for attitudes towards the world. In the phases of construction and destruction, two principal human tendencies come out. One is the tendency to crystallize units, to secure points of rest, definiteness, and absence of change. The other is the tendency to obtain a continual flow, a continuous change. These differences are reflected in the ideas of eternity and transitoriness. In a similar connection, James has referred to the formed and unformed elements in psychic life. The same entities come out in the conception of the quantum in physics in opposition to a continuous flow of energy. We have conceived the passing and the stabile as phases in creative construction.

We have spoken of the changes in the body-image. But the body is certainly not only where the borderline of the body and its clothes are. In an automobile accident I sustained a rather severe injury to my hand which was for some time connected with painful sensations. In the early days after the accident every approaching car seemed to involve a particular danger element which encroached into the sphere of the body, even when it was still a considerable distance away. In other words, around the body there was a zone closely interrelated with the body-image which was in some way the extension of the body. Later on this general zone diminished in size until finally there remained only a zone around the painful hand. These experiences induced in me the conviction that the body-image is surrounded by a sphere of particular sensitiveness. This is true even in the physiological sense, since the smell of the body goes further than the body itself. From a psycho-logical point of view the surroundings of the body are animated by it, and we could say that psychologically there exists something which corresponds to what Reichenbach has called the Od (he believes that everybody emanates a specific substance which scintillates in the dark). One sees again that every actual change in the postural model of the body also changes the surrounding zone, makes it asymmetric according to the specific life situation. We feel these zones especially when somebody else tries to come nearer to us. We feel even that when somebody comes near us he is intruding in our body-image even when he is far from touching us. This emphasizes again that the body-image is a social phenomenon.

PART III.

SOCIOLOGY OF THE BODY-IMAGE

(1) *Space and the body-image*

The discussions in the previous chapters show clearly that the body-image expands beyond the confines of the body. A stick, a hat, any kind of clothes, become part of the body-image. The more rigid the connection of the body with the object is, the more easily it becomes part of the body-image. But objects which were once connected with the body always retain something of the quality of the body-image on them. I have specifically pointed out the fact that whatever originates in or emanates out of our body will still remain a part of the body-image. The voice, the breath, the odour, faeces, menstrual blood, urine, semen, are still parts of the body-image even when they are separated in space from the body. (Cf. Roheim). The patient who felt torn by anxiety felt the parts of his body flying around. All these instances, different though they may be in detail and in their deepest mechanism, have one thing in common; the space in and around the postural model is not the space of physics. The body-image incorporates objects or spreads itself into space.

Anna R., 42 years old, admitted to Bellevue Hospital on May 6th, 1932, had, according to her own and her daughter's report, already been in the hospital seven years ago. A year before this first admission one of her children had been run over by a truck. After the accident she heard people talk about her and believed that they knew everything that was going on in the house. She then came to Bellevue Hospital and a little later was for a year and a half in the State Hospital. She was never quite free from hallucinations. This time she entered the hospital voluntarily because she felt that she was being hounded by enemies who talked about her and sent electricity into her. In the clinic she complained in a vivid and often agitated manner about the persecution she had to stand. But one could always establish good relations with her. " Everybody knows what is wrong with me. They say that I was in a ' Crazy House.' I did not like my husband ; I threw him away. He sold me to the government and to the public. He gave me out of his power. This was ten years ago. They nagged me wherever I went. I had spells of shivering. I got feelings in my heart like ' I love you.' A man passed me and smiled at me ; I thought I loved him and that he might be a good husband. My child of 9 got killed by a truck. I saw a man at the trial and I thought I loved him. I cried and said, ' I must have that man.' The man never paid any attention to me. It was only my craziness. I asked my husband to divorce me ; he took me to Bellevue seven years ago."

" I was there for a year and a half, then my husband took me home. I said that I did not love him. I left him and went to work. They used to call me names in the street and where I worked. The Jews especially hate me. They say I must die. A woman from downstairs said that she would spoil my food. She would make it bitter and sour. She could make it as she liked. It would never taste right to me. Funny smells like stinking fish, very disgusting. I don't know how she does it. She started a year and a half ago."

"When the street-cleaner used to sweep the street I felt as if he was sweeping over my genitals. It felt as if he was tearing me. It was terrible pain. It made me shiver. I was on the fifth floor and he was in the street. They were killing my girl. She began to shiver; her face had red streaks and her eyes turned up. I saw a man from the street. He upset my nerves with electricity. I don't know what it means. He was in front of my face. He took my breath. He hurt my heart. He breathes my breath. Right now, it hurts me here (pointing to her pelvis); it is in the womb. Anyone in here does it; anybody here can kill me. This morning a doctor walked on top of me; he was stepping on my body (he was not near me, but it hurt me). They break my legs with electricity. They stop my thinking, my breathing, my eating. Whatever I say here everybody knows. They even hear what I think. They come and call me S. O. B. They show me a man's action when they pass on the street. When a man passed he looked down and said 'look'.

He did not take out his genitals but I could see them as if he was naked. People in the street were running after me to kill me. When you talk naturally it is all right. But when you talk unnaturally you hurt me here and there. You just coughed on me and you touched me with your cough (the patient coughs). When I cough I do not do it on you. When you move your shoulder I feel it too. There is electricity all over where I am. I had a neighbour who left a smell in my house. They used it again on me in another house. It was killing my blood. They used to make me stink. A boy used to make on me a dirty woman's smell. I smell now a fresh green smell like a tree-smell. That woman (pointing to the street) makes signs as if I want to go to the toilet. Everybody works on me...men, women, children, crazies. They used to let people into my bedroom and they tore my sex organ. And they burn me. They used to put a sort of red paint in me. Maybe they worked on me. I am like a radio. They can work on me. When a kid makes a grabbing motion of pointing I feel it in my blood and bones. They say such dirty things all day. Whatever I do, for instance if I buy meat, they talk all day and night about me and make jokes. The butcher comes at night and he talks hard words at me which kill and stick. I could not eat anything. Every butcher did it. He put his hands on me like electricity and tore my sex-parts. He made my stomach swell. They used to stop up my bowels. When somebody laughed it went through me like an electric machine. A policeman told him to do it. Through my knees and everywhere I get it. They do the same thing in the Ward. I don't go to the toilet; they locked up my womb. A boy of 14 used to live with me as man and wife. He was downstairs; he did it through electricity. It was terrible, I had pain, I was ashamed. For years my faeces do not smell right. When I walk they make me vomit if they want to".

We see that the patient connects herself with everybody. When a person breathes it is her breath. When a person moves his shoulders she feels it in her shoulders. In other words, she takes the postural models of others into her own. Their spatial difference does not exist any more. By magic she is forced to imitate. It is passive imitative magic. When a man sweeps the street she feels the movement on her genitals. When somebody walks by she feels him walk on herself. The actions which go on in the outside world are felt in her body-image. The difference in space between her body-image and the outside world has been changed. One may say that her libido attracts other persons nearer to her. A boy who lives downstairs has sexual relations with her, "by electricity".

Magic action is an action which influences the body-image irrespective of the actual distance in space. It influences, not only in this case, the sex organs in particular. It seems that the psychological space around the sex organs has its special characteristics.

In the obsession neurosis case mentioned on page 157, the patient felt his penis crushed in the street by a passing car. His penis and his bladder were separated from him.

The specific space round the body-image may either bring the objects nearer to the body or the body nearer to the objects. The emotional configuration determines the distances of objects from the body.

(2) On curiosity and on the expression of emotions

In the previous chapter I dealt with sexuality and libidinous tendencies. I spoke about genital sexuality and the part-steps of sexuality. I considered libido from the point of view of the body-image of the person who experiences this desire. Such a discussion must necessarily be incomplete, since libidinous tendencies are always directed towards the body-image of another. Libidinous tendencies are necessarily social phenomena; they are always directed towards body-images in the outside world. Even in the narcissistic stage there is a direction towards something present which is living and in the outside world. Optic experiences which lead to the construction of one's own body-image lead at the same time to the construction of the body-images of others. The same holds true for tactile experiences. As the discussions in the first part of this book have shown, we have to do with perceptive processes of great complication. But every separation between perceptive and emotional (libidinous) processes is artificial. We not only see, but we also have a tendency to see our own body as well as the bodies of others. There is also a desire to get knowledge by touch. In other words, we may talk of sex curiosity, voyeuristic tendencies, and optic part-steps of sexuality. There is curiosity concerning the surface of the body, its skin, and its complexion. But there is also curiosity concerning the inner parts of one's own body and the inner parts of the bodies of others. Furthermore, there is an interest in the sexual action of others. Although this curiosity is mainly based on vision, it is not exclusively due to optic tendencies; tactile tendencies also play a part which will be more or less important according to the situation. When we are curious about another person's body, optic will generally precede tactile curiosity.

In his three papers on *The Theory of Sex*, Freud discusses exhibitionism, the tendency to show one's own body and especially the sex parts to a person of the other sex. He comes to the conclusion that the exhibitionist shows his body and his genitals to the person of the other sex because he expects a satisfaction of his curiosity in return. But I am of the opinion that the desire to be seen, to be looked at, is as inborn as the desire to see. There exists a deep community between one's own body-image and the body-image of others. In the construction of the body-image there is a continual testing to discover what could be incorporated in the body. When we look at our own body we are curious about it too, not less curious than we are about the bodies of others. When we have satisfied the eye, we use tactile experiences, and we want to intrude into every hole of our body with our fingers. We want to expose our body to ourselves. The body-image should be known to ourselves and to others. Voyeurism and exhibitionism thus have the same root. Both want to be satisfied. The body-image is a social phenomenon.[1]

If one wants to see another person's face and body and the body in its nakedness, one sees necessarily a body which is moving and in action. And a body in action is either expressing something

---

[1] The nudist movement gratifies this libidinous tendency. But since it is only the satisfaction of a partial desire, it remains necessarily incomplete even when the genitals are exposed freely, which is after all the real nucleus of the nudist movement. I have mentioned that we never come to a clear perception of the skin and complexion of our fellow human beings. I see in that the expression of the impossibility of satisfying libido in this way only. The great problem of integrating the sex desires is not solved when humanity dispenses with clothes and runs about naked. (Cf. Lorand's paper on Nudism).

or doing something. A body is always the body of a personality, and the personality has emotions, feelings, tendencies, motives, and thoughts. Even sex curiosity is not only a curiosity concerning sex parts and their actions but also a curiosity about the sex organs and sex activities of a person. Just as one sees and understands the body of another person, one understands immediately the action of this person expressed in movements. The perception of the body of others and their expression of emotion is as primary as the perception of one's own body and its emotional expression. We come also from this point of view to an objection against Lipps' idea of 'Einfühlung.' It is not true that we are instinctively forced to imitate another person, that we then experience what he experiences, and that we project it into him. (Cf. the following chapter.) Of course, we are not only curious about the body, we are no less curious about the emotions of the other person and their expression in face and body. We want also to know what he thinks, what his ideas and representations are. But we also have the urge to make known to the other person what emotions and thoughts are going on in ourselves. We not only express emotions, but we want to express them.[1] Even the emotion of the lonely person is an emotion directed to an imaginary onlooker.

Emotions are directed towards others. Emotions are always social. Similarly, thinking is a social function even in the lonely person. Humanity is the unseen listener to his thinking. We may expect that pathology will show us these mechanisms more clearly.

Austin O., a tall, slenderly-built man of aesthetic habits, came on April 19th, 1932, to the psychiatric station of Bellevue Hospital of his own accord. Somatically, he showed signs of severe alcoholism, his body was shaking all over, and he had marked alcoholic tremor in his hands. He confessed freely that he was a heavy drinker, that he had been drinking all his life, but that he had drunk more during the last week. He sought shelter in the hospital because of voices which called him bad names and

[1] Donald Hayworth has suggested the interesting theory that the main function of laughter is to advise one's fellows that there is no danger; that they may now relax, feed, or play. We show our emotions to others and take them back into ourselves.

accused him of being a degenerate and a homosexual. These persecutions had been going on for several weeks. He felt haunted by these voices, and because of them had left St Louis where he was living; he had also left a hospital in which he had been for a short time. It is not necessary to follow the complicated route he had taken in order to escape his persecutors. It is sufficient to know that the patient continued to be bothered by voices for more than three weeks in the hospital. Sometimes he talked quite clearly and coherently, but at other times his thoughts seemed almost disconnected. He actually hallucinated, but he also misinterpreted voices of real people. These misinterpretations played the most important part. I propose to give some examples of his utterances during this phase.

"I heard a confusion of voices, noises. I was in the hospital in St Louis for drinking. I left the hospital because the noises and voices sneered at me. They said, "You Red, you thief, you are a stool-pigeon", and finally, "you are a degenerate". My thought was that they wanted to pick me to pieces to determine whether I was a degenerate or not. My feelings were that they had something on me and wanted to get the rest of the information that I have. As I walked down the street, these noises seemed to follow me. I still feel that it is real. They say that I broadcast and that they are able to read my thoughts. In the car, in which I was coming here, there were five or six men sharing the car. They kept on mumbling and sucking their teeth and making noises and chattering their teeth. On looking through the glass in front, I could catch one and he would turn round and give me a look. He seemed to be making signs to the man next to him. I felt that these people were very much interested in every move I made. I noticed that at each stop there was one man who wasn't a railroad worker, and I thought this man was to play up from town to town. I heard them say, "Well, we got your eyes, we got your nose, we got your teeth, we got your hands, we got your feet". Then it came, "You are a degenerate". I thought that I had bad teeth, that they were picking them to pieces. They got my lips, that means that they could read my lips. Then my teeth, that meant that they could read my thoughts in my teeth. Everything that happened provoked thoughts against my will. You passed by me; I tried to concentrate on the wall; I couldn't help saying, "There goes the dirty rotten Jew". When I ate food, I was forced to think about penis and punk. I wanted to know why Negroes were introduced into the Lindbergh house. I thought it might be because they might read thoughts, because their sense of feeling was more acute than in white people, so that they could catch the nurse. If they could read thoughts, they could read the thoughts of the nurse and if the nurse or anybody else in the house was implicated they could read them".

Sometimes his utterances were still more disconnected. He had to think that gelatine was blubber. "That came since I have been here. This play, that seems to be going on, is about this needle business they have pulled, I don't know anything about it. I understand that there is such a thing; you needle a person, you read his thoughts. People make remarks to one another and if you listen you turn around and the first thing you know is that they are talking about you. When they put their hand on their throat that means 'hot under the collar'. That business about needling is so that you can be read. These people know what you are talking about. Little by little it came to me that walking along the street I am saying something. I am not uttering, I am just trying to go along straight ahead, not paying attention. These people came along, people passed and looked at you. Right in here it starts every night, and more and more so. It comes to me, like this morning, with castile soap, I rubbed it and washed my hands and something seems to say, 'Oh, he is talking Spain now', and my thoughts go to Spain. This kind of business, whether it's real or not, seems to have taken me to Ross Sea, and that means that I am a bully dagger, a spear, or something that goes into a whale. There is a blow, there is a whale, and I spear it. And it isn't mine—all like that. That means that they take you all around the globe and you either go to the North Pole, that means one thing, and the next thing it is farther South, that's the Ross Sea. If I think about anything in the past, people seem to mention it. For instance, one of the coloured fellows out here says, 'I know you, I have seen you before, you got very thin'. At that time I am concentrating on Florida, Seminole Indians, and at that time the Negro says that I am not looking at him at all. If I do look at him associations of Indians and Negroes come. I don't know what he means by that. I don't want to talk to him. They walk along in rhythmic motion, slow, people singing, sucking. When it gets up to the business of boxes, things, clocks, then suction is suggested. Then my lips finally say 'sip.' If you look at the clock, it is supposed to carry out signals. Time seems to mean that they want my thoughts at a particular time, take me back to something at a particular time. When it is two o'clock I am supposed to say, 'two o'clock'; and then my thoughts go back to two o'clock and there is an association of ideas. Little by little, when they get your thoughts over a period of time, they get your life story."

After the twelfth of May the patient became completely clear. He lost his suspiciousness and apprehension and was no longer secretive. His psychosis was discussed with him, and he was able to explain his disconnected remarks. He now believed that he did not hear real voices, but that he only misinterpreted what other people said, and their movements and thoughts. (But it seems to be much more probable that at least the remarks, 'thief', etc. (cf. above), were real hallucinations.) The objects he saw and the movements of other people provoked thoughts in him which others could read. When he saw the broken wing of a chicken in his food, it represented to him that he was a stool-pigeon. Frankfurt sausages reminded him of the male organ. (This was probably a memory of childhood. "Kids called the penis frank-furters, hot-dogs, red-hot, etc., when I was seven or eight years old.") "Odours of the toilet would stay with me for hours. At first a cigarette tasted like Chinese punk. Everybody was smoking Camels and I got the taste of punk. When I was a child, four or five years old, we would take punk and smoke it." When they made signs about him, it seemed to provoke in him thoughts of 'degenerate', 'stool-pigeon', etc. When his thoughts were provoked in this way, he felt that all eyes were concentrated on him, and that his fingers were contracted and formed letters which other people could read. They provoked his thoughts in him and then read them on his fingers.

But the psychosis of this patient cannot be fully understood without at least a short insight into his personality and development. He came from a family in which there had not been any psychosis. The first six brothers and sisters died in childhood. Three of his brothers were priests, and one older sister a nun. The father and mother were rather strict. The mother used to spank all the children. The father drank all his life, but was not a drunkard. Sex was never discussed in the family, and sex topics were strictly forbidden. He slept in the same bed as his brother till he was five years old, but he never saw his genitals. "I trained myself not to notice such things ever since I can remember. When I was very young I saw a girl defecating, I saw her buttocks; it nauseated me." The patient liked his father as well as his mother. He was very clean. The mother insisted on scrupulous cleanliness. He was rather religious when he was about five years old. It was not till he was ten years old that he found out the difference between boys and girls. But from his sixth year on he started to become curious about other people's affairs. He began to smoke at six and to drink beer at eight. When he was about twenty, he became interested in a murder case and worked as an investigator with some success. He was at that time a reporter. When he was in the navy, there was much talk about homosexuality. The 'fairies' were staging a show. Some society woman had witnessed the performance and complained. He helped to trace these men and to get them discharged from the navy for medical reasons. He is still interested in investigations. He has a disgust for all kinds of perversions, especially for homosexuality. In his conscious life he has never had any particular relation to his defecation. His sex life consists in intercourse with prostitutes. He would think it wrong to have sex relations with a decent girl. Sometimes one or two months pass without his having intercourse. The sex urge does not bother him, especially when he drinks. He drinks heavily, mostly in company.

We have here a typical alcohol hallucinosis in which delusional elements prevail. The psychosis brings to the foreground traits which were fundamental for his personality. He was always curious. We may suppose that this curiosity was to a great extent sex curiosity. With the repression of the sexual curiosity, his interest in the affairs of others and especially in their criminal activities increased. He never fully developed his heterosexuality. The zeal with which he conducted the investigation of homosexuality in the navy proves a strong latent homo-sexuality. In his psychosis, his sexuality and his anal and oral tendencies came out openly. But the outstanding point in this observation is that others were able to read his thoughts and his activities in exactly the same way as he investigated the activities of others before. People induced the forbidden thoughts in him by gestures. Free associations came which led to perverse thoughts. He had to express them either by the motions of his mouth or through his hands, and so reveal his infantile tendencies to others. He understood others, he understood their bodies and his body, and his thoughts were subsequently understood by others. Their gestures and his gestures, their thoughts and his thoughts, communicated freely. Generally, we want to under-stand the thoughts and gestures of others, but we also want our own thoughts and gestures to be understood. The expressive movements of our patient are communication. We may suppose that they are generally communications which we direct to others.

(3) *Preliminary remarks on the relation between body-images*

The observation we have just discussed shows clearly what can be observed in a great number of psychoses. In one of my pre-vious cases (*Seele und Leben*, p. 78), the patient complained that a picture of his body had been taken, and was kept in a far-distant town under the influence of an investigator. Whenever a per-ception was offered to this picture, it went to him. His thought went into this picture. The investigator could then read whether the patient was a pervert or not. According to Tausk, machines symbolize the body. The picture of the patient is just such a machine. It is like a picture in the mirror, a part of himself out-side. There is a community between my picture, my image in the mirror, and myself. But are not my fellow human beings outside myself also a picture of myself?

A simple experiment may emphasize again that the community between the body-image outside and the body exists already in the sphere of perception. I sit about ten feet away from a mirror holding a pipe or a pencil in my hand and look into the mirror. I press my fingers tightly against the pipe and have a clear-cut feeling of pressure in my fingers. When I look intently at the picture of my hand in the mirror I now feel clearly that the sensation of pressure is not only in my fingers in my own hand, but also in the hand which is twenty feet distant in the mirror. Even when I hold the pipe in such a way that only the pipe is seen and not my hand, I can still feel, though with some difficulty, the pressure on the pipe in the mirror. This feeling is therefore not only in my actual hand but also in the hand in the mirror. One could say that the postural model of the body is also present in my picture in the mirror. Not only is it the optic picture but it also carries with it tactile sensation. My postural model of the body is in a picture outside myself. But is not every other person like a picture of myself? One sees again how strong is the influence of the optic sphere on the postural model of the body. We meet again the dependence of the image on the body which we encountered in our discussion of Stratton's experiment and experiments concerning the doubling of one's own finger by double vision.

The sensations felt in the above experiment cannot be attributed to projection. The experience of the sensation in the mirror is as immediate and original as the experience in the real hand. It is at least very probable that part of these experiences are given when we see the bodies of others, especially when one considers how little the optic experience concerning one's own body-image differs from the experiences we have concerning the optic image of the bodies of others. Further, one may compare the important investigations made by Landis and his co-workers with the conclusions deduced from our own experiences. Landis has found that the expression of emotions is very often misunderstood. He has taken photographs of persons in actual emotional situations. People who looked at these photographs often misinterpreted their meaning. But it is not justifiable to select one part only out of a whole situation. The emotion cannot be separated from the sequences of motility, and the object which provokes an emotion is a part of the emotional situation. Landis' interesting investigations show therefore that we understand emotional situations only as wholes and not in parts, even when the snapshot catches the climax of the emotional situation. (Landis himself comes to very similar conclusions.)

The close relation between one's own body and the bodies of

others also comes into the foreground in a series of interesting investigations made by David Levy. He has studied body interest in children. All the children examined presented evidence of physical disease. There were many responses indicating special interest in or sensitivity to a part of the body, which they considered inferior. The problems were chiefly aesthetic. Only three can be interpreted as interfering with the functions (knock-knees, flat feet, squint). Many of the children complained about the skull; its funny shape; its being big, long, and narrow. But particular interest was also displayed in length and strength, for instance in the length of the fingers. Of all parts of the body the visible area was most productive of sensitivity. A number of boys under the age of 12 objected to the idea of body hair, one accepted it only on the face, another had no objection to body hair if light.

It is of special interest in this connection that sensitivity to a discovery on one's own body may draw special attention to the corresponding part in the bodies of others. A boy with inverted nipples was especially observant of women's breasts. But in Levy's material it comes out clearly that children find out about their own body by the talk and observation of others. The attitude of the parents towards scars and the observation of others provoke a great interest in the child's own body. Family conversations about health, appearance, or illness in the family may also increase the child's interest in its own body.[1]

It is obvious that interest in particular parts of one's own body provokes interest in the corresponding parts of the bodies of others. Between one's own body and the bodies of others there exists a connection. We may emphasize again our previous observation that patients found out about their own bodies with the help of others. It is remarkable that interest in others and interest in oneself run in some way parallel to each other. In a case in which a mutilation of the hand took place, the patient at first took an enormous interest in the people with whom he came into contact. But his interest in his surroundings soon decreased and with it also his self-consciousness concerning the change. A person's own interest in the body and the social interest of others

[1] In a further paper Levy has studied these attitudes in connection with the individual life problems of the children.

concerning the body run parallel to each other. When we try to assess the value of Levy's material we have, of course, to take into consideration that he does not deal with primary changes in a postural model of the body, but that we deal with special interest in the body and the adjustments which are based upon this interest. There is also the intellectual and emotional interest of others concerning the body of the child.

We should not forget that the postural image of the body, although it is primarily an experience of the senses, provokes attitudes of an emotional type, and that these emotional attitudes are inseparable from the sensory experience. The judgment concerning the body is derived from both sources, and is only possible on the basis of the underlying sensory and emotional factors. The same levels can be distinguished when we see the body of another person. We first get a sensory impression about the other person's body. This sensory impression gets its real meaning by our emotional interest in the various parts of his body, and finally we come to a judgment relating to the different parts of the other's body. But even this threefold sub-division does not give the full importance of the body-image. Just as one's own body-image gains its full meaning only by its motion and by its function, which expresses itself again in a sensory way, the motion of another person's body-image, its changes concerning function, and its prospects concerning action, give the body-image a deeper meaning.

The alcoholic hallucinosis case reported above opens the way into still another field. Motion and function of the body-image are after all closely related to the aims and tendencies of the individual, and motion and function are also an integral part of the body-image of others as an expression of the personality. Body-image and emotion are very closely connected with each other, and just as our own body-image is the expression of our own emotional life and personality, the bodies of others get their final meaning by being the bodies of other personalities. The perception of the bodies of others and of their expression of emotions is as primary as the perception of our own body and its emotions and expressions. Our own body, as all the previous discussions show, in sensory perception is not different from the sensory perception of the bodies of others. We find our own libidinous body-image very often by the libidinous tendency of others directed against us. Just as we have rejected the idea of ' Einfüh-lung ' we have to reject the idea that we arrive at the knowledge of the bodies of others and their emotions by projecting our body and our feelings into other personalities. But it is true that there is a continual interchange between our own body-image and the body-image of others. What we have seen in others we may find out in ourselves. What we have found out in ourselves we may see in others.

(4) *Erythrophobia* (*fear of blushing*) *as an instance of a social neurosis*

The 31-year-old S. L. complains of blushing and sweating when he is in the presence of others. If he does not actually blush and perspire he is afraid of doing so. This fear hinders him in all his social contacts and makes him afraid of meeting anyone. His self-consciousness goes back to his very early childhood. He was very tall for his age and was always afraid that other people would look at him and wonder why he played with children so much smaller than himself. But his real troubles began later at the age of about 13 when he took to masturbating and his hair began to grow. He felt that the masturbation provoked the growth of the hair and that people looking at him would realize that he masturbated. He was also afraid that his erection might be seen.

Besides this fear of blushing and sweating there are obsessions that he may strangle other people, that he may throw bottles in their faces. This fear especially concerns his wife. But he is also afraid of hurting his 5-year-old child and also of hurting people who are sitting in front of him at the cinema. He regards his blushing and sweating as a sign of weakness and femininity. He wants to be strong and wants to be a man. His sex development was a very slow one. Urged by his brother, he occasionally had sex relations with a girl for whom he had no affection. In his marriage his wife had played the more active part. His sex activity in marriage was not only limited, but he avoided any preliminary sex play; he had never seen his wife naked before the first analysis started. He often felt attracted to other women but never made any active attempt to make love to any of them. In the year preceding the analysis he was attracted by his sister-in law, but there were only occasional touches and verbal plays.

Before he came to the analysis he had been analysed for a year by another analyst to whom he developed a very great positive transference. This analyst was for him an ideal of masculine strength. He admired him extremely. He made considerable progress, especially during the time he spent in the summer with his sister-in-law when he also allowed himself a greater sexual freedom with this sister-in-law. On his return to his original home his old difficulties started again and, in agreement with his analyst, he broke up the analysis and tried to get along alone, but soon felt that he needed somebody.

He chose the analyst because he had heard that he had a high pitched voice. He supposed this analyst would be more feminine and therefore more suitable to him. This leads immediately to one of the central problems of his neurosis—the relation to his father. His father was a man who had started in rather limited circumstances but had attained considerable success, and had built up with a partner, a factory in which the patient also worked. His father was always a rather grouchy person. The patient complained that from his early childhood he had never had any praise and encouragement from his father, who always blamed him and told him that he would never amount to anything. His father never beat him, but from his earliest childhood (the remembrances go back to about his fourth year) had scolded and terrorized him. He was especially afraid of his father's angry look. His hatred against his father was clear in his consciousness. His father was for him a very masculine type. Coupled with this hatred was an enormous admiration which remained more or less unconscious but came out in the analysis.

The situation became more complicated for him since there were two older brothers. The eldest one especially was wild and tyrannical. This brother, who was seven or eight years older than the patient, died of tuberculosis, was of a violent temper, and once tried to hang himself when he could not get what he wanted. Whereas the two older brothers resisted the father openly, the patient thought he would try to win the appreciation of his parents by giving in and by being obedient to his wishes. He also did a he could to please his mother—washing walls and doing all kinds of housework for her. But at the same time he felt that all this giving-in was hypocritical. He nursed a strong feeling of revolt against his father as well as against his brothers. To give in, to be subservient, was for him a proof of passivity and femininity which he felt in himself and against which he revolted. In one of his first dreams in the analysis, he dreamt that a detective or gangster asked a telegraph girl to give up a secret telegram. In the association he brought out that detectives, policemen, and gangsters are courageous. He did not like to have anything to do with them. He associated both analysts with them. As a child he was interested in telephones. He liked to play at telephones, and telephoned to a friend across the street. He identified himself with this girl. He did not want anybody to know about his masturbation. He is afraid of others knowing something about him.

His disposition to identify himself with women was apparently connected with his strong anal tendencies. When he was about five or six years old, he was very much afraid that someone might see him on the toilet, especially when defecating. In the later phases of the analysis it came into his memory that he may have put match-sticks into a boy's anus, but he was not sure whether he did not put them into his own. His mother had always been very modest, and had warned him against showing himself naked. It is among his early remembrances that he saw mothers holding up their babies to perform their natural functions. These memories went back to a very early age, between three and four. There was also the memory of a stoop under which there were faeces. Anal components and femininity were closely connected for him. In about his eighth year he played 'family' with a neighbour's child, and an important part in the play with this girl was that he spanked her on her naked buttocks. His anal tendencies assumed a new and stronger expression when he was about eight years old and his brother's temperature was taken by the doctor *per anum*. When he started his masturbation he imagined that the doctor was taking a woman's temperature and that he would smell the thermometer. Later on, he put the thermometer in his anus as the doctor would do to a female patient. He then put his phallus between his legs and looked upon himself as a woman, at the same time imagining that he was lying besides a woman and having intercourse with her. He had similar sexual phantasies about the wife of his father's business partner. In his relations with his own wife touching her anus played a great part.

Boys told him about sexual intercourse when he was about ten years old. He always felt that he did not really want to have sex relations with women. He was always very much afraid of having erections. He slept in the same bed with his two older brothers when he was a boy. He never wanted to sleep between them, being afraid that he would get an erection and they would find out. He was not interested whether his brothers had erections or not. Also when he went into his father's bed he was afraid of having an erection. Through all his later life he did not like to have erections, and was afraid that others might realize it.

His sadistic tendencies against the father were strong. He sometimes imagined him lying in a coffin and was afraid that his thoughts might have an effect on his father. But he had immediate aggressive impulses against his wife, his child, and persons sitting before him at a show. These thoughts made him suffer. In his consciousness he wanted to be friendly towards everyone. He was very much afraid that people might take revenge on him when he was not friendly towards them. It was very difficult in the analysis to make him bring forward any word concerning negative transference. He was afraid of the revenge of the analyst (father). He was afraid of death and dead people. He felt he would not like to see any dead person; he thought he could not get the picture out of his mind. He was afraid to look in a mirror in the evening—he might see dead people in it. He would not have liked to be in the same building with a dead body. He was often afraid that he might strangle another person.

In childhood he had a nightmare that a substance might come out of his mouth and enshroud him completely; the substance might become solid and choking. There were other fears concerning his mouth. He might put dirty things into his mouth; dead animals, even faeces. These ideas also came as a compulsion.

Closely related to his first anal experiences and fears was the fear of being seen when defecating. There were some associations that he felt he would like to see his mother and other people on the toilet. In his early childhood he saw his mother on the chamber. In his sixth, seventh, and eighth years he used to urinate in company with other boys. Once they played 'burning house' and he urinated on another boy in order to extinguish the fire. Soon after that the weight of repression started in and with it the special fear that his erection might be seen by others. At that time he was also self-conscious about his size. He was angry when the other boys called him 'chink'. He felt that he was very much the centre of attention to others. He did not want to be seen and yet felt that other people were looking at him. When he masturbated, he felt that the masturbation would make his beard grow. Even at the time of the analysis he felt especially self-conscious when he was at the barber's. He was very much interested in his face. He thought that his nose was too long. He liked to look into the mirror and watch what he was doing. He also watched other people carefully when he was blushing and perspiring. He felt that other people were looking at him and thought that he was inferior. He also felt that they were laughing at him. He could not talk, but blushed and perspired. He would have liked to be a public orator. He admired people who came in free contact with others and who were able to talk freely. He would have liked to be a salesman, a buyer, or an actor. He was extremely resentful when others ridiculed an actor; he felt that they should not do so. In his dreams he again dreamt about actors and theatres. Here is one of his dreams.

"I am at the theatre sitting in the front row. The show starts and a young boy about 18 years of age is the leading actor. He has a dark complexion. He says that I won't like the show and tells me to come on the stage, which I do. I am surprised that I go so easily without any fear. The boy performs tricks of magic and makes me float into the air horizontally around the stage and then through the audience. The feat is done without any wires and I am fully conscious. In the audience are my brother-in-law and his wife. When I get back on the stage the people in the audience laugh. I think they are laughing at me and I am only a trifle uneasy as I have my back to them. I find an old hat in my pocket and I don't know whose it is and I ask the actor. He calls a member of the audience on to the stage to watch what he is doing.

I remain on the stage and later I go off and forget my Derby, so I go back and get it."

In this dream his desire to be the centre of attention, to be in close contact with everybody, is in the foreground. At the same time losing his hat is a fear of castration. He was afraid that people might harm him (castration) when they looked at him. They obtained an advantage over him by looking at him. He said indeed that he felt more at ease when he was in the dark.

He wanted to be with people. His ideal was to have as many friends as possible, but he felt so self-conscious that he never visited his friends.

His eyes hurt him. When he looked at bright lights, tears came into his eyes. He had a queer sensation in his forehead between the eyes. Looking was for him a strong social relation which he desired and feared and which was connected with dangers (castration). He was very much interested in the perspiration of other people, in their looks, in their attitudes, and in their way of talking. He was continually observing and felt continually observed. He was extremely self-conscious about his whole appearance—about his hair, his beard, and his size. In his relations with others he was always afraid that they might take advantage of him.

The patient was dominated by his fear concerning his father. He was afraid of being seen, of being looked at by his father. It came out very clearly in the analysis that this fear was a fear of being castrated by his father, of becoming feminine through the anger of his father. But there was not only this fear, there was also the primary wish of being passive, of being the passive love-object for the father. We generally consider phenomena of this kind, which we meet in almost every analytic case, more or less from the point of view of the libidinous situation of the patient. But we should know that we have here before us a very important social relation. Generally one does not give much consideration to the facts on which the social relation is based, but the social relation is not only a relation between two personalities but is also always a relation between two bodies. The question of the body-image therefore goes into every situation of this kind. We have to ask what is the body-image of the father. The patient's fear of his father's look was of special importance. Of course, the look was at the same time an expression in the father, and also an expression in the body-image of the father. There were also the actions of the father, his scolding, his nagging; but for the patient they became the expression of virility. There is again the question what virility means in this connection. We have reason to believe that virility means something connected with the physique, especially with the sex-organ of the father. This latter point does not come out so clearly in the analysis of this case. In another patient, who was often severely beaten by his father, ideas about the father's genitals and his large nose played an important part.

Erotic relations are therefore relations between two bodies, and depend upon our attitude towards our own body and also our attitude towards the bodies of others. We should not forget in this connection that the discovery of our own body is often made by observing the bodies of others.

Our patient started with the fear of being seen when he was defecating. It seems that defecation is an attitude where one is passive and active at the same time. The patient was apparently afraid of his passivity at this moment. The analysis does not give any hints whether his fear of being seen during defecation was preceded by the castration dread or not. We have reason to believe so, but there is a possibility that we are dealing with an over-emphasis of the anal zone which is prior to the castration complex and only secondarily increased by the castration threat. At the same time anality meant for him to be passive, to take the place of the mother in the relation to the father. The fear of castration must necessarily lead to an increase of interest in the actions and expressions of the father and of substitutes for the father. His emotional relation to the persons around him must therefore be increased. The tyrannical attitude of his two brothers was bound to increase the psychological trends which we have described.

When the patient saw the temperature of his brother taken *per anum*, he was prepared to answer with an increase in his anal tendency. It is characteristic that again something which was going on in the body of another person increased his tendencies concerning his own body. It is obvious that there is a particularly close relation between the parts of the body-image of different persons in the erogenic zones. In a short clinical examination the patient with an obsession neurosis reported that whenever his mother gave him an enema he felt a sexual satisfaction in the anal zone and supposed that his mother did also. The anal irritation caused by the thermometer brought the patient immediately into a passive and feminine situation. That was why, as mentioned above, he hid the organ between his legs. The situation during his practices was characteristic as well as complicated. He was at first himself. He also played the doctor who took his temperature *per anum*. At the same time, he played the part of a woman whose temperature was taken by the doctor. Finally, he played a woman who had intercourse and a person lying beside himself, and who was himself, who had intercourse with the woman. No better instance could be given of the fact that in an individual's own postural image many postural images of others are melted together. But in order that this may take place these postural images must have been perceived and built up beforehand. We are not interested here so much in the problem of the so-called identification with other personalities; but we can follow up the process by which the postural model of one's own body melts together with the postural model of others under the influence of an erotic need. The patient projected himself out of his own body but took others into his body. He was living at the same time outside and inside his own body. But his own body had amalgamated the bodies of others. The fundamental philosophical problem of Ego and outside world appears under a new aspect.

(5) *Social relations of body-images. The social distance*

There now arises the question what is our own body and what is the body of others? Which does one perceive first? Is the one secondary to the other? Do we perceive them at the same time? According to the dogmatic formulation of analysis, the child knows first about his own body. But our whole discussion shows clearly that our own body is not nearer to us than the outside world, at least in important parts. The optic impressions concerning our own body, which are so important for the formation of the body-image, are in no way different from the optic impressions we have concerning the bodies of others. It is not possible to say that we gain our knowledge of outside bodies and their images by projecting our own body into the outside world. But we are also not justified in taking the opposite view, and saying that we gain the knowledge of our own body by introjecting the body-images of others into ourselves. The body-image is not a product of the appersonization of the bodies of others, although we may take parts of the body-images of others into our postural model. It is also not gained by identification with the body-images of others, although we may enrich our body-image perception by such identifications. There is no other way out than to formulate that our own body-image and the body-images of others are primary data of experience, and that there is from the beginning a very close connection between the body-image of ourselves and the body-images of others. We take parts of the body-images of others into others, and push parts of our body-images into others. We may push our own body-images completely into others, or in some way there may be a continuous interplay between the body-images of ourselves and the persons around us. This interplay may be an interplay of parts or of wholes.

There is no question that there are from the beginning connecting links between all body-images, and it is important to follow the lines of body-image intercourse. We meet here the question of the way in which distance in space influences these lines. There is no doubt that the far-distant body will offer less possibility of interplay. If we put our body into an imaginary centre we may measure the spatial distance of other bodies when we want to determine the relation between the body-images. To be close in space increases the possibility of an interrelation between the body-images, and besides other things contact between two bodies must afford a greater possibility of the melting together of the body-images. We must also consider sexual contact between two bodies from the point of view of spatial nearness. It is true that when two bodies come very near each other, optic distinction becomes more difficult and there will be a greater possibility of a complete melting and reconstructing of one's own body-image as well as the body-image of the other person. It must also not be forgotten that every touch given or received will, as the discussion in the first and second parts show, immediately produce new and interesting problems concerning the structure of one's own body-image as well as of the body-image of the other person. The factor of spatial distance is at first an optic factor and becomes finally a factor of touch.[1] Besides the factor of spatial distance we have to consider that every emotion concerning the other person brings the body-image of this other person nearer to us.

We have therefore the factor of the emotional distance. Language throws considerable light on this relation. We say of a person with whom we are in emotional relations that he is near to us. We could describe the relations between the body-images of different persons under the metaphor of a magnetic field with stream-lines going in all directions.

But it would be wrong to conclude that the metaphorical distance between the various images of the body is the same in the case of all parts of the body. Parts which have an erotic interest are nearer to each other than parts which are less important from an erotic point of view. It might almost be said that the erogenic zones of the various body-images are closer to each other than the other parts of the body, or that the intercourse between the body-images takes place especially through the erogenic zones. I purposely use this word which has a double meaning because sexual intercourse is certainly a very complete melting together of body-images, and if we ever have a psychology of intercourse (we are pretty far from that) it will be based on the relation of body-images in intercourse.

In the masturbation phantasies of our patient, the point which connected the various body-images and attached them to each other was certainly the anus, in view of the whole psycho-sexual

[1] It is a well known trick on the vaudeville stage for two comedians to intertwine their legs so closely that they are apparently unable to determine the ownership.

I was once present at a conference in which the question was discussed with a friend of a patient whether the patient should stay in the hospital or not. The patient was present. The friend took the patient's part. I wondered what was the connection between these two? Why was this other man so much interested in the fate of this other person sitting nearby?

structure of our patient. But the observation teaches us something else. The patient had at the moment of his masturbation not
only one body-image but at least four. Somehow the melting
together was not complete; it might rather be regarded as a
summing up. One may have as many body-images as clothes.
One may be enshrouded by various body-images. They cannot
form a unit, but they may form a sum. It is possible that we have
in the relations between body-images two different types, the one
completely integrating his own body-image with the body-image
of others, and the other having the various parts of the body-
image not integrated into a whole. Actually these types will not
always emerge clearly; summation and integration will be present
in various proportions.

In the case we have been discussing the patient soon developed
the fear that his masturbation might be noticed by others. It is
remarkable that he was afraid that an increased growth of hair
might be a sign to others that he had masturbated. We have here
a transfer from below to above, from the genito-anal region
into the face. This fear that masturbation may be seen in the face
is a very typical one. Body-images should not exist in isolation.
We desire the relation of our body-images to the body-images of
all other persons, and we want it especially concerning all sexual
activities and their expression in the body-image. Masturbation is
specifically social. It is an act by which we attempt to draw the
body-images of others, especially in their genital region, nearer to
us. The super-ego interferes with this tendency, and represses it,
and it then comes out in another part of the body-image. It seems
that the face has here a special significance. In the face the
secondary sex characteristics are manifest by the different growths
of hair. (We know that hair is a rather common symbolization for
sex organs. A patient of mine, who had resisted intercourse and
had thereby provoked an ejaculation of her partner outside the
vagina, afterwards fell asleep and scolded a servant maid for
spilling the expensive hair oil.) But persons who masturbate are
particularly afraid that it may be seen in their eyes that they have
practiced it and that everybody knows about it. The desire to be
seen is transformed into the fear of being seen.

One's own eyes and those of others thus become the tool of the

body-image intercourse. The eyes grant the possibility of estab-
lishing social relations with another person. It is remarkable that
our patient who was so much afraid that others might see him
complained of a queer feeling between his eyes, of weeping and an
inability to look into the sun. We are reminded of the great part
the optic sphere plays in the construction of the body-image.

In the later phase of the development the patient was afraid of
sweating and blushing. Blushing is, as is analytically well known,
a substitute for erection. We should have mentioned that both
masturbation and also erection as such are extremely social
phenomena, and concern the body-image of others as well as
one's own. Our patient strove frantically to hide his erection and
his phallus (a very common phenomenon in neurotics). The
blushing was again a transfer into the face. This time the transfer
was not only in what one usually calls the psychic sphere (the
patient's obsession about the growth of his hair is merely a
psychic phenomenon), but we are also dealing with a change
going on in the somatic sphere, or, in other words, the processes
concerning the body-image may also be processes which change
the body as such. It is remarkable that the face now became the
centre of his body-image which attracted the attention of all the
other people. It was the tool by which he brought the body-
images of others nearer to himself. Everybody looked at him,
saw him, and gave him attention. This was the attention which he
primarily wanted for his defecation and for his erection.

There is reason to believe that we are dealing here with a very
typical phenomenon which leads to the psychology of blushing
and the psychology of expressive movements generally. Every
change in the expression, either by vasomotor changes or by
changes in attitude, also immediately becomes a change in
our social relations to others. Every expression or change in
expression is always directed towards the people around us and
has the function of drawing other people nearer to us. There are
no expressions of an isolated individual, and the blushing (in the
case of our patient, the sweating also) only shows more clearly
principles which we may meet in almost every human activity.

The face has, of course, its special importance in the body-
image as a whole because it is the most expressive part of the

body and is the part of the body which can be seen by everybody. We communicate by means of our faces, and there is also a psychological significance in the fact that the mouth, one of the principle organs of communication, is in the middle of the face. The blushing of our patient thus says, "See my erection (defecation), be excited with me, and come nearer to me". It is a method by which he comes nearer to other people than he would come otherwise. The blushing thus increases his social relations or decreases the social distance between himself and others. It is not surprising that this illicit satisfaction by blushing is not tolerated by the ego system and provokes repressive mechanism. The patient now avoids other people and is afraid of them. His fear that his blushing will make him defenceless against others and that they may castrate him is connected with this. To be seen means to be the object of a sexual attack and to be castrated. This basic relation reflects itself in the patient's fear that others may take advantage of him. On the other hand, he wants to help others as much as possible. He does not want to hurt anybody because he fears their revenge. It is in connection with this fact that the patient wants to have as many friends as possible and that he wants to be as close as possible to as many people as possible. In reality he is finally farther from this aim than anybody else, but at least he is near them in his phantasy.

It is a matter of course that the patient, in these conditions, must be extremely interested in his body-image. It will make a great difference to him what kind of clothes he wears, how he looks, whether he is tall or not. He will finally aim at being the centre of attention for all the people around him. To be an actor would be the fulfilment of all these wishes, or to be a public orator would serve similar purposes.

It will perhaps be of interest to consider the peculiar situation of the actor in the light of this discussion. While the actor is the emotional centre of the attention of many other people and they draw his body-image near them, yet he is separated from them by an invisible but insurmountable barrier. There is no way which leads nearer from him to them. The onlooker identifies himself with the actor, but the actor is unable to reciprocate this identification in the same way. There is a queer relation between being near and far in relation to others at the same time. The actor's appearance and his words try to draw others nearer to him. It is a great question whether we can come from this point of view to a clearer formulation of narcissistic tendencies. In the case of the actor, in the case of the patient, we see that the narcissistic interest in oneself is more closely interrelated with the attitude of others than we usually suppose.

The final result of the neurosis of our patient is that he is actually more isolated and more interested in himself and that it does not matter to him who others are. The individuality of others no longer plays an important part for him: they are merely human beings, body-images without a particular individuality. Or in some way he has changed the individual relation to other body-images as the expression of human personalities into a general and unindividual relation. All human beings are threatening or admiring. He is in a closer relation to others, but the relation has lost the individual trends. He blushes before everybody. It is true that he is especially afraid to meet people with whom he is acquainted. It is worthy of remark that he, like all who suffer from fear of blushing, wants to hide his blushing and does not want others to know about it. He does not dare to confess his difficulties. There is also another trend which is common to a great number of these cases. They are always afraid that others may look at them and not only look at them but also make remarks about them and laugh at them.

When we try to come to more general formulations we can make the following propositions: (1) Body-images are never isolated. They are always encircled by the body-images of others. (2) The relation to the body-images of others is determined by the factor of spatial nearness and remoteness and by the factor of emotional nearness and remoteness. (3) Body-images are nearer to each other in the erogenic zones and are closely bound together in the erogenic zones. (4) The transfer of erogenic zones will reflect itself also in the social relation to other body-images. (5) Erotic changes in the body-image are always social phenomena and are accompanied by corresponding phenomena in the body-images of others. (6) Body-images are on principle social. Our own body-image is never isolated but is always accompanied by the body-images of others. (7) Our own body-image and the body-image of others are not primarily dependent upon each other; they are equal, and the one cannot be explained by the other. (8) There is a continuous interchange between parts of our own body-image and the body-images of others. There is projection and appersonization. But in addition the whole body-image of others can be taken in (identification) or our own body-image can be pushed out as a whole. (9) The body-images of others and their parts can be integrated completely with our own body-image and can form a unit, or they can be simply added to our own body-image and then merely form a sum. (10) We have always emphasized that the postural model of the body is not static, that it changes continually according to the life circumstances. We have considered it as a construction of a creative type. It is built up, dissolved, built up again. An important part in this continuous process of construction, reconstruction, and dissolution of the body-image, is played by the processes of identification, appersonization, and projection. When the body-image has once been created according to our needs and tendencies it does not remain unchanged; it is in a continual flow, and a crystallization is immediately followed by a plastic stage from which new constructions and new efforts are possible according to the emotional situation of the individual. Moreover, there is not only the continual change in our own body-image but also the continual changes in its spatial relations, emotional relations of the body-images of others and the construction of the body-images of others. Also the social relation of the body-images is not a fixed 'gestalt.' But we have a process of forming a 'gestalt,' 'gestaltung,' or creative construction in the social image.

Our previous case has already shown us how near we come with these formulations to the problem of paranoia, in which the individual comes into changed relations to all other people. Schulte has called paranoia a difficulty in the 'Wirbildung' (change in the experience of WE). Stockert calls attention to contact neuroses, in which he includes stammering. But we should place more emphasis on the important part bodies play in the 'WE', and we should never forget that the 'WE' is not a rigid unit but is under the continual influence of a purposeful, emotional creation.

Q

A short time ago I saw a patient who had shot her husband of whom she was jealous. She said that she had only threatened him in order to get a confession from him. His confession would have relieved her. The patient felt that many of her husband's friends were hostile to her. In the hospital, where pretty soon definite paranoic symptoms developed, she also felt that the people round her were either particularly hostile or particularly friendly. According to her feelings, the attitude of the group towards her changed. In other words, there was an exaggeration of her social feelings and a diminution of what we might call the social distance. According to her emotions, individuals came nearer to her. In the observation as such there was no change in the relation of the postural model of the body, but from our experiences in analyzed cases and especially from our knowledge of jealousy, we may suppose that these attitudes towards the bodies of others are at least in the psychic background.[1]

We have come to the connotation of the social distance of body-images. Sociologists now speak of race prejudice and other prejudices between groups as social distance (Folsom, p. 316). But it is obvious that social distance, as we have used the term, is based upon the emotional reaction, and it does not matter whether this emotional reaction is love or hatred. Both bring the other person nearer to us. In the formulation of sociologists, hatred and prejudice mean a greater social distance. I would like to emphasize that social distance diminishes whenever there is a strong emotional reaction, and it does not matter whether this reaction is a plus or minus reaction. Bogardus has devised a method of measuring social distance by asking whether one would like a member of a special group admitted: (1) to close kinship by marriage; (2) to one's club as a personal chum; (3) to one's street as a neighbour; (4) to employment in one's occupation; (5) to citizenship in one's country; (6) as a visitor only to the country; or, (7) would one exclude him altogether from the country?

It is clear that social distance is partly concerned with the question of how near to ourselves we want to have the body of

[1] Spinoza wrote that jealousy consists in the obsessing thought of the connection of the excreta of another person with the beloved object.

the other person concerned, and that the whole conception of social distance gets its real meaning only when we consider the postural model of the body in its relations to the postural model of the bodies of others.

(6) *Imitation and the body-image*

In social psychology, imitation and the important function imitation has in the building up of the social structure are often mentioned. Tarde especially has based this social psychology on the laws of imitation. Tarde used the word imitation for three processes: the imitation of conviction, of feelings, and of actions. The child is led by imitation from an animal's instinctive life to a life of self-determination and deliberation. Imitation can act in a competitive way. The qualities of every social group are based upon their mutual imitation. In this way the peculiarities of language, the religious, moral, and political convictions, are created as well as the habits of eating, dressing, dwelling, and recreation, all the routine activities which make up the great part of the lives of men. But imitation may be an agent of progress as well. Its operation as a factor in progress is of two principal kinds, the spread of imitation throughout the people of ideas and practices generated within it from time to time by its exceptionally gifted members and the spread of ideas of imitations and practices from one people to another. (This is MacDougall's formulation of Tarde's ideas.) According to Tarde, the imitation of convictions is prior to the imitation of expressive movements, the imitation of aims prior to the imitation of the method to reach the aim. In his opinion belief in religion precedes the performance of the cult. A person who imitates somebody else in dressing and entertainment has previously taken over his feelings and desires. Imitation goes therefore, according to Tarde, from inside to outside, but it also goes from above to below. Defeated nations imitate the victors; the nobility, the court.

MacDougall does not use the term 'imitation' when there is an induction of emotions. He points to the spread of fear and its flight impulse among the members of a flock or herd. Many gregarious animals, on being startled, utter the characteristic cry of

fear. When the cry is emitted by one member of the flock or herd
it immediately excites the flight impulse in all of its fellows who
are within hearing of it. The whole herd, flock, or covey, takes to
flight like one individual. Human sympathy has its roots in
similar specialization of the instinctive dispositions on their
afferent sides. The sympathetic induction of emotion and feeling
may be observed in children at an age at which they cannot be
credited with understanding of the significance of the expression
that provokes their reactions...the sight of a smiling face, the
expression of pleasure provokes a smile. Laughter is notoriously
infectious, also crying, and this, though not the truly instinctive
expression, affords the most familiar example of sympathetic
induction of an affective state. In the adult also sympathetic
reactions of this kind are present. A merry face makes us feel
brighter. "In short, each of the great primary emotions that has
its characteristic and unmistakable bodily expression seems to be
capable of being excited by way of its immediate sympathetic
response." Imitative actions of this sort (which are not true
imitations) are displayed by all the gregarious animals and are the
only kind of which most of the animals seem capable. They are
displayed on a great scale by crowds of human beings and are the
principal source of the wild excesses of which crowds are so often
guilty.

There exist, however, real imitation actions which are due to
the fact that the visual presentation of the movement of another
apt to evoke the representation of a similar movement of one's
own body, which, like all motor representation, tends to realize
itself immediately in movements. Many of the imitative
movements of children are of this class. Some person attracts a
child's curious attention, it becomes absorbed in watching him
and presently imitates his movements. This kind of imitation may
be in part voluntary and so merges into the third kind of deliberate, voluntary, or self-conscious imitation. MacDougall mentions
among other kinds of imitations very young children's imitation
of movements that are not expressive of feeling or emotion.
MacDougall, Allport, and Folsom deny that imitation is
instinct. This is more important from the point of view of Mac-
Dougall, who uses the term 'instinct' rather freely for man-

activities. But we owe it to Watson and his behavioristic approach that the term 'instinct' has lost a great deal of its magic. We are more interested in the description of attitudes and actions than in the classification of instinctive and not instinctive. If the term 'instinct' means that there are actions which are not dependent on the total situation and developed automatically and in a rigid way, instincts do not exist. If the term 'instinct' means an action of primitive character with comparatively little variability, then instincts do exist. I do not see then why one should not speak about an instinct of imitation in all the cases in which MacDougall speaks of imitation of actions and sympathetic induction of emotions.

According to Bühler, the child imitates what it hears. It may imitate its own sounds and its own babbling. It is not easy to find out when the first imitations of others start. A real imitation can only be supposed when one succeeds in making the quiet child, by talking, produce a sound similar to what has been pronounced to it. The Sterns have observed this in their children in their first half year, others found it much later, and it is certain that the repetition of everything that the child hears is very obtrusive in the second and third year. The child becomes almost an echo of all speech and natural sounds which it hears around it. The imitation of sound produced by others is apparently very difficult in the beginning, and very often it is only after prolonged exercise that the child is able to repeat by imitation combinations of sounds which it has brought forward with ease spontaneously.[1] Brain pathology shows that there is an imitation which, if inner needs exist, succeeds, whereas it fails when such an inner need is not present. Aphasics show this fairly frequently.

Laughing and crying and emotions of any kind provoke similar reactions in others. This is especially obvious in laughing, crying, and yawning. Allport and Folsom are inclined to deny imitation even in those instances. Allport in particular argues that it is very difficult to provoke an imitative reaction in a baby under 18 months; that, when imitative reactions finally occur, they can be explained by the process of conditioned reflexes; that

[1] But Preyer reports the case of a girl who could imitate correctly a tone struck on her piano when she was nine months old.

many apparently imitative acts are due to the fact that several people are reacting in the same way; and finally, that when they try to imitate some act of skill they require much practice before they can copy it perfectly.

Folsom thinks that the imitation of yawning is in reality a conditioned response (p. 321). "Many times in the past we have been stimulated to yawn by long speeches and hot air...and at the same time have seen others yawning. The sight of the neighbouring yawn has become a conditioned stimulus which now automatically produces our own yawn. But the only inborn stimulus was the warm air or the prolonged strain on the attention." I do not think, however, that we are justified in making such complicated interpretations. There is no question that the emotion of others and its expression induces in ourselves this very emotion and leads to a very similar expression. But Allport is quite right in emphasizing that this imitation is not a blind instinct, a blind force. Certainly imitation, like every other activity, is dependent upon the total situation, and the human being as a totality always has motives which are a part of this general situation. The instinctive and the purposive imitation are in their nucleus identical. We finally believe that an organism is, in all its expressions, a purposive being.

But what goes on when we see an expression in a face or any other expressive movement, or even when deliberate action takes place? There is always a person acting and it is always in the structure of experience that living beings, personalities, are acting. And when we imitate the single action, the single expression, do we not rather imitate another person in his actions and expressions? Our own emotions and those of other persons and their expressions are never isolated. In the language of the 'gestalt' psychology, every expression of the face and of the other parts of the body is a configuration, a 'gestalt.' In Lewis Carroll's *Alice in Wonderland*, the Cheshire cat disappears and only its grin remains. This is true in so far as the 'gestalt' of grinning may be present, even when no single parts of the face are perceived. But the grinning will always be connected with an image of the body, and it will be connected with the personality. It may be the personality of a human being, it may be an animal; but it must be something living endowed with a body-image. The optic and kinaesthetic factors we have studied in the construction of the postural model of the body will be of fundamental importance not only for the building up of one's own postural model of the body, but also for the building up of the body-image of others. It would be still better to say that my body-image and the body-images of others are primarily very closely connected with each other. Other persons' actions also have a relation to my own actions. When I imitate another person's actions and doings, I acknowledge only the deep-lying factor of the partial community of the body-image. This is a basic sensory factor. The emotional tendencies are attached to it and use the sensory construction of the body-image. There is, of course, the rich world of motives and strivings which determine what we want to imitate in another person.

MacDougall seems to have similar problems in mind when he discusses the imitative actions of simple ideomotor type. "And all of us, if our attention is keenly concentrated on the movement of another person, are apt to make, at least in a partial incipient fashion, every movement we observe, e.g. on watching a difficult stroke in billiards, the balancing of a tight-rope walker, the rhythmic swaying of a dancer. In all these cases the imitative movements seem to be due to the fact that the visual presentation of the movements of another is apt to evoke the representations of a similar movement of one's own body which like all motor representations tends to realize itself immediately in movement."

I have only to emphasize again that movements are always connected with the body-image and underlie all the laws concerning the body-image that we have already discussed. We come now to a deeper understanding of the sympathetic induction of emotions. Laughing is indeed common to all of us. It is immediately the affair of a social group, like the cry of panic, senseless as the panic may be. It is wrong to call this induction. Emotions are in themselves connected with expressions and are in themselves connected with the emotions of others. We perceive the body-image of others, we perceive their expressions which are expressions of emotions, and emotions are emotions of personalities. These are primary data. They are not secondary to the building up of our own postural model of the body, and I have shown in detail how much the postural model of the body is dependent on what we see and experience in others.

We are very far from Lipps' formulations concerning 'Einfühlung.' 'Einfühlung' is, according to Lipps, a projection of one's own feeling into another person or another object. "The threatening gesture of the other person provokes in me the instinct of imitation, and by this imitation I experience the threat and project it into the other. It is true that there exist tendencies to imitation and that they are of very primitive type. One can see that in children, and also in adults.... One is justified in agreeing with Lipps about the instinct of imitation. Pathology shows us the same phenomena in a clearer picture. There are hallucinated patients who repeat everything that they hear. Others do what they hallucinate optically, and even become the picture which they see. It may be said generally that every picture, every sensual experience, brings with itself the tendency to an action; and one may distinguish two possibilities. Either we act as if we wanted to be the picture ourselves, or we take action against the picture, acknowledging it as an object. It is doubtless of enormous importance to know these tendencies of co-acting and imitation" (*Medizinische Psychologie*, pp. 276 ff.). "But it is doubtful whether we could ever come in this way to the acknowledgement of the personality of the other, because when I imitate instinctively it is again I myself who have the experiences, and the task still remains to find out how these experiences can become the experiences of another.... 'Einfühlung' does not lead us out of the circle of the ego, and we come back to the claim that there must be an independent experience of outside egos and outside personalities." I have only to add that the personality of the other person is based on his body-image.

Imitation is a term which comes to us from descriptive psychology. It is a term which indicates the fully conscious psychic life. The attempt made by Tarde and others to give some insight into the formal structure of imitation and its motives remains on the surface, since they do not consider the 'unconscious' psychic life. I may repeat that, according to Freud, psychic processes in the system of the unconscious have special characteristics. In the unconscious sphere, reality and representation are not separated from each other. Symbolization and condensation and transpositions take place. Psychic investment of one representation may be transferred to a similar one which then becomes the symbol for the primary representation. Unconscious experiences not only remain but also become efficient in the present. Whereas our conscious thinking does not stand for contradictions and tries to come to a unification of contradictive tendencies, the tendencies in the unconscious do not contradict each other. In this sense, doubtless, no degree of certainty and assurance, no relations, are of importance in the unconscious thought. Freud speaks of a system of the unconscious when he means this particular way of psychic action. Although he is of the opinion that psychic processes of that kind are generally not in the field of psychic awareness, he still thinks that occasionally psychic processes of the unconscious may become conscious, but may retain the systematic character of the system of the unconscious. The child, the primitive person, and the schizophrenic may, for instance, have unconscious processes in the field of awareness. I have gone a step further. I do not think that there are any psychic processes which do not possess the quality of awareness. Nor do I think that we can speak of a psychic unconscious if unconscious is to mean that there is no awareness.

(7) On *identification*

There are many psychic processes which remain in the background of consciousness as thoughts, atmospheres, 'Bewusstheiten' (Ach), and as germs of thoughts and pictures. Modern psychology and especially the thought experiments of Külpe and his School have enlightened us about the psychic background. Germs of thoughts are directions which we experience and which give their full meaning in the subsequent development of the thinking processes. I have characterized this psychic background of our experiences as the sphere. Psychic processes in this sphere certainly show the qualities which Freud ascribes to his system of the unconscious. His discovery of the *system* of the unconscious is indeed of enormous importance. But I do think that the processes in the psychic sphere also remain in the field of psychic awareness. When I developed the connotation of sphere, I intended also to show that there is a continual development in the process of thinking. Thought processes in the sphere are at first a general scheme, a mere diagram. Under the urge of an actual situation to which we want to adapt ourselves, we take out of the reservoir of our experiences those parts which fit in with the actual situation. There is a continual testing-out in the development of the thought-processes. Thought-processes are in this respect constructive, and a construction is guided by our system of strivings and desires, which are directed towards a single part of the reality. Psychology which neglects the system of the unconscious, the sphere, necessarily remains incomplete and superficial. Freud has already shown in his book on *Dream Interpretation* that many instances of so-called imitation can be interpreted in a deeper way. He uses the same instance with a riper interpretation in his book on *Mass Psychology*.

"When, for instance, one of the girls in the boarding-school has received a letter from the secretly beloved, which provokes her jealousy and to which she reacts with an hysterical attack, some of her friends who know about it will take over this attack, as we say, in the way of psychic infection. The mechanism is therefore identification on the basis of the possibility and tendency to put oneself into the same position. The others would also like to have a secret love affair and accept, under the influence of the feeling of guilt, the suffering connected with it. It would not be correct to assert that they appropriate the symptom out of sympathy. On the contrary, a sympathy originates out of the identification. This can be proved, since such infection and imitation occur under circumstances where there is still less sympathy present between the two persons than there usually is among boarding-school friends. The one ego has perceived an important analogy in one point—in our instance, in the preparedness for the same feeling. An identification in this point follows and, under the influence of the pathogenic situation, the identification transforms to a symptom which the one ego has produced. The identification through the symptom thus becomes the sign of a point of coincidence of the two egos which has to be kept repressed."[1]

I have little to add to this classic description. But I would prefer to use the term ' appersonization ' in cases in which the individual does not want to play the rôle of the other person, but wants only to adopt a part of the emotions, experiences, and actions of the other person. But in the instance given, a part of the body-image of the other person is also taken. The appersonization is an appersonization by body-image. The motives for appersonization can remain unconscious. We have, therefore, to do with imitation derived from unconscious motives.

But what is identification in its strict definition? In identification the individual identifies himself with persons in his actual or imagined surroundings, and expresses his identification in symptoms, either actions or phantasies. He plays a rôle, enriches himself by the experiences of others without knowledge of the procedure.[2] The identification takes place with persons whom we admire and with whom we are in love. In the development of infantile sexuality the little boy admires the father and wants to take his place. We may be dealing with a conscious wish. But often this wish will never come to a clear inner conception. He will only betray it by taking over gestures, habits, and trends of the father, which then become symptoms of identification. Since he does not know about his tendency to take the place of his father, he may not feel changed at all in his conscious personality. The imitation remains again in the unconscious, but is not so much imitation as taking the place of another person. But the fact that identification is in the unconscious makes it possible to identify oneself with several persons at the same time. We know that in the little boy there are not only tendencies towards identification with the father, though they may predominate, but also tendencies towards identification with the mother. This tendency

---

[1] Our previous discussion shows that I am unable to follow Freud when he states that sympathy originates from identification.
[2] Cf. my paper on homosexuality.

towards identification with the mother may come into the fore-ground in cases of homosexuality. But the boy may also identify himself with his nurse, with his uncle, with the footman, and with any one else in whom he is interested. By identification one may play the part of an enormous number of persons at the same time. We know that this is not only a possibility, but a psychological fact which is typical in every psychic development.

The process of identification is deeply based upon the emotional life of the individual. We identify ourselves with the love-object, though not completely, for if we do it completely, the love-object in the outside world has become superfluous and does not exist any more. Complete identification with the mother leads the boy to homosexuality: he himself is the woman, he does not need any other. Complete identification with the father will give him independent heterosexuality. The most important processes of identification take place in early childhood before the fifth year, but they never cease throughout our whole life. There is a continual 'unconscious' wandering of other personalities into ourselves. They may come nearer us, they may melt completely into us, or, as in the case reported above, the melting process may also remain incomplete from the point of view of the consciousness. But there is a continuous movement of personalities, and, we may add, of body-images towards our own body-image. I have shown above that when we take personalities and body-images of others into ourselves, we may try to get rid of our own personality and body-image and project them into others. A homosexual whose case I observed, and who identified himself with his mother, chose his boy lovers as images of his own personality before he identified himself with his mother. By the complete identification with his mother, he now attracts the same libidinous feelings which he himself primarily lavished on his mother. By the projection of his own personality into the boys, he assures for himself the full amount of love he once gave to his mother.

Freud rightly emphasizes that every identification is in the end ambivalent. The little boy not only wants to be like his father, but also wants to take the place of the father and become the father himself. The complete identification is the removal of the love-object, as is shown clearly by the instance of the homosexual given above. But we may add that just as conscious imitation does not secure a complete melting together of the body-images, in identification also the melting together of one's own personality and the personality of others is as incomplete as the melting together of the body-images in the conscious. They always retain some independence; they never form a complete unit and a new rôle, but the body-images of others remain as parts in the unconscious of the individual. We have known for some time that parts of the incorporated father and mother may retain their independence. The voice of conscience is the voice of the father, whose image has remained partially independent. We should also bear in mind that the unconscious body-image is built up by summations which do not lead to a complete unification. We are dealing with relations between totalities which do not lose their independence completely.

It may be asked how far the tendency to identification goes. Markuszewicz reports the case of a child who had lost a kitten of which it was very fond. It presently started to act like a kitten and to assert that it was the kitten itself. A similar observation was made by S. Ferenczi. A little boy aged $3\frac{1}{2}$ identified himself so far with a rooster that he started to crow and was interested only in chickens and other fowls. We need not go into the analytical meaning of this identification which has been clearly interpreted by Freud, we only wish to emphasize that the plasticity of the postural model of the body makes it possible to have the postural model of the body in common with animals.

It is fascinating to follow the remote possibilities of identification. They descend from the animal of the mammalian type to everything which is animated, thence to plants, and beyond that to the inanimate world, especially in so far as it moves. And the world is primarily a moving world. Rest is only a special type of movement. When we are connected with the world by identification, we derive from it the feeling of unity with the world. But at the same time the world remains different. It is an object towards which we are acting.

We have reached the final problem of identification. What type of action is based on identification? In the final analysis it can be only the action of another person towards the world, so that the direction and action of the individual remain the basic attitude. Actions are directed towards objects. Sometimes the identification helps in this direction towards the object. Identification is therefore not, as Freud states, the earliest and most original type of emotional cathexis.

Our primary emotional cathexis is directed towards objects. Before the boy identifies himself with his father he has an interest in him. It is true that he has to construct his own body and the father's body out of similar material. There will be a tendency to treat this material as one and to answer to every action of the other with an identical action of his own. But at any rate, even if we concede that, this tendency is not more primitive than the tendency to act towards objects. Freud contradicts himself when he says that, where identification exists, the aggression towards the person with whom one identifies oneself is restricted, and the person will be spared and helped. When there is an aggression, is there not already an object relation? Are not aggression and identification at least equals? Another passage of Freud's also contains the same contradiction.

"The study of such identifications which are, for instance, at the basis of the clan organization, leads Robertson Smith to the surprising conclusion that it is based upon the acknowledgement of a common substance (*Kinship and Marriage*, 1885) and can therefore be created by a meal which is taken in community with others. This trait allows us to connect such an identification with the primeval history of the human family as I have construed it in *Totem and Tabu*."

When the common substance is created by a meal, there must be a strong primary interest in the meal. But the meal is a substitute for the father. There is the need to devour the father, to kill the father, and to eat him up. But there is at least the primary tendency towards the object which is followed by the act of eating (identification).

Hoff and I have arrived at the formulation, based upon neurological studies, that there exist two types of actions, one based upon identification and the other based upon reactions towards the object. It is not possible to construe a greater primitivity of the one or the other type. It even seems that in many respects more primitive reactions towards objects are possible.[1]

In Gamper's case, in which the brain-stem was present, there was grasping and sucking. In Trömner's anencephalus grasping was preserved. But there is no hint of imitative movements. Also when we go deeply into the study of primitive organisms, there is little proof of mere identification and actions based upon it. I do not doubt that deeper study will probably prove that the identification tendency and movements based upon it are as primitive as movements directed towards an object. I consider that we are dealing with two original types. The facts at present available do not prove this contention; but they do prove definitely that the identification type is not more primitive than the objective type of action. Human beings are acting in the world and they are primarily acting in the world. This means that they are acting in relation to objects, either taking them or pushing them away. But strong as the tendency may be to act towards the world as we see it, there is also the tendency to unite the body-image with all other body-images. We deal with basic and conflicting tendencies.

We may even try to push the discussion further. We have seen that the little boy wants to become like his father and mother by

[1] Every function of an organism is connected with a direction of the organism to the place where this function occurs. The whole body is directed towards the stimulus. This being directed, a primitive reaction of reception or defence, is dependent on the muscle tone. But the tonic state of our body is of importance not only for the reaction of the organism but also for our experiences for the structure of our world in spatial, temporal, and qualitative relation for our conscious action and also for our thinking. So far Goldstein, with whom we agree completely. But there is no doubt that the changes in tone belonging to the induced tone are only a sector of the motor possibilities of the organism. Besides these mass reactions, which act mostly with one half of the body, there are more specific ones which are based upon this primitive function. In this group belong all reactions of grasping, taking, the ingestion into the body, as they appear in the primitive grasping reflexes. Here belongs also the sucking reflex which appears after special brain lesions. But here belong also a series of primitive defence reflexes. One is justified in opposing to the induced tone all those functions which have their central points in the striopallidar system and the pyramidal tract, all quick attitudinal movements, the primary automatism of C. and O. Vogt, and voluntary action in the narrower sense. One is justified in assuming that to every perception belongs a double series of motor actions—the kinetic and the tonic, the latter being doubtless the more primitive one. The kinetic functions have many levels. We may distinguish two important types, one being directed towards the object (object type), whereas the other imitates the movements of the objects (identification type). The tonic type seems to be only an object type. Identification and imitation do not appear to play an important part in the tonic reaction.

identification. He wants to have the same power, the same rights, and the same ability to conquer the world. Identification thus becomes, as I have pointed out elsewhere, merely a method by which we become better able to act in the world. I have already, in accordance with Freud, drawn attention to the idea that identification means taking the other object into one's self, and would interpret this as an action towards the outside world. If this discussion is on the right path, identification would be of service in acting in the world. When it conflicts with the action directed towards objects, we should not be dealing with a conflict between equals, but one between the world and the tool which has become of too great an importance. But, even so, identification and imitation cannot be derived from actions towards objects. Identification remains an inborn human drive of primary importance.

Freud has used his connotation of identification especially for the study of mass psychology, in which, like Le Bon, Sighele, and Tarde, he is especially interested. He recognizes that the relation between the hypnotizer and the hypnotized person can be compared with a mass in which only two persons play a part. The hypnotized person identifies himself with the hypnotizer. We may add that in this identification the body-image also plays some part. But it is questionable whether the fully developed body-image of the hypnotizer wanders into the hypnotized person. We shall meet later on the problem whether the body-image might not be much more primitive than the actual body perceived. But in order to decide this problem we must know more about the relation between soul and body. There cannot be any doubt that identifications are basic for human society. But identifications are not the only basis for human relations nor the only relation between body-images. It must be repeatedly emphasized that when we have construed the body-image of others as the expression of their personality, we act towards them as towards equals, and all the human relations take place between bodies. Identifications and imitations are only one part, although an important one, of these manifold human relations. It is true that every individual is social in his core, but this is only partially due to identification. Individuals see other individuals and bodies also independent from themselves. The following quotation contains, therefore, only a limited truth.

Bukharin (quoted by Kornilow), a noted Russian Marxian, describes in the following way this dependence of man in his social conditions. He says, "If we examine separate individuals in the process of development, we observe that essentially they are packed with the influence of their environment to the same extent that a sausage is filled with meat. A man is bred in his family, in the street, in the school. He speaks the language that is the product of social development, thinks with the conceptions worked out by a number of previous generations, sees around him other people with all their ways of life, sees before him the whole order of life, which influences him every second. Like a sponge, he continually absorbs new impressions. On this material he forms himself as an individual. Every individual, therefore, is social in his core. Every individual is a conglomeration of social influences, tied in a small knot."

It seems that the appreciation of the body-image of others is not far developed in animals. But the material we have on this point is very incomplete. Köhler observed that a group of chimpanzees got into an enormous state of excitement when one of its members was attacked, and that friends or the whole group would start a passionate defence. In adult animals this tendency is stronger. But our knowledge about these phenomena is too incomplete for us to venture to talk about the social image in animals. The studies made by Alverdes on the sociology of animals furnish some material. But there is no question that animals behave in a different way towards members of the same group and species than towards members of a different species. Our knowledge of this subject is, however, too incomplete to allow of further conclusions.

(8) Beauty and body-image

A. M., 29 years old, came to be analysed with the complaint that he was too ugly and that no girl who was in any way attractive ever fell in love with him. He had had several disappointments which upset him greatly. About two years before he started this analysis he had been analysed for about one year. He

R

was at that time refused by a girl named Anne. Since he felt that his ugly features were responsible for his rejection and the analysis failed to give him any particular relief, he decided to let himself be operated on and had a plastic operation on his nose. His nose was particularly offensive to him since it was in his opinion too Jewish. Since his disappointment about two years ago he had not had any deep love interest. Several months before the analysis started he had met a Christian girl in whom he was deeply interested. Shortly before he came to be analysed, he felt that this effort would also be a failure. One of the reasons why he wished to be analysed was that he wanted either to prevent this failure or to assure success when he fell in love next time. He was a young man, tall, with a comparatively small head, rather attractive, certainly not ugly in any way. Since the author had not seen him before his operation it is difficult to state what change the operation made. The patient did not express himself clearly on this point; he quoted others who said that before his operation his face was more characteristic than it was now, but seemed on the whole rather contented with the result. The analyst who analysed him the first time considered that the operation had indeed improved his appearance.

His family situation was as follows: his mother was 52 years old, and apparently very concerned about him. His father had died about seven years before of heart-disease. His mother had told him that she married his father after a serious disappointment. She considered herself engaged, but the man whom she really loved married another girl and she married for convenience' sake. After the death of his father, his mother had, according to the patient, tried in vain to attract other men. She felt elated when she could obtain the attentions of men and complained bitterly when she failed. The patient felt that the same lack of sex appeal which marred his life also spoilt his mother's life. He thought that she was not attractive and had to make an effort to attract married couples and friends. She had to give many invitations in order to get invited herself. In the patient's opinion there was a curse of unattractiveness and misery which afflicted his mother's family.

He hated his father's family because of their very semitic

appearance and specific Jewish qualities. There had always been a deep antagonism between the mother's and the father's family, especially his grandfather. His mother had been very ill after the birth of the patient, her only child. She blamed the family physician and especially her husband's father for her illness. She had to be treated for several years, was often in bed, and went several times to Europe. Whereas she was now on good terms with the physician who had treated her, wrongly according to her opinion, she had never pardoned her husband's father and his whole family. She always felt superior to them. After a few years she herself recovered, but then her husband started the heart-disease, to which he finally succumbed. She asserted that in the course of the marriage a deep feeling for her husband developed and that there were several contented years between her illness and his. The patient never acknowledged this part of his mother's statement, but remained firmly convinced that his mother's life was a failure because of her unattractiveness. In his childhood he had considered her a beautiful woman and especially admired her hair.

There were not many remembrances about his early life. (They did not come out in the analysis either). There were some vague remembrances concerning his mother's illness—presents brought home by his father when he came back from business trips. There was also a vague remembrance of a German nurse, who held him under rather rough discipline when he was three or four years old. He was rarely punished by his parents. He remembered only a few instances when he was deprived of his evening meal or was forced to stay alone in his rooms. The analysis made it more than probable that he had an extremely strong attachment to his mother, and that he accepted her hostile attitude towards his father and grandfather. His dislike for his grandfather especially was rather obvious and fully in consciousness. The grandfather died when the patient was seven or eight years old. Later difficulties in his life made him more and more dependent upon his mother. In spite of the fact that he wanted to be independent he stayed with his mother and told her almost everything, confided to her his failures in love affairs, and got excited when she got excited. She blamed him severely for being only interested in girls he could not get and threatening suicide when he was gloomy. When she got too excited about his being depressed, he said that life did not mean anything to him, and so filled her with despair. He felt compelled to talk over his sex affairs with his mother. His mother had always been against the analysis, and made considerable difficulties during the first analysis. The patient, who was not very successful in business, was also financially dependent on his mother. When he complained, she gave him a considerable sum, which he invested in stocks and lost almost completely.

When he was about four or five years old an important relation started with a male cousin who was older, stronger, and more independent than himself. Sex relations soon started. The patient was passive. These practices did not take place very often. At about ten or eleven, he started to go to a camp for several years. He had stopped his masturbation (connected with phantasies concerning his cousin). Whereas he had so far been considered as outstanding and clever, especially in reciting poems, the boys laughed at him in camp and treated him as greatly inferior to them. He accepted their attitude and felt miserable about it. But still he got on very well in High School and College, and there formed some intimate friendships. In his life generally, friends played an important part. He admired them very much. He thought that they were not only better-looking than he was, but that they also had more sex-appeal and more success in life. One of the girls in whom he was later interested married one of his friends. His other friends married attractive and beautiful girls whom he himself could never, in his opinion, have attained. He envied his friends very much, but often thought that his married friends looked down on him and sneered at him. He responded with a more or less open hatred, but still remained dependent upon his friends. He must always have somebody to whom he could complain about his erotic difficulties.

The analysis brought out that his relation to his friends was the continuation of his early dependence on his cousin, and that he assumed towards them the same passive and masochistic attitude as he had towards his cousin. It seems that his masochistic attitude, even before he met his cousin, derived nourishment from the illness of his mother who apparently was fond of complaining. There were therefore present not only an erotic, probably genital, sex relation to his mother, but also the tendency to identify himself with her, admiring not the father who, like the grandfather, was the object of a hatred which came from the Oedipus complex, but his mother's first lover who had rejected her.

The anal components in this relation already came to the foreground in the relation to his cousin which has been mentioned. In addition to that his mother often gave him enemas to which he strongly objected. These remembrances went back to his fourth year. He was therefore passive towards his mother, but he was also passive towards her supposed love-object, and then he became identified with his mother. It is understandable that before he came to the first analysis his bowel-movements were very irregular. He had a particular distaste for all dirty things; the smell of excrements was especially repulsive to him. In the same category was decay and the smell of corpses. He thought with disgust of the menstruation of women and of the body odour of women after intercourse. He felt revulsion when a woman went to the toilet. He had a horror of the word 'stench'. He was also horrified when he heard about cancer, mangling, and operations. He hated everything which might disturb the symmetry of the body. He was afraid of freaks in the circus.

He himself was very much afraid of being mangled and operated upon. When he was young he saw his father's sex-organ which seemed too big to him. A few years later the thought came to him that his own organ was too small. But this thought was provoked by the question of a physician. On several occasions he had had a fear that his phallus might be cut off. It was obvious that his castration complex was strongly developed. The specific childhood situation did not come out in remembrances. Reconstruction was also impossible. Connected with the castration complex was the feeling he sometimes had that he was hollow. When he was a child he had a strong feeling of guilt in connection with his masturbation and the fear that he might be found out. He also felt that it would be terrible if others heard anything about his sex activity. He had a general tendency to strong fear reactions, probably connected with early unremembered experiences when he was scolded for sex activity.

His special horror concerning operations led him to wonder how one could survive operations. When he was operated on for appendicitis at the age of seven or eight, he was especially afraid of being put to sleep, for he felt he would never wake up again. He often thought about death as an easy solution for his problems. He often talked of suicide, but felt that his suicide would also mean his mother's death. He had phantasies about a suicide-pact with her. (This would be the final union with her and at the same time a self-punishment for the illicit relation). Yet he was afraid that he might be knocked over by a car when crossing the street. He nursed the phantasy that he would die at the age of 31.

(His father married at the age of 31. This death-phantasy was a death-wish against his father whose place he wanted to take).

He had strong sadistic phantasies against those who treated him badly. He was dismissed from a previous position because some of the customers disliked him. He wished them dead. He was delighted that one of them failed in his business and that the other was abandoned by his wife. He also had phantasies of shooting his former employer. A murder case made a great impression on him when he was ten years old. When he was jealous of the girl with whom he was then in love, he developed the phantasy of disfiguring and killing his rival. But he went further in his phantasy and imagined that the girl he loved gave herself to the man to whom she was betrothed and then drowned herself when he left her. He imagined that he killed her former fiancé at the funeral. He was thoroughly ambivalent concerning this love-object, who during the analysis refused definitely to marry him. One of his dreams read as follows:

"We were coming out of the house with R. (his love-object). A perverted man holds us up. It is some kind of spell. It is a dark figure. Maybe he wants to kill me and do something to her (assault). Feeling horror, I get afraid and ask him to let me go and then to let her go. I go and pick up stones. We ran. We threw stones through the windows in order to get help.

"In the next part of the dream we tried to get into a taxicab.

The taxicab went on, the driver was like one dead. We both fall in the mud."

The first part of the dream shows the fear of castration and death in connection with the sexual wish. In the second part of the dream the idea of the suicide-pact with his mother comes back. The common suicide means at the same time an illicit sex relation which is forbidden and ugly. He liked to read poems about lovers riding to death together. On the other hand he was afraid that his mother might harm him and herself when she got into a rage.

It was a compromise between his fear of death and his wish for life that he drank and smoked a considerable amount and felt that he might die in this way.

His destructive death-wish and suicidal tendency also came out strongly when there was a failure in his love-life. He felt then that he was nothing, that he was not alive at all, and cursed his body because of its ugliness. He often had the feeling that he was not alive. His childhood remembrances seemed insubstantial to him. His ideal was complete beauty. He thought only about beauty. In his opinion, human beings are ranged in a strict line according to their beauty. He thought that only a beautiful man could get a beautiful woman. Beauty was in some way the central idea of his life. He did not want to marry a girl who was not really beautiful, but he felt that he could never attain his wish. He was afraid that he might die before he had reached his aim. He badly wanted to be married. But he fell in love with beautiful girls after they had indicated that they would refuse him. He had a strong idea that one should marry when one is very young. He was terribly disappointed that he had not yet married. He admired his friends who were married. Marriage seemed to him to be an almost final attainment. It is remarkable that only the beauty of women appealed to him. If he could not attain it, nothing seemed to be worth while at all. He thought he had already lost eight or nine years of his life. He was afraid of the competition of other men, and felt that he could not compare with them. It was his misfortune that his friends were especially handsome and successful in marriage and love affairs. He defended his point of view ardently from an intellectual point of view. In spite of the fact that he did not consider himself gifted he was proud of his intellectual reasoning. His narcissism came out in this particular way. It was difficult to bring him from intellectual reasoning to free association. It was therefore very difficult to get the transference which was necessary to enter into the deeper layers of his personality. He tried to use the analyst as friend and adviser in his peculiar love difficulties.

Under those conditions the analysis was certainly an incomplete one. But the case does not interest us so much from a purely analytic point of view. We are interested in the problem of beauty in its relation to the body-image. It is clear that for our patient, beauty meant beauty of the body. Freud writes in *Civilization and its Discontents*, p. 35: "The science of aesthetics examines the conditions under which we experience beauty. It could not give an explanation of nature and genesis of beauty. As usual, the lack of results is hidden by a display of full-sounding and empty words. It is bad that psycho-analysis also can say the least about beauty. Only its origin out of the field of sexual feelings seems assured. It is an exemplary instance of a tendency which has not reached its aim. Beauty and charm are primarily qualities of the sexual object itself. It is remarkable that the genitals themselves, the look of which is always exciting, are almost never considered beautiful, but it seems that the character of beauty is connected with certain secondary characters of sex."

We must emphasize that sexual excitement and its derivative beauty must therefore be connected with the postural model of the body. Our case does not help us to say what beauty is. He was very vague and indistinct about this question. But it is remarkable that he saw beauty only in the body of others and missed it in his own body. It is worthy of remark that his sexual drive was strong, but that in spite of this his sexual activity was rather limited. At the age of puberty a servant girl interfered with him and he had a few incomplete sex relations with her. He then became afraid that her husband might find out about it and kill him. He also felt ashamed and degraded about it. He had a few casual sex relations afterwards, two or three before he came to the analysis. He never got any particular pleasure out of it. Sex organs did not interest him very much. When he came to the analysis, his knowledge of the female sex organ was rather limited and incorrect. He never dared to think about sex activities with his real love object, although he dreamt occasionally about it. In sex contacts to which the analyst forced him, he had a tendency to detach this sexuality from his other sexual life. He never actually felt sexually excited in the presence of those women with whom he was deeply in love.

The philosophers who are interested in aesthetics have always emphasized the absence of an immediate interest when we are enjoying from an aesthetic point of view, and see in some way, in the detached attitude, an important characteristic of the aesthetic attitude. This may be true from a merely descriptive point of view, but when we consider the beauty of the human figure, we see immediately that aesthetic interest is certainly closely connected with interest in sex and therefore with a very urgent and very actual need. The beauty of the human figure does not provoke the desires immediately, but it contains in itself the germ of the development of desires. When we remain purely in the field of aesthetics we repress the immediate urge. The individual feels that he can command his desires; that he is not forced to follow them. I have written elsewhere: " It is remarkable that it was a long time before the beauty of landscape was discovered, and we may suppose that the original aesthetic values are to be found only in the animate world. This is therefore important, because the beauty of the human figure has an open relation to sexuality. It is clear that the aesthetic influence disappears when the sexual desire becomes stronger, and we arrive at the conclusion that the aesthetic object elicits instinctive attitudes, but that these attitudes are prematurely inhibited and interrupted, so that aesthetic enjoyment, although it offers rest and relaxation, does not bring a full satisfaction of desires, and remains, therefore, distant from the object. When we consider the fates of human beings near us, we may remain in an aesthetic attitude. But we shall never enjoy a tragic event in an aesthetic way if we do not have an inner distance to this event. Therefore we shall never have an aesthetic enjoyment concerning our own experiences unless we depersonalize them and put them before us like the experiences of strangers."

"The aesthetic object thus offers a promise and a half-satisfaction of desires, and these desires are characterized as incompletely satisfied and unfinished by the fact that in the aesthetic picture more than one desire seeks expression and satisfaction. One may say, in accordance with this point of view, that the aesthetic object provokes experiences in this sphere. The aesthetic effect consists in the fact that instinctive attitudes are provoked but not despatched. Aesthetic experiences are unfinished and cannot even be finished. Schopenhauer's view that the essence of aesthetic is in the abolition of will and striving is therefore partly true. The aesthetic object gets its colouring through the damming up of the instinctive energy. The person who enjoys aesthetic experiences enjoys the free play of his desires without the appropriate responsibility."

But there is no question that aesthetic enjoyment is empty if it does not point beyond itself and does not point to the final possibility of action with the full responsibility which every action carries with itself. When Plato in his *Republic* has only a very limited estimation for art and the beauty of the single object, he expresses a feeling which is based upon the final dissatisfaction of aesthetics.

It is worthy of remark that in our case the extreme appreciation of the beauty of the female is the result of very complicated psychic processes. His mother's early illness and his hatred against his father provoked in him the ideas of beauty which were erected against the father. He wanted to take the place of the uglier father, but was always afraid that he would not be able to do so. The identification with his father, his ugliness, and later on his weakness and illness and his mother's lack of love for his father, increased in him the fear of castration, and the fear of being put into an inferior rôle. All these elements thrust him into a situation of identification with his mother who was ill. This passive and masochistic attitude was increased by the enemas his mother gave him. The passive anal homosexuality with his cousin was a natural consequence of the earlier infantile situation. The Oedipus complex in his ramifications became the motor for the development of his ideal of beauty. It is remarkable how strong the anal components are in this picture—his particular fear of rotting, faeces, death and decay. Since castration is irregularity, he was afraid of everything which might disturb the symmetry of the body. His adoration of beauty meant therefore a desire to take the place of his father, to be different and superior to his father, not to be castrated, not to be passive, not to have to take the place of the diseased mother, not to indulge in his anality, not to be passive in an anal way. It is obvious that such a history was bound to hinder his approach to beauty, and to make his endeavour to come nearer to the beloved object a futile one.

We come, at least in this case, to an insight why the adoration of beauty checks the action. The patient's attitude towards the beauty of others was closely related to his attitude concerning his own body-image, and the adoration of the beauty of others was closely connected with the depreciation of his own postural model of the body. We thus understand that the actual change in his appearance by the operation on his nose did not bring about a great change in his attitude and his success. Our own body is, as we have stated before, an image, and is built up in ourselves in accordance with our instinctive attitudes. An actual change in the appearance can therefore only have a limited result. It is true that a cosmetic operation may occasionally change not only the body but also the body-image. We may build up the body-image again. We may look into the mirror and project the mirror-image into ourselves. We may also study the changed attitude of others and transfer it to our body-image. But all these factors will not have a decisive influence when they are not able to change the psychic attitude of the individual. These considerations also explain the special difficulties in plastic operations, which will set in motion so many of the deep-lying pregenital activities.

We should not underrate the importance of actual beauty and ugliness in human life. Beauty can be a promise of complete satisfaction and can lead up to this complete satisfaction. Our own beauty or ugliness will not only figure in the image we get about ourselves, but will also figure in the image others build up about us and which will be taken back again into ourselves. The body-image is the result of social life. Beauty and ugliness are certainly not phenomena in the single individual, but are social phenomena of the utmost importance. They regulate the sex activities in human relations, and not only the manifest hetero-sexual activities, but also the homosexual ones which are so important for the social structure. In the case of our patient, the admiration for his friends who were, in his opinion, better endowed than himself, plays an enormous part. Our own body-image and the body-images of others, their beauty and ugliness, thus become the basis for our sexual and social activities. We like to believe that our standards of measurement of beauty are absolute.

The unprejudiced study of the ideas of beauty of the human body in different societies offers considerable difficulties for this point of view. When we leave the borders of our own cultural race, it is very difficult to keep up the standards of beauty. It is sometimes impossible to appreciate the beauty standard of primitive races, but even when we compare our own beauty standard with the beauty standard of the yellow, brown, or black races, the integration into a general law is not a simple task. It is difficult for us to understand that the crippling of the feet in the Chinese is considered by them to increase their beauty. We need not even go so far for an example. It is hard for us now to under-stand that the crippling of the female figure by a tight corset ever conformed with the general ideas of beauty. Tattooing, pulling out the lips, and many other disfigurements which are supposed to be decorations in primitive societies are other instances of this kind.

We understand the actual changes which different societies perform on their bodies when we study the instinctive desires and drives. The ideal of beauty and the measurement of beauty will always be the expression of the libidinous situation in society. This libidinous situation is necessarily changeable. I do not want to give the impression that I adhere to a relativistic idea of beauty. There are laws of libidinous structures, but the libidinous structure changes its manifestations according to the whole social situation, and in this way the manifestation of beauty will also change.

Body-images and their beauty are not rigid entities. We con-struct and reconstruct our own body-image as well as the body-images of others. In these perpetual processes we interchange parts of our images with the images of others, or, in other words, there is a continual socialization of body-images. It is one phase in the continual stream of libidinous desires, a phase where we feel that no immediate responsible action, either social or sexual, is forced upon us, where the action can remain an un-accomplished germ, or where the action may be a play. The treacherous character of beauty is based upon this. We are, after all, not able to perceive without acting. We are not able to main-tain the attitude of merely perceiving without acting. Action is not something added to the passive reception of the experiences of the world; action and reception are an inseparable unit. There is no play which is only play, there is some responsibility in every play. We like to deceive ourselves with the thought that we may dispense with actions and that we may act not as personalities as a whole but may reserve our final inner commitment. But we know in the core of our personality that the real beauty of life lies in its inexorability and seriousness. This is in some respects the same idea as that expressed by Plato in his *Republic* (Plato, *Republic*, Book v).

"And this is the distinction which I draw between the sight-loving, art-loving, practical class and those of whom I am speaking, and who are alone worthy of the name of philosophers. How do you distinguish them? he said.

"The lovers of sounds and sights, I replied, are, as I conceive, fond of fine tones and colours and forms and all the artificial products that are made out of them, but their mind is incapable of seeing or loving absolute beauty.

"True, he replied.

"Few are they who are able to attain to the sight of this.

"Very true.

"And he who, having a sense of beautiful things has no sense of absolute beauty, or who, if another lead him to a knowledge of that beauty is unable to follow—of such an one I ask, is he awake or in a dream only?

"Reflect; is not the dreamer, sleeping or waking, one who likens dissimilar things, who puts the copy in the place of the real object?

I should certainly say that such an one was dreaming.

"But take the case of the other, who recognizes the existence of absolute beauty and is able to distinguish the idea from the objects which participate in the idea, neither putting the objects in the place of the idea nor the idea in the place of the objects—Is he a dreamer, or is he awake?

"He is awake."

Absolute beauty lies beyond beauty in action.

In discussing the beauty of the body, we have so far only considered the body at rest. But this is a great schematization of the problem. The fact that we have so far considered the beauty of the form more than the beauty of the function has a deeper meaning. As soon as we leave the state of rest and start movement, it is much more difficult to remain in the attitude of what Kant has called, 'Interesseloses Wohlgefallen'. We are immediately stirred up to a more energetic action. It is true that when we build up our own body-image and the body-image of others, we always tend to build up something static and then to dissolve it again. We always return to the primary positions of the body. When we think about a person running, we see him changing from one primary position into another primary position. Primary positions are positions of relative rest. The positions in between the two primary positions are neglected and even the movement is neglected as such. To use a simile taken from physics, we may say that we are less interested in what is going on in the field, we are not interested in the continual flow, but more or less in the quantums, the crystallized units of the postural model. We should, however, realize that our own body-image and the body-image of others is not only a body-image at rest but a body-image in movement. But beauty is especially connected with the body-image at rest. It is owing to this that we are so astonished when we see a single phase of any movement in a photograph. It does not seem to be natural. The process of the human being in motion is reconstructed by ourselves according to the laws of the body-image.

It is conceded that the main object of art is the human body. Joachim Winckelmann says in his *Erinnerung über die Betrachtung der alten Kunst*, "The highest subject of art for thinking man is man or only his outer surface, and this is as difficult to explore for the artist as its inside is for the sage. And the most difficult subject is beauty, although it seems paradoxical. But beauty, properly speaking, is not subjected to number and measurement." "If someone asked me to determine the sensual connotation of beauty, I would not hesitate to construct it according to the single parts taken from the most beautiful human beings in the place where I am writing. But I would restrict myself to the face, because of shortness of time."

Winckelmann has emphasized that the chief outstanding sign of the Greek masterpieces is a noble simplicity and acquired greatness, in the posture as well as in the expression. "As the depth of the sea remains always quiet however much the surface may rage, the expression in the Greek statues shows a great and determined soul in spite of all passions. The more quiet the posture of the body is, the more apt it becomes to describe and express the true character of the soul. In all postures which deviate too much from the state of rest, the soul is not in its proper, but in a forcible and forced state. More recognizable and characteristic is the soul in violent passions. But it is great and noble in the state of unity and rest" (*Gedanken über die Nachahmung der Griechischen Werke in der Malerei und Bildhauer-kunst*). It is well known how strongly Winckelmann has influenced the art-theory of Goethe and Schiller. It is the classicistic theory which is based upon the body-image at rest. One knows that in all romantic and baroque epochs, the interest is transferred from rest to motion. The expression of passions comes more and more into the foreground and the states in which the body-image is in danger of being disrupted move more and more into the centre of the artist's attention. Epochs like these will always be inclined to sacrifice the abstract idea of beauty. They will be more interested in the phases of change in the postural model than in the states of rest where the postural model is undisrupted and stabilized. It would be of interest to find out what factors led Winckelmann to regard Greek art from this particular point of view. Modern investigations have made it at least probable that Winckelmann has misrepresented the spirit of Greek art and that he has overlooked its wild striving and wrestling for expression and motion. We may suppose that

Winckelmann himself was trying to escape violent sexual desires and that he fled from action into the world of beauty which was for him rest. It appears that Winckelmann suffered as much from his homosexuality as Schopenhauer from his heterosexuality. Art was for Schopenhauer a method of throwing off the pressing power of will and life and escaping into the realm of relative inactivity.

Plastic art necessarily neglects the colour of the human body. But there is no question that colour is of enormous importance in the image of the human body. Although one might think that it should be very simple to know the colour of the human body, yet nothing is more changeable, more elusive, than this very colour. It is true that the configuration of the human body, the changing lights will provoke many variations. But there is, in addition, the ever varying play of movements, which gives an additional life to the surface of the body. There are also the continual variations of the tone of the skin, its turgidity connected with the variation in the blood supply and the water absorption. But even when we consider these factors, it remains unexplained why the colour of the human body is again and again a surprise to us. Painters have incessantly tried to catch this colour. The nude body and bathers are the eternal problems of painting. They reflect the surprise we feel again and again when seeing the various colours of human bodies. It may be said that this is due to our social habits which generally hide the body. But the colour of the human face is not less mysterious. And when one sits in a stadium and looks about, one wonders about the mysterious appearance of the faces of thousands.

The same difficulties that we have in building up the postural image of the body arise when we try to build up a deeper knowledge of the colour of the human body. There is no question that an explanation is only possible when we keep in mind how many interfering libidinous tendencies are attached to the image of our body. And the uncertainty concerning the colours of the body, our never flagging curiosity concerning the body, emphasize the dynamic character of our knowledge of the human body and of our body-images. It would be a fascinating problem to go through the history of painting and study the various ways in which the different ages have seen the human body and especially its colour. All these different interpretations reflect our change in attitudes towards the body and its colours and different stages in our libidinous development. Our own body is in no way better known to us than the bodies of others. We should not use the mirror so eagerly if it were otherwise. The interest we have in mirrors is the expression of the lability of our own postural model of the body, of the incompleteness of the immediate data, of the necessity of building up the image of our body in a continual constructive effort.

(9) *Variability of the body-image*

We regard beauty as being primarily connected with the beauty of the human body. The problem of beauty is therefore closely linked with the problem of the body-image. But I have shown that the body-image has great variability and derives its parts not only from other human beings but also from animals. We have mentioned the deep connection which the primitive man feels between himself and everything that is animated. But is there not a stage in which we see body-images everywhere? Is there not a stage where the soul and the body-image are practically all over the world? Is there not an animistic phase in human development? Identification exists between ourselves and our fellow beings. There are identifications with persons of the same sex and with persons of the other sex. These identifications triumph above differences in sex, age, and race. We could even go further, as the previous deductions have shown, and say that all these persons outside ourselves are necessary to build up the picture of our own body. When we have built up our own body we spread it again all over the world and melt it into others. It would be wrong to conclude that collective processes go on. There is no collective body-image; but everybody builds his own body-image in contact with others. There is, however, a constant giving and taking so that it is true that many parts of body-images are common to persons who see each other, meet each other, and are in an emotional relation to each other. Lévy-Bruhl has interpreted this as the law of participation and primitive collective representations. "I should be inclined to say that, in the collective representations of primitive mentality, objects, beings, and phenomena can be, though in a way incomprehensible to us, themselves and something other than themselves. In a fashion which is no less incomprehensible they give forth and they receive mystic powers, virtuous qualities, influences, which make themselves felt outside without seeming to remain where they are.

"In other words, the opposition between the one and the many, the same and another, etc., does not impose upon this mentality the necessity of affirming one of the terms, if the other be denied or vice versa. This opposition is of but secondary interest. Sometimes it is perceived and frequently, too, it is not. It often disappears entirely before the mystic community of substance and entities which, to our way of thinking, could not be associated without absurdity. For instance, the Trumai (a tribe of Northern Brazil) say that they are aquatic animals—the Borroros (a neighbouring tribe) boast that they are red Arraras (Parakeets). This does not merely signify that Arraras are metamorphosed Borroros and must be treated as such. It is something entirely different. The Borroros, says Von den Steinen (who would not believe it, but finally had to give in to their explicit explanations), give one seriously to understand that they are Arrarars at the present time, just as if a caterpillar declared itself to be a butterfly. What they desire to express by this is actual identity, that they really can be both. They are human beings and birds with scarlet plumage at the same time. All communities which are Totemic in form, admit of collective representations of this kind implying similar identity between the individual members of a Totemic group and their Totem."

It is impossible for us to grasp the real meaning of participation unless we study the laws of identification, and we are especially interested here in identification from the point of view of the schema of the body. If we follow carefully the way in which body-images communicate between various persons, there can be no doubt that there exists, not a collective image of the body, but a collection of the various images of bodies. This collection is not in the full light of consciousness. In the terminology of psychoanalysis this would be called unconscious identification. I prefer to talk of the background of the consciousness or to use the term ' sphere.' Identifications are spheric experiences. I do not want here to go deeper into the question whether Jung's collective unconscious does exist or not. I merely express my belief that Jung's conception is erroneous when it implies that there is a real identity in the unconscious of various persons. It is true that the deeper we go into the structure of the personality, the more the similarity between the various persons increases, and identification and projection play a more and more important part. It cannot be denied that a further-going uniformity in actions and feelings may result when the deeper layers of the personalities break through. Then in these deeper layers, identification and projection continually take place. But there is no question that even the expressions of the deeper layers of the personality are expressions of personalities. A collective unconsciousness as an entity does not exist, but deep similarities exist in the deeper layers of the personalities, which are increased by the give and take of projections and identifications.

We are, however, less interested here in the general question than in the question of body-images. There exists an individuality of body-images besides their close interrelation with the body-images of others. The quotation taken from Lévy-Bruhl shows clearly that identification takes place not only with human beings but also with animals. We may add that some primitive tribes believe themselves to be descended from plants and therefore consider themselves plants too. But we have seen how plastic the postural model of the body is. The plasticity of the postural model of the body makes multiple identification possible also with shapes which are very different from the fully developed body-image. But does this identification stop with the animate world, and is there not a possibility of identification with everything which moves? It is a great question whether primitive races do not see life in every movement and whether the world to them consists primarily in motion. It is indeed an opinion widely held by anthropologists that some primitive peoples believe that the working powers in the universe are of a psychological type. Tylor writes in *Primitive Culture*, vol. 1, pp. 428–9, 4th edition, 1903:

"It seems as though thinking men, as yet at a low level of

culture, were deeply impressed by two groups of biological problems. In the first place, what is it that makes the difference between the living body and the dead one? What causes waking, sleep, trance, disease, death? In the second place, what are those human shapes which appear in dreams and visions? Looking at these two groups of phenomena, the ancient savage philosophers probably made their first step to the obvious inference that every man has two things belonging to him, namely, his life and his phantom. These two are evidently in close connection with the body, the life as enabling him to feel and think and act, the phantom as being his image or second self; both, also, are perceived to be things separable from the body, the life as able to go away and leave it insensible or dead, the phantom as appearing to people at a distance from it. The second step...merely the combining the life and the phantom. As both belong to the body, why should they not also belong to one another, and be manifestations of one and the same soul?...This, at any rate, corresponds with the actual conception of the personal soul or spirit among the lower races, which may be defined as follows: a thin, unsubstantial, human image, in its nature a sort of vapour, film, or shadow; the cause of life and thought in the individual it animates, independently possessing the personal conscience and volition of its corporal owner, past or present; capable of leaving the body far behind, to flash swiftly from place to place; mostly impalpable and invisible, yet also manifesting physical power, and especially the appearing to men, waking or asleep, as a phantom separate from the body to which it bears a likeness; continuing to exist and appear to men after the death of that body; able to enter into, possess, and act in the bodies of other men, animals, and even of things.... These are doctrines answering in the most forcible way to the plain evidence of men's senses, as interpreted by a fairly consistent and rational primitive philosophy." (Quoted in Lévy-Bruhl's *How Natives Think*, pp. 80–81.)

A similar view is taken by Frazer (*The Worship of Nature*, vol. 1, p. 6):

"When man began seriously to reflect on the nature of things, it was almost inevitable that he should explain them on the analogy of what he knew best, that is, by his own thoughts, feelings, and emotions. Accordingly he tended to attribute to everything, not only to animals, but also to plants and inanimate objects, a principle of life like that of which he was himself conscious, and which, for want of a better name, we are accustomed to call a soul. This primitive philosophy is commonly known as animism. It is a childlike interpretation of the universe in terms of man. Whether or not it was man's earliest attempt at solving the riddle of the world, we cannot say. The history of man on earth is long; the evidence of geology and archaeology appears to be continually stretching the life of the species farther and farther into the past. It may be that the animistic hypothesis is only one of many guesses at truth which man has successively formed and rejected as unsatisfactory. All we know is that it has found favour with many backward races down to our own time."

A newer development of anthropology has, however, discarded Tylor's view. Preuss insists that magic is prior to animistic theories. Vierkandt expresses this view in the following way: "Magic actions are primarily and in their nucleus free from the representation of supernatural beings in their co-operation. They trust only in the power of the man who exerts them, who is convinced that he can get the result he wishes. Representations of the direct or indirect help of supernatural beings are secondary. The representation of such supernatural beings, especially the belief in souls which can exist outside the body, proves that the so-called animism is subsequent to the magic art and originates only in connection with it. There is a preanimistic age of religion."

Lévy-Bruhl has put forward similar ideas. In a previous book I showed that in psychotic patients of the schizophrenic and paraphrenic group the idea of magic is prevalent—and a magic which is not connected with the ideas of soul. But, at any rate, the acting power in the universe is, in the opinion of primitive peoples, of a psychological type. I wrote: "The connotations which in primitive peoples point to the magic substance of Orenda, Manna, and Wakan, are closely related to the connotation of energy of nature. We have considered that whatever inspires adoration and fear is called Wakan. The idea of acting powers derives a part of its importance from the fact that these acting powers are significant for the individual."

Whenever we study primitive magic we see that it is connected with specific parts of the body and especially with those which have a libidinous significance. In Case 5 of my publication, the magic influence is due especially to ' Wünschelchen ' (wish-beings) which are a span long, which one can carry in the pocket, and which come out of the pocket of a man down his trousers. They push a needle into the private parts of the patient. There is no question that they symbolize the magic power of the phallus. In other words, magic power is connected with parts of the body-image. We thus arrive at the formulation that animism supposes a complete body-image, whereas magic power and magic art are connected with an incomplete or undeveloped postural model of the body. Animistic theories are thus partially justified. Will and will power, acting psychic forces, are by their innermost nature bound to the body-image and especially to those parts of the body-image which have a special libidinous significance. But guided by the ethnological material, we must give renewed attention to the problem of the soul. I have emphasized that the body-image is not confined to the borderlines of one's own body. It transgresses them in the mirror. There is a body-image outside ourselves, and it is remarkable that primitive peoples even ascribe a substantial existence to the picture in the mirror. Witchcraft connected with mirrors is in this respect of great significance.

The same is true of the shadow. "Often the savage regards his shadow as a reflection of his soul, or, at all events, as a vital part of himself, and, as such, it is necessarily a source of danger to him, since it may be trampled upon, struck, or stabbed. He will feel the injury as if it were done to his person, and if it is detached from him entirely, as he believes it may be, he will die" (Frazer, *The Golden Bough*, part II, pp. 77 ff.). "At critical periods the life or soul is sometimes temporarily stowed away in a safe place till the danger has passed."

We have indeed seen how easily a phantom may leave the confines of the body. I do not think that the physiological data concerning the postural model of the body can explain the beliefs of primitive peoples. After all, the body-image is only a part of our whole life. But it is important to study the facts here from this one-sided point of view. The physiology and psychology of the body-image doubtless form the basis of the belief of primitive peoples. It has often been pointed out that dreams are one of the sources for the primitive peoples' belief in souls. But I have emphasized that dreaming is also a state of mind in which there is an enormous change in one's own body-image as well as in the body-image of others. The changeability, plasticity, and transportability of the body-image thus lead us to a deeper understanding of the belief of primitive people. But is not this primitive thought also a part of our own thought, and do we not find more clearly in the mind of the primitive person that which in our own life remains in the background of experience?

Magic thus becomes the influence of complete and incomplete body-images upon each other. In this respect the observations quoted above to the effect that the paranoic often feels influenced not only by the body of others, but also by his own body take on a new significance. From a psychoanalytic point of view the whole body-image often symbolizes an important part of it, especially the genitals. When the primitive person and the paraphrenic feel that the world is directed by psychic substances, the image of the body in its ramifications is behind it. In primitive thought the world becomes an interrelation between body-images. When the body-images are in any way complete we may talk of souls, otherwise we may talk of magic.

The problem of being possessed must also be connected with the problem of the postural model of the body. Another body wanders into the body of the possessed person. In an interesting observation made by Bender,[1] the persecutors spoke out of the body of the possessed person. They entered primarily through the rectum. They were the father and mother and the aunt. But the drawing the patient made rendered it probable that the persecutors were really parts of her own body and especially her faeces. The patient also said that they smelt. She said at the same time that they were like ether, electricity, or souls. The observation shows clearly the ambivalence towards the excretions which one wants both to keep in the body and to expel from the body. They are parts of the body-image, but they become independent.

[1] It will appear in the *Psychoanalytic Review*.

And since they have once been parts of the body-image, they may have the same value as the body-image itself.

One last remark about the dead body in its relation to the body-image. Since the body-image is a creation which uses raw experience only as material, death does not destroy the body-image of another person. We build up also in the dead person the body-image of a living person. Since the body-image and its parts are so often interchangeable, we understand that every part of the body of a dead person remains connected with him. Even his clothes retain a part of his personality. It has often been emphasized that dreams about dead persons add to the belief in their immortality. I have mentioned that the body of a fellow-being is built up and constructed like a picture of imagination and like a picture of a dream. The continuation of the body-image in dream and phantasy retains, therefore, an important part of what we actually perceive in fellow human beings. The dead, therefore, do not disappear from the community of the living. They remain in this community as long as their pictures are revived in any members of the community.

I have repeatedly emphasized that every isolated psychological study is necessarily artificial. The body-image does not exist *per se*, it is a part of the world. And even if we suppose that in some stages of development the whole world consists of parts of bodies, still the outside world is also there in a less structured form. This outside world becomes, however, clearer in the developed experience of the fully conscious mind. On the other hand, there is not only an outside world of a structure different from the body-image, but there is also a personality, the whole world of psychic life, as far as it is the expression of an ego, of a subject. But it is true that in every experience the body-image is present. It is one side of the full experience which comprises the personality (the true ego), the body, and the world. We have merely taken the body as one of the three spheres of experiences which constitute life and existence.

So far we have followed up the body-image through the realm of perception, through the realm of sociology and aesthetics, fully conscious of the one-sidedness of the methods. We have to emphasize it again when we approach the field of ethics. Moral laws can only find an application to human beings with a body, and moral phenomena are therefore closely interwoven with our own image and the image of others. It is, according to our previous discussion, not a mere figure of speech when we emphasize that the pain and suffering of one person can never be an isolated phenomenon. The laws of identification and of communication of body-images make the suffering and pain of the one the concern of everybody. This may be called psychic infection, but the term is not quite appropriate to the facts explained above.

The same is true of joy. Emotions which find their expressions in the postural model of the body in the tone, in the motility, in the vaso-vegetative system, necessarily pass over from one person to others. When we have the primary intention of helping another person, of showing him some degree of kindness, we do it out of the same spirit by which we desire our own preservation and satisfaction. When we are troubled by the hunger and misery of our fellow-beings, we base this immediate and primary tendency upon the deep communication of the body-images. There is no reason why we should neglect, as Freud does, these primary tendencies concerning others. They will be different according to the variations of the emotional and spatial distance of the body-image of the other person. It is true that there will certainly also be aggressive and destructive tendencies against the body of that other person, since our own body is torn and recreated and torn again. There is no reason to believe that one of the two tendencies is primary. But the constructive forces are always present, even if the destruction is in the foreground of the scene.

There is also another fact of enormous importance. Our own body-image gets its possibilities and existence only because our body is not isolated. A body is necessarily a body among other bodies. We must have others about us. There is no sense in the word 'ego' when there is not a 'thou'. We not only tolerate others; their existence is an inner necessity for us. We may need to destroy them but we must also have the tendency to preserve them and to build them up. We are interested not only in our own integrity but also in the integrity of others. Just as the integrity of our own body and its preservation is a moral value, the preservation of the bodies of others is a moral value too. But the body-image is not only destroyed and endangered by pain, disease, and actual mutilation, it is also torn and endangered by every deeply-lying dissatisfaction and libidinous disturbance. We come therefore to the conclusion that there is a moral law not only to preserve the form of the body of another as we perceive it with our senses, but also to preserve or to restore his libidinous structure, the regulated function of which is the only basis for a full and harmonized postural model of the fellow human being.

This formulation is very one-sided. It formulates the problem only from the point of view of the body-image. There is no body-image without personality. But the full development of the personality of another and its values is only possible through the medium of the body and the body-image. The preservation, construction, and building-up of the body-image of this other thus become a sign, signal, and symbol for the value of his integrated personality. In this respect the study of the psychology of the body-image may lead to a system of ethics and a system of morals. Pain, joy, destruction, mutilation, death, are thus the concern of those who are near to us, but a magic stream connects the nearest with those who are farthest, and goes from there even to the animal, to the plant, and to the inanimate world.

It would, however, be erroneous to say, "Do not hurt others because by identification you will suffer". We have the same immediate interest in the absence of suffering and the destruction of the body-image in others as we have in our own body-image. We want to help others; we have primary interests in them, not less dear than the interests we have in ourselves. We act freely towards our fellow human beings. There are deep connections between our actions and interests towards ourselves and our actions and interests towards others. The preservation of the body-image of another person is an ethical value in itself. It is true that there is again a tendency to destroy our own body-image as well as the body-image of the other. But is not destruction merely a way to renewed construction, which is, after all, the meaning of life?

CONCLUSION

When one looks through the older text books of psychology, one can hardly find anything else but descriptions of sensations. These sensations are considered partly in connection with the outward senses like hearing and seeing and partly in connection with irritations coming from the inside of the body, body sensations. But in the voluminous books by Wundt and Titchener there is no mention of the body as an entity and as a unit. In this book we consider the body as a unit and as an entity. We are here in better accord with the philosophers, especially with Scheler, who emphasizes the unit of the body and considers it necessary to differentiate between the body as we perceive it with our outward senses and the body based upon the inner consciousness which is not present concerning the inanimate. He uses for this inner body the German word 'Leib'. In his opinion the 'Leib' is independent of the sensation of the inner organs; it is different from single sensations and different from any other object. He emphasizes that our body (Leib) is always given to us as a unit with some more or less vague structure. It accompanies all organ sensations. I am unable to follow him when he tries to differentiate the inner sensations constituting the 'Leib' and the other body. There is only one unit. It is the body, and there is an outside of the body and a substance of heavy mass which fills this body. But it is true that the body in this sense is always present; it is not the product of sensations, but is co-ordinated with the sensations which get their final meaning only from the unit which is one of the fundamental units of our experience.

It belongs to these *a priori* data of our experience that there are other units present like the unit of our own body, and finally that there are also units outside this body, which are, at least for the fully developed consciousness, different from the unit of the body. It is true that it is problematical whether such inanimate units are data of primitive experience. But we cannot doubt that they are data of fully developed experience. There is a world partly animate, partly inanimate, there is our body, and finally there is a personality which has this close and specific relation in the body. These structures are given from the beginning. No analysis can go beyond them. And it would be wrong to try to dissolve them into an aggregate of single parts. We have the three specific categories of world, body, and personality. It is one of the main functions of philosophy and psychology to determine the relations of these categories to each other.

It is true that the world is not a unit in the same sense as the body and the personality are units. The structure of the world is much looser, less closely knit than the structure of the body. The world as a whole has many parts which are separate units, as, for instance, other human beings, animals, objects. There are also many gestalten around us. The psychology of experience would have to determine the relation of these gestalten to each other and to the gestalt of one's own body. It would not have been worth while to undertake this task if the structure of this gestalt, which has certainly a deep importance for the meaning of life, did not help us to an insight into gestalten generally. The contention of the gestalt psychology is that gestalten simply exist in an external world. They are already present in the objects of physics. They wander from there to the perceptive apparatus, i.e. through the optic sphere.

In the optic sector physiological processes develop which immediately correspond to the psychic experience of gestalt. The question whether there exist physical gestalten, which originate immediately from the nature of the nervous system, is called the Wertheimer problem by Köhler. "Als Wertheimer Problem soll kurz die Frage nach solchen physischen Gestalten bezeichnet werden, welche aus der Natur des Nervensystems abzuleiten, also jedenfalls in ihm möglich sind, und welche den Eigenschaften phaenomenaler Gestalten entsprechen." According to Köhler, the physical gestalten which occur in the nervous system and there gain psycho-physical significance, must have analogies or parallel qualities, like the gestalten in the phenomenological experience. "We consider that the contrast between physical world and consciousness and especially between nervous functions and phenomena is generally represented in an exaggerated way."

"...Müssen wir uns sagen, dass der Gegensatz von physischer Welt und Bewusstsein, besonders aber der von nervösem Geschehen und Phänomenen, gewöhnlich etwas übertrieben dargestellt wird." Köhler comes to the conclusion: "Denn was innen ist, ist aussen" (What is inside, is outside also). He also writes: "Wir sahen, dass phaenomenale Gestalten nächste Verwandte in bestimmten anorganisch-physikalischen Gebilden haben, und finden jetzt, dass gestaltete Geschehens—oder Zustandsarten im optischen Sektor des Nervensystems, an denen wir die Eigenschaften jener anorganischen Vorbilder voraussetzen, in wesentlichen Zügen mit der Konstitution des zugehörigen optisch-phaenomenalen oder Gesichtsfeldes übereinstimmen dürften".

"We found that phenomenal gestalten have their nearest kin in certain inorganic physical structures, and find now that shaped occurrences and states in the optic sector of the nervous system, in which we suppose the qualities of those inorganic examples, probably coincide in essential features with the constitution of the corresponding optic-phenomenal or visual fields." But Köhler has protested against Woodworth's formulation: "Finding configuration to exist outside the organism, they suggest that it passes by some continuous flux into the organism, so that there need be no unfigured stage in the organism's response".

There are innate gestalt tendencies; there is a tendency to experience gestalten in their pregnancies; there is a tendency to perceive circles; there is a tendency to complete incomplete gestalten. There are good and bad gestalten ('gute' and 'schlechte Gestalten'). All these phenomenological experiences are based on the actual physical process and on the configuration of the processes in the optic sector. That the right angle is a 'good gestalt' and an angle of 80° a 'bad gestalt' has nothing to do with experience. Gestalten are given by their own value and not by experience. When a chimpanzee finally finds out that he can get a banana from outside his cage by using a stick or a branch of a tree, one is dealing with an insight, the creation of a new gestalt. This new configuration takes place when the inner tension has become overwhelmingly strong. It is a reorganization of experiences, not a simple learning. There are also inner tendencies to the development of gestalten and tendencies in the gestalt to dissolve out of inner reasons. Sander speaks of form emergence. If, for instance, an observer is presented with an irregular interrupted linear figure, lighted up on a dark surface, in extreme miniature, but gradually growing to normal size, he will often experience, with an intense emotional participation, a process of form emergence as out of the continued light nebulae. At first, figures arise, as a rule circular, which in comparison with the end figure are distinguished by greater wholeness, compactness, and regularity, and approach the irregular final figure only step by step.

"...we may gather the trend of the psycho-physical substructure which we are considering. The trend is towards close contours, towards compactness, in short, towards geometrical regularity, symmetry, softening of all curvatures, parallelism, towards general as well as detailed conformity to the primary, spatial axis, the vertical and the horizontal, finally towards an optimum of configuration on the level of geometrically primitive, non-connotative, purely aesthetic significance." But Sander means also that inner processes are going on, in which the general activity of the person is more or less negligible.

Let us compare these theories of gestalt psychology with the experiences of the body image. It is true that there is an immediate experience of something we call the body or the bodyimage, but this first experience is incomplete and far from distinct; and even for this very primitive postural model the contact with external reality is indispensable, and experience already modifies the most primitive body-image which can be thought of. But experience is not accepted in a passive way; parts of it are taken and rejected again. The image of the body is constructed, and, as in every construction, there is a continual testing to find out what parts fit the plan and fit the whole. The individual will try to get more and more impressions, because he wants to come to definite formations. The gestalt will be built up not in a continuous flow of experiences, but in distinct levels and layers, and a higher layer will contain a new element of structuralization or organization. Motion and action are necessary for this development. For this construction and organization not only the present experiences are used, but also the past, and the function of memory is to have material ready for new organization. Memory, learning, and experience are based on the fundamental psychological fact that past experiences do not disappear from our mind and can therefore be utilized for new organizations. Gestalt psychologists have tried to prove that only the process of organization is of importance, but they have neglected the fact that memory and learning are basic for the possibility of organization.

Gestalt psychology takes little account of the value and importance of attention. On the other hand, Köhler refers to the reorganization of the field of experience under the stress of a given situation. But what else is attention than being directed towards a situation by emotional needs? Such a direction, due either to the situation itself or only to the inner needs, will necessarily have an enormous influence on the organization. (Cf. my *Medizinische Psychologie*). Attention and action are not very different from each other. The individual is actively directed towards the acquisition of data concerning the world and his own body. The knowledge of our own body is the result of a continuous effort. There is no development of the postural model of the body which is only due to inner factors. It is true that maturation takes place. We do not know exactly when it stops. But maturation is not mechanical development. The development is guided by experience, trial and error, effort and attempt. Only in such a way can we gain the organized knowledge of our body.

There are tendencies which try to make the body-image complete, but it cannot remain so without a renewed effort. There are opposite tendencies as well. There is a tendency towards the dissolution of the body-image. When we close our eyes and remain as motionless as possible, the body-image tends towards dissolution. The body-image is the result of an effort and cannot be completely maintained when the effort ceases. The body-image is, to put it in a paradoxical way, never a complete structure; it is never static: there are always disrupting tendencies. With the changing physiological situations of life new structuralizations have to take place, and the life situations are always changing.

I am inclined to wonder if what is true of the body-image is not also true of gestalten in general. I consider that the connotations of gestalt psychology are too static and do not acknowledge sufficiently the never ceasing psychic activities. The body-image is based not merely on associations, memory, and experience, but also on intentions, will aims, and tendencies. It is now almost generally accepted that the connotation of association is only a theoretical construction. Associations do not exist in reality. The mind is never a mere slate. There are always processes of arranging and re-arranging the actual experiences according to the needs of the total personality. We could talk of associations when these active processes have been reduced down to a minimum. They can never disappear completely, and therefore real associations do not exist. We have found constructive and destructive tendencies in the psycho-physiological structure of the perception of the human gestalt, but one finds the same principle in the emotional and libidinous life, which is necessarily connected with every perception and especially with the body-image. Since I have the conviction that the emotional life is the nucleus of psychic experiences and the immediate expression of the life forces, we have to expect that in the emotional life the principles we have discovered concerning the sensual perceptions will stand out in a more distinct way. We find, indeed, the drive to renewed experiences, the drive to completion of the experiences, the drive to build up the total libidinous structure, and finally the tendency towards the destruction of what has just been created in order to create and construct again ; and all these developments are the expression of changing attitudes of the personality and its motility. The personality stands in varied situations of life which make changing adaptations necessary. Emotional attitudes directed by the life situations direct the construction of the libidinous half of the body-image as well as its sensual part.

In a paper on complexes I once wrote: (1) Every complex has as its basis instinctive attitudes which are given by the factors of coherence in the living situation and by the facts of the libidinous constitution. (2) These situations are very typical. Out of this typical situation originate, for instance, the Oedipus complex, the castration complex, and the complex of the integrity of the whole body and dismembering. (3) There are always new developments in the complexes. On the basis of primitive complexes, new complexes are based. In such a newly developed complex the previous parts of the complex remain. Finally, every complex of an adult is a new attitude based upon prior primitive attitudes which remain as parts in the whole of the complex. (4) Complexes which were incomplete tend to become complete. Complex parts tend to bring the whole complex again into being. (5) The architectonic structure of a complex which reaches back to the earliest age is dependent upon the instincts and desires which only in the minority act in the full light of consciousness. Voluntary attention (by attention I mean the dynamic factor of the instinctive attitude and not the resulting clearness of the experience) has only a limited significance. (6) The final development of a complex is dependent upon the individual experiences and attitudes, and therefore upon the experience. (7) The laws which occur in experimental studies of the memory and in experiments concerning thinking are the same as those which come out in a study of the real, more complex attitudes of life. The problems of gestalten and complexes can therefore also be studied by the psycho-analytical method.

I wrote these sentences in a study which was devoted to the problems of emotional life, to the problem of complexes in an analytical sense. Those experiences of great emotional value will determine our actions and feelings, even if they are not in the full light of the conscious personality. In this study also I met the fact that there are entities which lie in the physiological constitution and in the immediate reality of the situations, factors one is entitled to call gestalten. This means that every child must come into a situation in which it is, from a libidinous point of view and from the point of view of instincts generally, dependent upon the adult person. The psycho-physical structure of the child will necessarily develop special psychic attitudes. We may regard such a situation and its additional libidinous attitude as a comparatively rigid unit which has to be considered as an entity. The different parts of the unit are closely related to each other, or, in the words of Bühler and G. E. Müller, there are strong factors of inner coherence in this situation.

But even such typical situations must vary according to the differences in the situations. We know, for instance, that the Oedipus complex takes another shape in communities in which

T

the mother is dominant (Malinowski). But it is obvious that the development and the laws which govern these complexes, which are, after all, gestalten in the realm of meaning and emotion, are dependent upon experience and actual situations. Wertheimer, Köhler, Koffka, and Lewin are inclined to disregard the fact that the organisms and the individuals are always struggling, that they repeatedly come into new contacts and change with every new contact. The conception of the gestalt theory is too static. It neglects the dynamic factors which we can only understand in connection with the actual problem of the personality.

This study has not, however, been undertaken to gather material for or against the gestalt theory; its aims are not critical but constructive. I wanted to know how human beings arrive at a knowledge of their own body, and this research was undertaken with the idea that the insight into the psychological sphere of the knowledge of one's own body must lead to an insight into psychological and physiological laws.

 Our experience of our own body is based upon optic and upon tactile impressions. The postural model of the body can therefore be disturbed by lesions which destroy or impair tactile sensations and by lesions which destroy or impair optic sensations. It seems that cortical lesions are more efficient in this respect than lesions of other parts of the nervous system. But the postural model of the body can also be disturbed by cortical lesions which do not immediately impair the tactile and the optic sphere. We have to do with immediate disturbances in the postural model of the body by cortical lesions. The point from which the postural model of the body can be disturbed is probably in the parieto-occipital region. The cortical apparatus is necessary for the final integration and utilization of the afferent impulses.[1] But it would be wrong to assume that peripheral lesions do not disturb the postural model of the body. We can have a postural model of the body only when we get sufficient data with the help of the peripheral apparatus. The peripheral apparatus, therefore, plays as important a part as the central apparatus. We should not draw too

[1] I agree with Köhler when he assumes that the impulses are not merely conducted in an unspecific way through the peripheral apparatus, but that there are already specific qualities and configurations in the outside world, and that also the conduction is also specific.

strong a contrast between centre and periphery, for ultimately they form a unit.

Head has emphasized the importance of posture in the body, and has therefore referred to the postural model of the body. It is true that in order to build the body-image we have to know where the different limbs of our body are. But beyond that there must also be a possibility of orientating ourselves about the relation of the different parts of the body to each other. It is not probable that the localization of sensations of the skin is given immediately. But the sensations are qualitatively different from each other. The final connection between these qualitatively different points on the surface of the body is found out by optic experience and by our continual activity in localizing on the body, either by touching it or by moving of our muscles. Even the tactile localization of a single touch is not an immediate gift of the outside world to our consciousness; it is necessary to work it out, to gain it by experience in an active effort. An organic lesion may make this effort difficult or useless. The whole constitution of the body goes into this primitive structure and experience. Symmetrical parts of the body are physiologically connected with each other. But the relation between the symmetrical parts is only an outstanding instance of the laws which govern the relation between the different localizations of the sensations of our body.

Investigations on alloparalgia and alloaesthesia make it probable that the connection of symmetrical points is guaranteed by sympathetic nervous elements as well as by spinal connections. The whole process of co-ordinating and using the data of the various senses and their correlation to each other, the production of the local sign of a touch ('Localzeichen'), is not based upon reasoning in the full light of the consciousness.

The structure of the body-image in its purely physiological sense is to a great extent based upon processes which remain in the background of the consciousness. It is there that an active construction of the image of the body takes place. It is true that a part of this construction is certainly completely out of the field of consciousness, but it is also represented by conscious and 'unconscious' psychic processes. In the experiment of the Japanese illusion, a clear insight is afforded into the way in which, with complicated methods and continual endeavours, we get a final orientation in relation to our own body. Movements give us new tactile impressions which help us to determine the relative localization of a point touched.

Anton and Babinski's studies on anosognosia further contribute to an understanding of the structure of the postural model of the body. Patients of that kind either do not appreciate a paralysis which they have suffered or they even completely forget one side of their body. When one side of the body is not acknowledged, a part of the sensations may be transferred to the feeling side of the body. The transfer can be, but need not necessarily be, connected with motor impulses. The neglect of impressions of one half of the body, the non-perception of one half of the body, may occur without a transferring of the impulses to the other side. It can be based upon mechanism of the so-called purely psychic type. But it can also be based on organic mechanisms. This organic repressive mechanism can be a general one, 'Korsakoff,' but it can also be a mechanism based upon a focal lesion. The organic repression may either lead to overlooking the hemiplegia or it may lead to a total neglect of one side of the body. It may also lead to illusions and distortions concerning the perception of this side. In the majority of those cases disturbances of the sensibility are present which point to a serious lesion in the central pathways; but there is a disturbance in the special parietal mechanism, the integrity of which secures the tactile postural model of the body. All these mechanisms must be undisturbed if we want to obtain a full insight into the postural model of our body.

Every phenomenon in the psycho-physiological sphere—and all that goes on in the body belongs to the psycho-physiological sphere—contains a multiplicity of factors. The nervous system in itself is built up in levels of different integration. The higher levels of these integrations become more closely related to the psychic layers and show an increasing similarity to the mechanisms of the psychic sphere. The mechanisms which we have called the mechanisms of organic repression are in many respects similar to psychic mechanisms, but neither conscious nor unconscious psychic processes are connected with them. In the normal function all these mechanisms are integrated and form a unit. In the pathological cases, a part of this mechanism comes into the foreground.

The various parts of the postural model of the body are differently assessed according to the needs of the individual. The middle line is of special importance. The relation between left and right is a relation in the postural model of the body.

Perceptions, in the whole field of psychology, only have a meaning as the basis for actions. The postural model of the body, the knowledge of the limbs and of their relation to each other, is necessary for the start of every movement. In all actions directed against one's own body the knowledge of one's own body is also necessary. When the knowledge of the limbs is not sufficient for the start of the movement, the individual will increase his knowledge by testing movements. Knowledge without movement is always incomplete. The space of our body has a special characterization, but in addition a spatial knowledge is necessary about the arrangement of the separate parts of our body, if we desire a successful movement towards the separate parts of our body.

In the phantoms of persons who have lost their limbs more or less suddenly the postural model of the body finds its clearest expression. The attitude towards the phantom shows that persons afflicted with the loss of a limb want to re-create the integrity of the body. They are especially successful in this re-creation when there are paraesthesias of peripheral type which help in the constructive process. The physiological structure of the phantom and of the postural model of the body generally is itself very similar to the psychological structures which are concerned with the body as a whole and its integrity. Psychological factors determine the final shape of the phantom and also the final shape of the non-perception of parts of the body.

In hysterical cases and in cases of so-called allochiria, the psychogenic part of our emotions connected with the postural model of the body provokes phenomena very similar to organic repression. Not only are voluntary and semi-voluntary active movements necessary for the building up of the postural model of the body, but also the whole tonic state of the body will shape the postural model of the body. It is especially the tone of the postural and righting reflexes which distorts the postural model of the body, and in the tone a correct postural model of the body will be built up. But among these changing attitudes and the various impulses, the postural model of the body is in danger of no longer giving any definite help. It is in danger of changing like Proteus. The only remedy is the building up of primary postures. These postures are motor as well as sensory postures. It is worthy of note that we tend to neglect deviations from these primary postures. The primary postures are creations and constructions which give us a firmer stand concerning external situations.

In the postural model of our body, not only an outline is given. There is also a surface. It gets its definitiveness only in connection with optic impressions, but there is also a perception of what is going on in the inside of our body. In the inside of our body we feel mainly the heavy mass. We feel the heavy mass of our own body in the same way as we feel any other heavy mass. We do not feel anything else but the heavy mass inside our own body. All other sensations are felt very near the surface. Our appreciation of mass and heaviness changes with the tone of the muscles.

It is a matter of course that an irritation of the vestibular nerve will change with the tone the postural model of the body. This is true for rotatory movements as well, but it can also be studied very clearly in progressive movements in quick elevators. Here there are dissociations in the heavy mass of the postural model of the body, and part of the heavy mass leaves the body in the form of a phantom. The vestibular nerve contributes to the unity of the postural model of the body, especially to the unity of the heavy mass with the optic part of the body.

Pain is always connected with the postural model of the body, but cerebral lesion can dissociate pain from the postural model of the body. But the pain distorts the postural model of the body. An enormous number of somatic factors contribute to the postural model of the body, yet it is still a unit with different parts of various significance.

There are some general aspects of the experience of one's own body. It is certainly not a given unit, but a unit in development. There are four general levels which continually interfere. The first is the purely physiological level which is sympathetic, peripheral, spinal. The psychological processes connected with this level cannot yet be formulated. There is a second level which is connected with the focal activities in the brain. The mechanism as such is physiological but it continually sends reflections into the consciousness. The cases of non-perception of one half of the body are in this category. A third level has to do with the general organic activities connected with the cortical region. This mechanism is, for instance, disturbed in the Korsakoff psychosis. It is in its nucleus organic in the common sense, but it is an organic life which is closely akin to the psychological life. The reflection into the consciousness is stronger in the second level, while the third can be understood from a psychological point of view. The organic process here seems to be like a frozen psychological process. And finally there is a fourth level in which the processes go on in the psychic sphere but influence what is going on in the somatic sphere. There is a continuous interaction of these four levels of the postural model of the body.

This formulation has a significance which exceeds the special problem of the postural model of the body. We may suppose that the whole psycho-physiological life is built up in similar levels and that the interaction of these various levels is characteristic of organic life. Of course, the idea of various levels, the nervous integration, is not new. It plays a great part in the writings of Jackson and also of Head. It would certainly be easy to show that there exist not only the four levels of the type characterized here, but many more.[1] I would not deny that. But here we are only interested in the four principal levels. The literature so far has considered these levels merely from the point of view of organic neurology and has not considered their psychological bearing. Only Adolph Meyer has considered the psycho-physiological integrations. We deal also with different physiological and psycho-physiological levels. It may be asked whether the implication is that the physiological level with no reflection into the consciousness is really the basic one from which the others originate. I think that such an idea would be totally wrong. It is generally

[1] Orton has distinguished three levels in the cortical function.

accepted that activities of organisms are primarily psychic activities. In the highly developed organism there are primarily psychic activities, which partially take place in the full light of the consciousness. They have the character of logical thinking and logical intention. But many of these psychic activities take place in the background of the consciousness and have, to put it briefly, a symbolic or a spheric character. They fall into the category of Freud's so-called 'unconscious'. But all these are psychic experiences. They belong to our fourth cortical and psychic level, and here we have the primary activities of the psyche.

When some of the organic functions lose immediate access to the consciousness, we have to do more or less with a process of changing the psychic attitude into a merely physiological one to make a tool out of something which has been primarily a function. I do not think, therefore, that the first level is in any way prior to the second, third, and fourth. If one wants to make a construction, it is certainly simpler to derive the physiological function from the psychic function than the reverse. We know at any rate that the psychic function of exercise and adaptation brings with it a change in the function of the central nervous system and in the muscles. It is generally accepted that the function primarily creates the form. It is true that when the form is once created it may also have an influence on the function. But it is at least probable that form and function belong necessarily to each other and that function is necessarily psychic, or has at least a psychic part. It is probably an essential characteristic of organic life that there are several levels of integration which influence each other and penetrate each other.

If we wish to understand the development of the postural model of the body, we are not justified in saying that the physiological level is a primitive one and the psychic level a complicated one. We must try to understand the postural model of the body from a purely psychological point of view. The primitive postural model of the body shows a lack of differentiation of the separate parts, the impressions of gravity prevailing, and we deal more or less with an undifferentiated filled bag which differentiates itself by continual contact with the outside world. Motility is an outstanding factor in this development. As the study of phantoms shows, the postural model of the child is never completely lost. There are different strata of body-images which are incorporated in the body. Even the so-called physiological investigation shows that our own postural model is not closely defined; it is changed by every object which touches the body, and it is related to the postural model of the persons around us. Besides its other qualities, space has qualities which are connected with the postural model of the body. Right and left, below and above, in space are extensions of the postural model of the body.

So far we have dealt with the somatic part of the postural model of the body, or, in other words, with the perception of the postural model of the body. But it is clear that even the perception of the postural model of the body does not lead to a rigid and clear-cut entity. There is nothing definite about the perception, there is nothing static about it. There is a continual struggle to reach a static picture and to model something which is continually changing into a structure.

I would like to emphasize that this is even true about the perceptive side of the body-image. The body which seems so near to ourselves, so well known to ourselves, and so firm, thus becomes a very uncertain possession. Investigations of this kind take away the ground from most philosophical speculations which try to base the experience of life on the knowledge of the body alone and, still worse, on the sensations. I have shown that sensations get their final meaning only in connection with the postural model of the body.

Vestibular experiments and observations of amputated people have shown that every body contains in itself a phantom (perhaps the body itself is a phantom) in addition. It is obvious that the phantom character of one's own body will come to a still clearer expression in dreams, which, like phantasies, show a particular variability. The study of the postural model of the body has so far been one-sided. Only the perceptive side of the postural model of the body has been taken into consideration. One may say that it is in some way the body from the point of view of the ego in psycho-analytic nomenclature. According to my terminology, I would interpret the body from the point of view of the perception ego. There is no question that there are emotional needs expressed also in the mere perception and the action based upon it. There is some emotivity connected with the perception as such. But we know that there exists a strong libidinous life besides the mere functions of perceptions and actions based upon it. We talk of the libidinous structures or, in a more general terminology, of the emotional instinctive drives and desires.

The emotional life plays an enormous part in the final shaping of the postural model of the body. Emotional influence will change the relative value and clearness of the different parts of the body-image according to the libidinous tendencies. This change can be a change in the surface of the body, but it can also be a change in the inner parts of the body. There may be a change in the subjective appearance of the skin, there may be a loss of sensation concerning any part of the body, there may be a forgetting of one limb of the body or of one side of the body.

There may be changes of the perception of the gravity of the body. The heavy substance of the body may be loosened, may become foamy and even permeated by holes, or there may be a consolidation in the inner parts of the body. The libidinous structure will express itself in the various accents given to the diverse parts of the postural model and a subsequent appearance in their shape. What goes on in one part of the body may be transposed into another part of the body. The hole of the female genital organs may appear as a cavity in other parts of the body. The male sex organ may come out as a stiffness (like a piece of wood) in some other part of the body. We call this the transposition of one part of the body to another.

One part of the body may be symbolic for another part. There must be a natural foundation for this symbolic substitution. The nose may take the significance of the phallus. Every protruding part may become a symbol for the male sex-organ. The cavities and entrances of the body are freely interchangeable. Vagina, anus, mouth, ears, and even the entrance of the nose belong to the one group of openings. Our body consists, after all, of openings, cavities, and protrusions. In hypochondria, the symbolic interchange of organs provokes sensations in the body. The symbolic interchange may determine sensations in an organ or attitudes concerning these particular organs. Our attitude towards the different parts of the body can be to a great extent determined by the interest other persons take in our body. We elaborate our body-image according to the experiences we acquire by the actions and attitudes of others. These may be words or actions directed towards our body. But the attitudes of others towards their own bodies will also have a great influence. Diseases which provoke particular actions towards our own body also change the postural model of the body. Early infantile experiences are of special importance in this connection, but we never stop gathering experiences and exploring our own body.

We may take parts of the bodies of others and incorporate them in our own body-image. This is called appersonization. But we also play completely the rôle of others, identify ourselves with them, and this may lead to a particular attention and attitude towards parts of our own body.

The emotional unity of the body can only be maintained when the Oedipus complex has been reached and full object relations have been developed. The prevalence of sado-masochistic tendencies leads to a disruption of the postural model of the body. Psychogenic pain is one of the expressions of sado-masochistic tendencies that change the attention concerning the organ which is in the centre of the sado-masochistic attitude. In hypochondria we have to do with a transposition of the genitals and their libidinous investments to other parts of the body. This transposition can take place on the surface or in the inner parts of the body. The genitals are experienced as isolated and not connected with persons.

In neurasthenics we find an anal sadistic attitude towards other persons and accordingly a disruption of the postural model of the body. Their relations to other persons and their individual life experiences accordingly play a very important part. Anxiety connected with sado-masochistic tendencies may lead to a far-going dismembering of the whole body. In depersonalization they fight against genitality, and object relations lead not only to the elimination of genitals but also to other parts of the postural model which symbolize the elimination of sex organs.

Identification and appersonization play an enormous part in

the building up of the body-image. When the changes in the body-image symbolize the sex organ, the sex organs which are meant are often the sex organs of other persons which are regarded as whole personalities. The disruption of the postural model seems to be less violent in cases of hysteria. According to the extent of the disruption of the libidinous structure in psychosis, the postural model undergoes very considerable changes. The violent sadism of melancholics leads to an almost complete dissolution of the libidinous structure and of the postural model of the body, with a consequent action which brings the change of the postural model of the body into the field of reality. The emotional and libidinous level leads, therefore, to the final shape of the postural model of the body. No other structure can help us so clearly to understand the emotional life and its influence upon the perception of objects.

The change in the libidinous attitudes is again closely related to the life experiences of the individual and can only be understood in this way. The attitudes towards the life situation, the inner life history, will lead either to a different accentuation in the postural model of the body, or to a different perception of it connected with different sensations in it. But it will finally change the body itself. The postural model of the body is not merely a psychic addition to the solid structure of the body, but also a physiological entity with physiological consequences influencing the functions of the organs and possibly also their form and growth. The postural model lies on the way to conversion. Its changes may occur in the sphere of images, thoughts, voluntary or involuntary actions, and finally, in actual vasomotor and vasovegetative changes in the organ. Conversion is based upon the constitutional factors, upon the somatic constellation which reflects into the postural model of the body and the libidinous situation which gives the final shape to the postural model of the body.

The problem of organic disease can only be understood when we go into the problem of the postural model of the body. A symptom may be organic or psychogenic and is always connected with the postural model of the body. The ways in which the postural model may be prepared from the organic side as well as from the psychogenic side for a symbolic transposition in the form of an organic disfunction of a particular organ, can be studied in the light of the postural model of the body. Organic disease and psychogenic disturbance lead in the same way to suffering. Suffering expresses itself necessarily in the postural model of the body. Mental suffering finds its way into a somatic expression, and somatic disease leads to mental suffering.

The mental problems and libidinous conflicts of the neurosis lie in the centre of the personality and flow from there to the periphery of the personality and into the postural model of the body. Psychogenic disturbance has necessarily a centrifugal character. It expresses itself in a neurotic symptom, or even in an anatomical change which is created by a centrifugal psychic process. In organic disease the process begins in the periphery of the experience and provokes the changes in the central attitudes. The organic process is therefore centripetal from the point of view of the psychology of the central ego and postural model of the body. The difference between an organic and a psychogenic disease is merely a difference in the psychic direction.

Beyond this formulation we come to the insight that one of the fundamental characteristics of psychic life is given in the continual change of experience concerning the imaginary centre of the ego. There is a continual wandering of experiences in centrifugal and centripetal directions. The postural model of the body can be attacked from outside as well as from inside. The libidinous conflicts continually change the body-image. There is an intake and an output; a tendency to keep the body-image within its confines, and to expand and extend it; to keep its parts together, and to dissipate it all over the world. The deepest inner forces of the human mind, unit and part, integration and differentiation, find their immediate expression in the postural model of the body, which is the creation and the creator of constructive and destructive tendencies.

Movement and expression belong to the destructive phases in the continual process of change in the postural model of the body. Already in the perceptive sphere we note a close interrelation between the postural models of the bodies of different persons. But they are still more closely connected in an emotional and libidinous way. Whenever there is a particular interest in special parts of the bodies of others, the interest is also given to the same parts of one's own body. Whenever there is an abnormality in one's own body, the same parts of others are watched. Social life is based upon the interrelations of postural models. Nakedness and shame are connected with the social importance of the body-images. Blushing and social fear become particular difficulties in relations with other human beings. Sexual irritations change the postural model of the body, not only in its isolation, but also in its social significance. By identification and appersonization, our own body-image becomes united with the body-images of others, which retain a relative independence.

A body-image is in some way always the sum of the body-images of the community according to the various relations in the community. Relations to the body-images of others are determined by the factor of nearness and farness and by the factor of emotional nearness and farness. Body-images are nearer to each other in the erogenic zones and are closely bound together in their erogenic zones. The transfer of erogenic zones will reflect itself in the social relation to other body-images. Erotic changes in the body-image are always social phenomena and are accompanied by corresponding phenomena in the body-image of others.

Our own body-image and the body-image of others are not primarily dependent upon each other—they are equal, and one cannot be explained by the other. There is a continuous interchange between parts of our own body-image and the body-image of others. There is projection and appersonization. But also the whole body-image of others can be taken in identification with others, or the whole body-image can be pushed out as a whole. The body-images of others and their parts can be integrated with the whole body-image and can form a unit, or they can simply be added to our own body-image and form then merely a sum. There exists a social image of the body. These processes between individuals may make them in parts identical. But they are still processes between individuals. When an individual has socialized his postural image it still remains his postural image. There does not exist a postural image of the community, or a 'we'.

Social psychology is always a psychology of individuals under the condition of social life. Social life will provoke the tendency to identify ourselves with others. Imitation is one part of it. Identification is closely based upon the identification of body-images. But social life is based not only upon identification but also upon actions, where the full object character of the other person is preserved. There are two conflicting tendencies, one which by identification takes others into ourselves, and another, not less strong, which needs others as independent objects. We deal here with a social antinomy of a far-going importance.

Beauty is a social phenomenon. The human body, its postural model, is the primary object of plastic art and painting. The beautiful object provokes sexual tendencies without satisfying them, but at the same time allows everybody to enjoy it. Beauty thus becomes suspended action, and it is understandable that the classicist ideal does not desire the expression of strong emotion and violent movement. Beauty is also giving up one's own final claim for the benefit of all. Beauty is again a phenomenon of enormous social importance.

Ethics also must be based upon our appreciation of others as human beings with human bodies. The laws of ethics are also based upon the tendency to identification, the tendency to projection, our inner need that others should exist, and, more than that, should be satisfied, integrated, and should have their full and undisturbed postural model of the body. When there is, concerning one's own personality, a tendency to destroy and to build up, to construct and destroy, the same tendency must be present concerning others too. The other self is not a projection of the own self, and the own self is not an identification with the self of the other. There is a primary experience that we live in a world where there are other personalities, other bodies, besides ourselves.

Ego or 'thou' are not possible without the other. Our own body-image is not possible without the body-images of others. But when they are created, they are created in a continual interchange. These are the outlines given by the facts of human organization and organization of life in general. One may call these facts *a priori* facts. Ego, thou, personality, body, world, are separate entities, but then there occurs the continual psychological process which changes the relation between the ego and the world, between the ego and the body-image, between the body-images of various persons. The *a priori* scheme, the empty shell of life, the symbolization of the general conditions of life, reaches its final complete meaning when life is not a general philosophical connotation, but an actual process of varied experiences and life situations. I am inclined to believe that the purely philosophical method is insufficient in view of the manifold and varied facts of actual experience and situations. And we cannot even understand the *a priori* data if we do not go through the varied experiences and actual details. Of course, whenever we go back to the actual facts and the empirical data, it is difficult to arrive at a formulation of laws and general rules. The facts always reach somewhere beyond the general formulations, and the general formulations do not exhaust the multiplicity of the varied experience. The merely phenomenological method is insufficient concerning the multiplicity of facts, and only the empirical method which goes back to the life situations, the libidinous and the emotional strivings, will lead to formulations which come at least nearer to the multiplicity of strivings and tendencies in the human psychological and physiological organization. My discussions of the problems are therefore imbued with an empirical and realistic point of view. The empirical method is preferable to mere speculation. But the empirical method leads immediately to a deep insight that even our own body is beyond our immediate reach, that even our own body justifies Prospero's words: "We are such stuff as dreams are made on ; and our little life is rounded with a sleep" (*The Tempest*). A discussion of a body-image as an isolated entity is necessarily incomplete. A body is always the expression of an ego and of a personality, and is in a world. Even a preliminary answer to the problem of the body cannot be given unless we attempt a preliminary answer about personality and world.

APPENDIX I

CASE HISTORIES OF ORGANIC BRAIN LESIONS[1]

*(a) Polyaesthesia and transfer of sensations from the left to the right
side of the body in a case of parietal and capsula lesion*

Barbara M., born 1880, in the neurological clinic of the University of Vienna, from December 10th, 1922, to March 23rd, 1923. Family history and previous history without importance. Lues 1911. Apoplectic insult on February 7th, 1931. On February 10th, according to the report of another hospital, hemiparesis on the right side, analgesia, and anaesthesia on the right side of the body. Right angle of the mouth drops, tongue deviates to the right side and can be moved to the left side only with difficulty. The patient is unable to look to the right. The eyes go to the left and upward. Pupils are narrow and fixed to light. Babinski, Oppenheim, Gordon plus on the right side. Patellar and Achilles tendon reflexes absent. Speech slurred. Patient is somnolent and yawns often. Inner organs normal. Wassermann negative. On February 11th, slight degree of stiffness of the neck. February 19th, spasms of the right lower extremities. February 28th, strong perspiration of right arm. March 1st, head turned to the right side. March 3rd, sensibility for pain and touch is improving. April 9th, hemiplegia improved, patellar and Achilles tendon reflexes are stronger on the right side than on the left. Sensibility almost normal.

In the meantime the patient had several treatments. My findings are based upon a series of examinations. A change occurred only towards the end of the long observation. Inner organs and bones are normal. Wassermann in blood and spinal fluid positive. Nonne-Apelt positive. Two lymphocytes. Neurologically; paresis of the lower facial on the right side; the protruded tongue deviates to the right; palate and swallowing normal; speech normal; ocular movements free; no nystagmus; the pupils react

---

[1] These case histories will have interest for neurologists.

sluggishly to light, but well to accommodation; corneal, conjunctival, palate reflexes normal; visual field, eye grounds, hearing, vestibular apparatus, smell and taste normal; the right shoulder droops. There is a severe paresis of predilection type. On the right arm, typical posture. But the spasms are very limited, although of pyramidal character. The range of movements is diminished in all joints. It it best in the shoulder, whereas a voluntary movement of the hand is impossible. The tendon and periostal reflexes of the arm are stronger on the right than on the left side. Examination of co-ordination and diadochokinesis impossible. Paresis of the muscles of the trunk. Abdominals present on both sides. The right leg shows a strong pronation of the foot. Otherwise there is paresis of the predilection type of medium degree (only the motility of the toes is diminished). The tone shows a very mild tension of pyramidal character, the foot is even hypotonic. No ataxia, no adiadochokinesis. Patellar and Achilles tendon reflexes stronger on the right than on the leftside. Ankle clonus on the right side. Babinski, Oppenheim, Rossolimo plus on the right side. When the patient tries to walk, her shoulder sinks forward and she is unable to walk even with the help of sticks. Bladder and rectum functions are normal.

The sensibility shows the following disturbances. There is spontaneous pain in the region of the right eye. The pain sometimes diminishes to paraesthesias, sometimes it is completely absent. Sense of posture; she gives prompt answers concerning the left side of her body. If one lets her imitate passive movements of the right side of her body with the left side, she makes almost grotesque mistakes. If one examines, in the common way, the perception of the direction of the passive movements, the disturbance is greatest in hand and foot, whereas the disturbance is much less in the proximal joints. Sometimes one has the impression that the patient perceives in hand and foot when a movement has taken place, but that she is not clear about the direction of the movement.

She hallucinates often and believes that movements with her fingers have been made even if no examination has been started. Passive movements which have been made on the joints of the left extremities often provoke, after from 4 to 10 seconds, fainter sensations of the same character in the right extremities.

Generally, the sensibility of the patient on the right side of the body is characterized in the following way; there is a marked disposition to hallucinations on the right side of the body, and sensations on the left side of the body provoke, a short time later (from 4 to 10 seconds), an analogous sensation on a symmetrical spot on the right side of the body.

Temperature perception; sensation for cold is intact, sensation for heat has disappeared on the right side.

Pain of the deeper parts and on the surface is preserved. The patient is less sensitive to the faradic brush on the right side. Itching is identical on both sides of the body. Tickling is mostly felt as a touch on the right side. Pallaesthesia and sensitiveness to deep pressure are identical on both sides. Weights are felt on both sides in the same way. Touch is localized on the right side in a grotesquely wrong way. The gentlest touches are felt correctly. When the patient is touched on the right side, near the breast, she feels it first on the shoulder, but after from 4 to 10 seconds later she has a second sensation near the elbow, a third on the upper part of the leg, and a fourth on the dorsal side of the foot. But the sensations, 2, 3, and 4 are duller and less distinct than the first sensation. This polyaesthesia is constant when the right side of the body is touched. But fairly often only two sensations are felt. The polyaesthesia is also present when the stimulus is applied to the left side. At first, on the symmetrical spot of the right side, weaker and fainter sensations appear, and, after that, another one more distally localized. The right sensation is not always absolutely symmetrical to the left one. A touch on the left hand may provoke a sensation at the same level on the trunk.

The same phenomena are present when pin-pricks are applied. A pin-prick in the right upper leg provokes an indistinctly localized pin-prick sensation which is followed by a sensation of touch. If one pricks the left upper leg, a duller pin-prick appears on an approximately symmetrical place on the right upper leg. Although the localization for pin-pricks and touch on the right side is generally poor, the patient occasionally gives correct answers. A pin-prick in the right big toe can be occasionally localized correctly. The mistakes differ in direction and size.

Sometimes they are only a few centimetres, but sometimes a touch on the trunk may be transferred to the foot or the face, in transversal direction. The mistakes increase with fatigue. When she has paraesthesias in the face, she localizes all touches in the face. Also the left-sided temperature sensations are generally transferred without qualitative changes to the right side of the body. A touch with a warm glass is felt first on the left, then on the right side, although a little less warm, and for the most part approximately symmetrical. The same is true about sensations of cold and of pallaesthesia. Even when objects are put into her left hand, she feels them in her right hand also. Sometimes a sensation of cold and heat on the left side provokes only a pressure sensation on the right side. A touch of the nipple on the right side is generally well localized. When the patient's right arm is touched with rough clothes or with a brush, she feels only a simple touch or a pin-prick, even when the touch is spread over a large area, and when extensive movements are made on the skin. Lines on the skin made with the finger are felt only as a touch, even if the line is as long as 20 centimetres. Sometimes it is felt as several touches. If the nipples are touched, the patient localizes the touch on the nipple. Sometimes the patient pretended to feel the movement as a downward movement when the line was drawn by an upward movement. When a movement on the skin was made, the patient very often stated that her finger joints were moved. It is also true that all sensible qualities are transferred from the left side to the right side and that they are polyaesthetic. The second sensation is always a sensation of touch when there has been a sensation on the right side.

The patient has no knowledge of the position in space of her right limbs, but she is quite well able to show a specific point on the trunk. The discrimination is a good one. It is impossible to examine the successive discrimination because of her polyaesthesia. The vasomotor irritability is increased on the right side. There were no particular feelings of pleasure and displeasure concerning the right side of her body. She has correct optic images concerning the right side of her body. After a prolonged treatment with salvarsan, the spontaneous hallucinations diminished. The left-side sensations are now only incompletely transferred to the right side, although the phenomena are identical in their essence. The disturbance in the localization is still outstanding, although correct localizations occur more often.

(b) Imperception of right hemiplegia.

Harriet C., 48 years old, family history without any importance. The patient ceased menstruation about a year ago. Her sister states that she suffered from pneumonia in December, 1930; she recovered from the pneumonia, but on December 28th, 1931, she had a stroke and she was found three or four days later. At first her speech was not clear, but she could read her prayer-book without any difficulty. She often said that she had a fracture or dislocation. She screamed with pain. The patient had always been peculiar and eccentric and was very religious and reserved. She was admitted on March 8th, 1932, to the psychopathic ward of Bellevue Hospital. The patient said, "I had a stroke and couldn't get up where I fell; this is Bellevue, I know where I am". On the 9th of March, she said, "I am paralysed in my right arm and leg; I fractured them on December 27th; I just came off the street and this happened; I wasn't being treated for anything; I didn't work, but the bank where I worked as a filing clerk gave me some money".

The patient was poorly nourished. Her heart-beat is rapid. No murmurs heard. Lungs negative. Abdomen negative. The blood chemistry is normal. No albumen in the urine. No casts. The Wassermann in blood and spinal fluid is negative. Globulin normal. No increase in cells. Colloidal gold curve is normal. The neurological examination showed right-sided facial paralysis, no nystagmus, staring look, no deviation of the tongue, no hemianopsia. The speech is slightly hesitant. Pupils are equal, slightly irregular; they react well to light and accommodation. The patient is unable to move her right upper and lower extremity. The extremities are flexed. The corneal reflex is absent. The reflexes are markedly exaggerated on the right side with positive ankle and knee clonus. There is positive Rossolimo and Babinski on the right side. The abdominals were absent on the right side. Hoffmann positive on the right side. The position of the right hand is unusual. The hand is flat, closely resembling the Simian hand.

There is only slight flexion of the proximal finger joints and extension of the distal joints.

The patient is sensitive towards passive movements in the joints. She shows marked sensory changes on the right side of the body, including the face, consisting of a severe impairment for touch, pin-pricks and temperature changes. The sense of posture in hand and foot is almost completely gone. It is also impaired in the elbow. Movements in the shoulder and in the knee and hip are at least partially appreciated.

In the further course of the examination it was brought out that when she is touched four times on the right side of the hand, she often feels only three or less touches. When pin-pricks are applied to one point several times, she tends to spread them along a curve. Instead of a cross drawn on her skin, she feels only one point. She has difficulties in localization. Also the discrimination is impaired. In the further course of observation spasticity developed, especially in the arm, but it is not very marked. She speaks rapidly and likes to talk. She rarely blinks. Her face as a whole gives impression of rigidity.

The patient is orientated in space and also orientated in time, although the time orientation is not always quite correct. She had a tendency to identify persons wrongly and to mistake strangers for her relatives.

On March 10th, she said, "All these people here look like people I know. Everybody in here looks like somebody I know. I can't place this woman or that, but most of them I can. This is March, 1932. My sisters have taken all my things from me: I have nothing now, but it is because I am religious. I have seen lights and flashes on the walls. I saw them before I came here and I saw them after I came here. There is something peculiar on the wall now".

On the 12th of March the patient said, "This is not my hand, this is not my ankle. It won't stand the way the other does. It won't connect with anything". But when her paralysed arm was raised, she said, "This is my right arm; it is not in order, it won't stay back in this way. They told me at first it was a fracture, but it wasn't. My knee won't stay like this one would. I was confused, they told me I wouldn't get well, I was paralysed". When her attention was drawn again to her right arm, she said, "It does not look like mine. I think it is mine, but I am not sure. I can't get my leg up to stand on it. When they first told me it was a stroke, I believed them, but now I think it is out of place somewhere, disconnected at ankle and knee". When she was asked to do something with her right arm she said she could not. She has no difficulty in naming the fingers on the right side. She also looks readily to the right side.

On the 16th she said, "The hand was funny. The shape was funny, it is better now". (Is that your hand?) "It does not look like it, it is too big and swollen, it does not feel like it either and it just won't." (Where is your arm?) "I don't know, you must have it here, I wish you would help me and give me my arm." (Are these your fingers?) "I don't know; they are so swollen." (Is that your face?) "It is paralysed too." (Perhaps it is your arm, but paralysed?) "No, it has never behaved like this before." (Is that your leg?) "It won't let me stand on it, it looks peculiar to me." (Is it yours?) "I don't know." She now looked at both her hands and said, "No, it doesn't look like the other, I don't think it is". When she is ordered to sit up, she says, "With this hand I can't get up alone". (What has happened?) "I had a stroke at home, I haven't been well since. The doctor said I was crazy."

The patient repeatedly expresses doubt whether her right arm is really hers. When she is asked about the fingers, she says, "The fingers look so big, they look swollen. There is so much confusion here. Perhaps it is mine, but it is thicker than this one". The patient has at the same time no difficulty in optic perception even when examined tachystoscopically. The perception for colour is good. She has no reading difficulties when the print is sufficiently large. Judgment and reasoning are good. She has no definite memory disturbances. Her memory quotient in Well's memory tests is 91 (100 is normal). In the Healy completion tests, for which good optic perception is necessary, the patient showed a low average adult performance.

The patient has suffered from a hemiplegia which is either based on an embolus or a thrombosis. The extension of the process which involves the sensibility and the motility makes a large subcortical lesion probable. The readiness of the patient to talk, the report about speech troubles, and her attitude towards the right side of her body, make a cortical involvement at least probable. A particular interest the case offers is her attitude towards the right side of her body. Very often she says that her hand is not hers. She emphasizes that it looks different, that it is swollen. It is true that the hand shows some slight change due to the paralysis, but when there is a change it is more in the direction of a slight atrophy.[1]

It must be emphasized that the patient has no optic disturbances, and that her memory is unimpaired in spite of a slight difficulty in forming new associations. It is true that she has a tendency to see acquaintances and relatives in other people. But all this does not explain the persistent doubt concerning her right arm. It must be connected with her focal lesion. We are dealing with a case of focal non-perception of one side of the body. It is remarkable that on this occasion it is the right side of the body towards which the patient reacts in this peculiar way. The patient has never been left-handed, and there is no left-handedness in the family. It is clear that Babinski's rule is not absolute; there are exceptions in which the patients react in a peculiar way towards the right side of the body. It is remarkable that the patient not only develops the illusion that her hand and fingers are swollen but also often complains of a fracture of her right arm and of her right leg. We have here an organic tendency to localized illusions.

(c) Imperception of the left side of the body and changes in the postural attitude in a brain tumour case

Michael F., born 1882, came to Dr Mattauschek's psychiatric ward in Vienna on November 13th, 1925.

The patient had worked since his ninth year more with his left arm than with his right. His right shoulder was dislocated at that time. Since 1916 he had had attacks in which he lost consciousness. His limbs were shaky. These attacks followed shell-shock

---

[1] Attention has recently been drawn to the atrophies connected with parietal lobe le ions. One may venture the hypothesis that what in one case comes out as atrophic disturbances, comes out in another as a feeling of queerness and change in the body.

and gas-poisoning in the war. Before coming to the hospital he was depressed, clouded, and distracted. He complained of head-aches. He felt that people looked queerly at him.

In the ward he was indifferent and dreamy and showed a definite lack of spontaneity. There was a tendency to persevera-tion. There were no aphasic signs, and no objective signs with the exception of a mydriasis. On November 15th he was confused and spoke about his wife working with wires. He wetted his bed. Sometimes he was completely mute. He had several attacks in which his whole body shook though he did not lose conscious-ness. During the attacks his pupils were wide and rigid. There was Babinski on both sides and involuntary urination. At the beginning of the attack, the right arm was abducted and flexed in the elbow joint. Hand and fingers were flexed also. After the attack the left pupil was still without reaction. The corneal reflex was diminished on the right side. On the 16th, the pupils were blurred, injected, and prominent. There was some exudation. The veins were enlarged. Wassermann in blood and spinal fluid negative. The pressure was 265. The X-ray showed an increase in the endocranial pressure.

On November 20th he was clouded in his consciousness, but still interested in his surroundings. His answers to questions were belated. He was vague and showed definite memory diffi-culties. On the 29th there was a serious disturbance of the sensi-bility in the right trigeminus, and the masseter was weaker on the right side. There were disturbances in the sensibility, in the right arm and right leg. The spontaneity was increased. Since the ven-triculography showed an obliteration of the ventricle on the right side, a trephine-opening over the right temporo-parietal region was made. There was a diffuse resistance near the ventricle. On February 22nd he showed the same psychic attitude. His memory retention was poor. His orientation was somewhat impaired. He said that he should have been operated on and pointed to his phallus. He complained of pressure over his eyes. His gait was swaying. In March there was a decrease in his visual acuity, especially on the right side. During the next months a secondary atrophy developed. With the right eye he could count fingers at 2 metres distance. On the left eye, only a strong light provoked a sensation. On being sent home he speedily developed states of excitement. He felt he was being observed by other people and threatened his wife. An X-ray treatment did not bring any change, but the patient quieted down.

On April 26th, 1926, he returned to the hospital with tonic flexor attacks in the left upper extremity. He spoke slowly and omitted syllables and words in test phrases. During the following weeks the orientation in space and time became worse. He was confused and delirious. In May the patient was continually falling backwards and felt that he was leaning forward. He was unable to walk without being paretic. He did not put one leg before the other. He regarded his right leg and right arm as left extremities, and shook hands with his left hand saying that it was his right. He was unable to imitate the posture of one side with the other side. He localized in the face pretty well. On the right side of the body there still remained hemi-hypaesthesia. The right masseter was still impaired. There was sometimes Babinski on the right side. No paresis. The hypaesthesia on the right side was not very pronounced. He was for the most part able to differentiate between sharp and dull, but he very often did not know whether his legs were moved or not. When the legs were flexed, he often said that they were extended. He repeatedly made mistakes about left and right. His stereognosis was comparatively good. There was no apraxia in gestures of threatening, waving, or saluting. He handled objects very awkwardly. When he tried to walk his legs seemed glued to the floor. He often crossed one leg over the other.

A more careful examination of his motility was now made. There were many spontaneous movements with the right arm. He scratched his head and made brushing movements. His body had a tendency to fall to the left side. The trunk sank down to the left side. The left arm was held stiffly, especially the flexed index finger. When he was told to sit straight, he fell still more to the left. Also the left leg was crossed over the right one. When he was ordered to stretch his hands forwards his left arm sank downwards. He kept his eyes tightly closed. (What did you do with the leg?) "With what leg? I didn't do anything." His left hand now made a spontaneous movement towards the right leg. There were no particular difficulties in showing the tongue. He could close his fists but he was unable to open the left hand. When asked to open it, he said, "Which hand, I am not pressing", and increased the pressure. He strongly denied afterwards that he had exerted any pressure. He was now told to show his right thumb and little finger, and succeeded in doing so. He could also show his left thumb; but, when asked to show his left little finger, he repeated the words and showed the finger of the right hand. When asked again, he pointed to his nose with his right hand. (Show your left arm.) He raised his right arm and insisted it was the left. (Where is your right arm?) He showed the left side of his body and insisted it was the right arm. (Where is your left leg?) He touched his right upper leg with his right hand. When asked again, he said, "I must think it over". (Where is your left arm?) He raised his right arm and pointed to the left side. At the same time he raised his right leg with a tendency to cross to the left side. (Where is your left eye?) "Probably I have it in my head." (Show it.) "I am not certain." He pointed with both hands to his right eye and to the base of his nose. When ordered to do so, he showed his right ear with his right arm.

The examiner now took the right arm of the patient so that he could not move it, and asked him to show his ear. He tried hard to liberate his right arm, made movements of crossing with his right leg, and said, "You must let me free so that I can move my hand". He thumbed his nose according to order with his right hand, and repeated it, but also brought his left hand near his nose. He took his left hand with his right arm and brought both of them near his nose. When asked where the left arm was, he repeatedly touched his nose with his right hand. (Where is your left hand?) "Who? I have not got it; you have it yourself", and he persisted in taking hold of his nose with his right hand. He was able to answer correctly how many ears and eyes he had. An object was now put into his left hand. (What have you got in your left hand?) He looked at his right hand and said, "Nothing". (What have you got in your right hand?) He raised his left arm, said, "Nothing", but transferred the object (scissors) from his left hand into his right. (What have you got in your hand?) "A shoe-horn." (In which hand?) "In my right hand now." But he put the object into his left hand. He made continuous movements with his right leg, flexing it at the hip and crossing it over the left leg. (What were you doing?) "I felt something in my left leg."

When pin-pricks were applied to both the left and the right hand, he at first gave correct answers. But later on, after being pricked in the right side, he said, "You pricked me in the right side", but pointed vaguely to the left side. (Where is the left side of the body?) He pointed repeatedly to the right side of the body. He repeatedly said he had been pricked in the right side when it was really in the left. But he often scratched himself correctly on the point where he had been pricked. When pricked in the region of the left knee, he pointed correctly to it, but said it was on the right side. When the right knee was pricked, he said, "The same". When he was ordered to push forward his hands, he made circular movements with his right arm, the left arm deviated inwards and was flexed at the elbow. He often grasped his right arm with his left. When his head was passively turned to the right side, the right leg, which was crossed over to the left side, was flexed at the hip. There was a strong tendency to turn to the right side. With the turning of the head to the left side the crossing movement in the left leg began. When the patient went back with his left leg, the right leg was crossed to the left side. The left hand often fell into a cataleptic posture. After several applications of pain on the left side, which he localized correctly, the right side of the chest was pricked with a needle. He said it was right, but pointed to the left side. After the patient had spontaneously crossed his right leg to the left side, he was asked where his right leg was (it was now on the left side), and showed his left leg. He was now asked "Where is your left leg?" He said, "I have my left leg between my legs".

In the following weeks the delirious episodes increased. But the patient was still orientated from time to time. On June 20th the trunk was mostly turned to the left side, but the head and left extremities were turned to the right. The left leg was usually crossed over the right, though occasionally the opposite position was assumed. The left arm sometimes rose spontaneously. The left arm was flexed at the elbow and the wrist. The fingers were extended and the arm was pronated. From time to time the head went slowly to the left side and the right arm showed a tendency to pronation. There was still a hyperkinesis (scratching, wiping) in the right arm. The left arm was akinetic. There were frequent slight movements in the knee of the right leg. During the 'finger-nose' and knee-heel tests the arms and legs were often cataleptically arrested. Passive turning of the head to the left side provoked a turning of the trunk to the left side, and the right leg was crossed over the left leg. The turning of the head to the right side did not change the crossing of the leg. (Where is your left hand?) Correct. (Show your right thumb?) Correct. (Show the left thumb?) Correct. (Show the left index finger?) Correct. But later on he made movements as well with the left as with the right hand. (Show the right ear?) Correct. (Show the left ear?) Correct.

A pin-prick on the right side was localized with approximate correctness. Another one on the left side he said was on the right although he could show correctly where it was. Pin-pricks on the face were always correctly named as to the side. A pin-prick towards the left upper leg provoked wiping movements. At first he said it was on the left and then on the right and then again on the left side. Asked where his left hand was, he showed his right. Right and left leg were named correctly. When given a pin-prick on the left hand, he said it was on the right hand. His right hand was almost always named and shown correctly. Asked where his left hand was, he again showed the right one. When he crossed his right leg over the left one, a pin-prick was applied to his right knee. He pointed to his left hand and said that he had been pricked on the right hand. A pin-prick on the left hand was localized correctly by touching movement. But he had the tendency to point with his left hand towards the right one. Once when asked where the left hand was, he pointed with the right one to the place where the left one had been before. Occasionally he pointed correctly when he was pricked on the left knee. Sometimes he pointed correctly, but called the left knee the right one. During the examination he sometimes turned his head spontaneously to the left side and his trunk followed. The left arm then usually sank. When he was ordered to turn his head to the left, he turned to the right. When he was asked to take his left thumb with his right hand he was completely helpless and said, "One can't take it with the left hand". When asked where his left hand was, he showed the right one, but on repetition he shook the left one. When he was asked to take his left thumb, he caught hold of the examiner's index finger and said, "Now I have both thumbs". When asked to show his left knee, he grasped his right knee with his right hand and said, "I have no knee on the right leg". (Show your left knee.) "I have none, please show it to me?" When the examiner then touched his left knee, the patient moved his right hand there and at the same time moved his left hand near his left knee. When asked to show his left ear, he first showed his right ear with his right hand. Later on he succeeded. Generally the left hand tended to come into the right field.

On June 24th the patient became more and more comatose. He died on July 30th, 1926. The autopsy showed a tumour of the brain, which infiltrated both frontal lobes and the corpus callosum. Under the ependyma of the lateral ventricles there were several tumorous masses connected with tumorous masses which fill out the whole ventricular system. But the whole ependymal grey of the ventricular system was infiltrated with tumorous masses. Histopathological diagnosis: Glioma.

There are many questions open in this observation. The state of the patient did not allow of a very careful investigation. He was blind at the time when the allochiria took place. Troubles in the general orientation were also certainly present. But there is no question that the patient had a very incomplete knowledge about his left side. He had difficulties in showing parts of the left side of his body. When asked to do so he very often showed the right parts or was completely helpless. When questioned after a touch or pin-prick on the left side, he often said that he had been touched on the right side. The important feature in the case is that he showed so many motor phenomena connected with the achiria. His left hand showed a marked akinesis; he did not like using it. There was a marked tendency of the left foot to cross over the right one. The left arm deviated inwardly. There is no question that tendencies in the tonic attitude of the patient to transfer the left side of his body to the right side of the body were prevalent. Especially remarkable in this respect is the crossing of the left leg over the right one. There was also an increase in the tonic neck reflexes. There is no question that the alloaesthesia and the disorientation about left and right on the body were closely connected with these motor tendencies. I draw attention again to the fact that the head and body of the patient were usually turned to the right side. When asked for his right leg he showed the left, which had been crossed over, and, when asked where the left one was, he said, "I have it between my legs".

The increase in the neck reflexes has been described by Hoff and Schilder as a parieto-occipital syndrome. Tendencies to turn the body around the longitudinal axis occur. This turning often starts with crossing of the legs. In these observations also, the patients did not realize the crossing of the legs and the turning which was then started. This also occurred in a case observed with Gerstmann in which the autopsy showed a parieto-occipital lesion.

The autopsy in this case did not give any definite proof of localization since the tumour extended through the whole ventricular system besides affecting the frontal lobes.

APPENDIX II

SOME REMARKS ON THE ANATOMY AND PHYSIOLOGY OF THE NERVOUS SYSTEM[1]

The human central nervous system is in its earliest stages of development a long stretched tube, the so-called medullar tube. The central canal is covered with the grey substance containing the ganglion cells; the outside of the tube is formed by white substance, containing the myelin sheets. The anterior end of the medullar tube starts to grow more quickly, becomes more bulky, and thus creates the primitive brain bag. The picture of the central nervous system of a seven weeks' old human embryo (Fig. 1) shows the effect of this growth. The structure which is seen in the picture gets its complications by the curvings the tube undergoes in the course of its growth. Several parts become more and more distinct in the course of this growth, and we may distinguish telencephalon (fore-brain), diencephalon, mid-brain, metencephalon (hind-brain) and postencephalon (after-brain). The fore-brain grows excessively, develops the cerebral hemispheres, and covers in the course of its excessive growth, diencephalon, mid-brain, and even a part of the hind-brain. Even in the fully developed human brain, the medulla oblongata originating from the after-brain is not covered by the hemispheres. The diencephalon develops a rather large bulk of grey substance, the so-called thalamus opticus. One of the most important formations in the mid-brain is the nucleus ruber.

The central channel broadens itself in the course of the development of the fore-brain and forms the complicated ventricular system, which can be understood when it is considered that the broadened central channel grows with the hemispheres of the brain and is so extended into the hemispheres which cover the other parts of the brain. The horizontal section through the fully developed brain (Fig. 2) shows this ventricular system which extends into the anterior part of the brain as well as in to the posterior

[1] These remarks are designed for those who are not in contact with the facts of brain anatomy, and are intended to help to the understanding of Part I. These remarks are necessarily elementary and schematic.

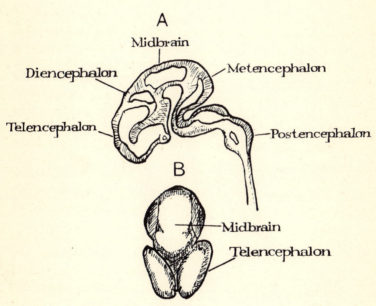

FIG. I. Brain of a 7 weeks' old human embryo, 3 times enlarged.
A. Lateral view. B. Top view. After Mihalkovics.

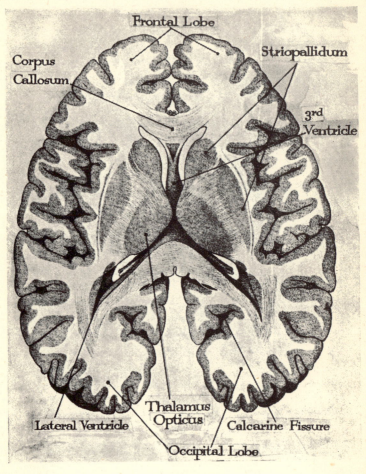

Fig. 2

and inferior part of the hemispheres. Some communication between this ventricular system in the hemispheres and the ventricular system in the centre of the brain remains. The ventricular system narrows down in the mid-brain and broadens out again in the region of the hind-brain and after-brain to the shallow rhomboid of the fourth ventricle, which continues into the central canal of the spinal cord. From the foot of the hind-brain develops the cerebellum, which is only partially covered by the occipital part of the hemispheres.

After-brain, hind-brain, mid-brain, diencephalon, are also called brain-stem. The brain-stem is covered by the hemispheres, which form a cloak up to the diencephalon. The nerve cells which form the grey substance remain in their original place around the opening of the medullar tube and its derivate in the fourth and third ventricles. But the grey substance does not remain in the immediate surroundings of the central canal; many changes take place, and in the hemispheres the grey substance wanders to the surface, which is now covered with grey substance. Parts of the brain which contain ganglion cells are grey. One is justified in believing that they are of especial importance for the function of the nervous system. The grey masses contain what one usually calls the centres. The white masses contain nerve fibres, covered with myelin sheets. They form the pathways which connect the different central units. Often the pathways are considered merely as electric wires which connect the stations. But it is doubtful whether this idea is correct and whether they have not a greater independence than one usually supposes. When one takes the brain out of the skull, one sees the surface of the hemispheres with its different sulci and gyri. The lateral view of the schematic figure (Fig. 3) shows the hemisphere, which does not completely cover the masses of the cerebellum. One also sees the medulla oblongata which continues into the brain-stem. The connection between spinal cord and brain-stem is more clearly seen when one turns the brain round and looks at its inferior surface. One sees (Fig. 4) the connecting part between cerebellum and brain-stem (pons), and the so-called pes pedunculi, an important part of the brain-stem. One sees, also, in this figure, the inferior surface of the hemispheres.

V

These remarks are necessarily very incomplete and give only a very preliminary idea of the gross anatomy of the brain. There is no necessity to discuss the structure of the brain and of the connective tissue, the blood vessels and the glia. The brain is, of course, an organ like any other organ, with a complicated nutritional and metabolic apparatus which makes its function possible. But we are more interested here in the function than in the way in which the function is secured.

The function of motility can, of course, as the whole tendency of this book shows, be only artificially separated from the other functions of the nervous system, and it is still more artificial to bring separate parts of the motor apparatus into connection with different aspects of the motility. But there can be no question that the lesion of particular pathways and centres causes a particular symptomatology and impairs one side of the motility more than the other. There can be no question that different lesions in the central nervous system cause different symptoms. There may be a lack and loss in the function. But we should not believe that when the function is impaired by the lesion of a particular part it is localized in this particular structure.

The pyramidal tract originates in the grey substance of the gyrus centralis anterior (Figs. 3 and 5). The schematic Fig. 5 shows the hemispheres connected by the white substance of the corpus callosum. The passage continues through the so-called capsula interna, which lies between the grey substances of the thalamus opticus and the lenticular nucleus, and goes from there through the brain-stem to the medulla oblongata, where it crosses partially to the other side. From there the fibres go to the anterior horn of the grey substance of the spinal cord. From the ganglion cells in the spinal cord the motor impulses are conducted towards the muscles. Lesion of the pyramidal tract provokes a paresis on the other side of the body. With this paresis muscular spasms are connected. The function of the flexor and adductor muscles of the arms and the extensor and adductor muscles of the legs is generally better preserved. A paresis of this type is called a paresis of the predilection type. The schematic figure shows the secondary degeneration of the pathway when a lesion in the capsula interna has taken place. But even when the pyramidal

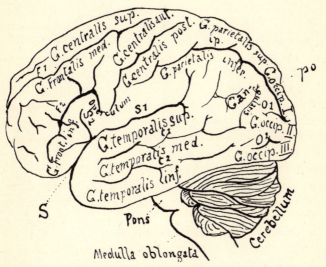

FIG. 3. Lateral view of the Brain.

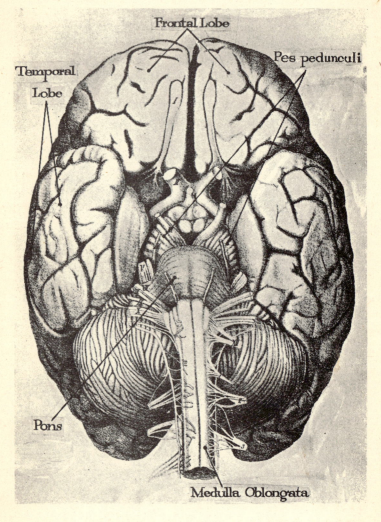

Frontal Lobe

Pes pedunculi

Temporal Lobe

Pons

Medulla Oblongata

Fig. 4.

tract is well preserved, the motor function is not guaranteed. Lesion of the grey substance deeper in the brain may provoke serious disturbances in the motility. The horizontal section (Fig. 2) shows parts of the striopallidar system, the lesion of which provokes a particular type of rigidity, tremors, and especially also changes in the motor impulses. The schematic Fig. 5 shows also a part of this important grey substance. The lesion of this organ disturbs the correct distribution of the tone and also impairs involuntary motor impulses.

In the mid-brain are further important centres for tone and motility. I mention the nucleus ruber and the substantia nigra. The schematic Fig. 6 shows the complicated apparatus which serves the muscle tone. One sees in this schematic figure that the nucleus ruber and striopallidar system are connected with each other and that passages also connect the cerebellum with the nucleus ruber. From the nucleus ruber passages go to the spinal cord. The figure shows clearly that the cerebellum has close relations to all the parts which have to do with the maintenance and distribution of muscle tone. The nucleus ruber as well as the cerebellum is under the control of the frontal lobe as well as the temporal lobe, the function of which is of importance for the muscle tone. The term 'tone' means the amount of tension in the muscle. But many complicated functions which serve the maintenance of posture are covered by the same term, so that many physiologists advocate dropping the term 'tone' completely. At any rate, in the medulla oblongata there exists also a primitive motor apparatus which serves the maintenance and regulation of posture. This apparatus extends through the medulla oblongata and mid-brain and ends in the nucleus ruber, which is the most outstanding part of this postural apparatus. But this primitive postural apparatus is controlled by the action of cerebellum, frontal lobe, occipital lobe, and parietal lobe. Magnus and de Kleyn in particular have studied the apparatus which serves standing, posture, and attitude, have described important postural and righting reflexes, and were able to prove that the primary centres for these reflexes are localized in the apparatus mentioned, extending from the medulla oblongata to the nucleus ruber. The vestibular nuclei are an important part of this apparatus. It is, of course, impossible to give more than a very superficial idea of this important part of neurophysiology. In every motor activity all the functions mentioned are necessary parts. But pyramidal and extrapyramidal systems do not constitute the motility, but serve the motility, which is always the result of the activity of the whole personality, which acts according to a motive and according to a plan. For the performance of this plan, the gyrus supramarginalis is necessary. Lesion of this part of the cortical region provokes apraxia. But motility cannot be separated from sensory experiences and sensory regulations. As pointed out above, lesions of the sensory system will necessarily affect the motor system.

The sensory passages (Fig. 7) originate in the peripheral nerve, go to the spinal ganglion, and from there into the spinal cord. A part of these fibres go without crossing upward through the posterior column. These passages are especially passages for posture and touch. Other fibres go into the grey substance of the spinal cord to ganglion cells, which send fibres to the other side of the spinal cord, especially to the lateral column. These fibres have to do with the conduction of touch, temperature and pain impulses. In Dusser de Barenne's experiment the transection of the one side of the spinal cord will block the pain sensation of the other side. When strychnine is applied below this transection, the pain impulses will be increased. Since they cannot pass the region where the transection has been made, the impulses will go to the side of the spinal cord which has not been injured, and the sensation will now appear on the side where the transection has been made. Strychnine applied to one side of the spinal cord in connection with blocking by transection will therefore provoke alloaesthesia. The stimulus applied to the side opposite to the transection will be felt on the side of the transection. The sensory impulses travel through the spinal cord and the medulla oblongata into the mid-brain. On their way, those fibres which have not yet crossed, cross the midline after having reached ganglion cells in the medulla oblongata. When the sensory fibres have traversed the mid-brain and have reached the diencephalon, they have completely crossed to the other side. They reach the grey masses of

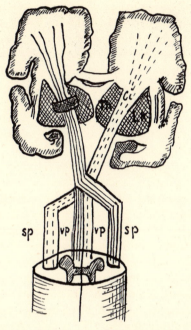

Fig. 5. Pyramidal tract in man (according to Edinger). Th Thalamus Opticus, L K nucleus lenticularis (part of the striatum) Ci capsula interna, sp lateral column part of the pyramidal tract, vp anterior column part of the pyramidal tract. The uninterrupted lines are the fibres coming from the left hemisphere, which degenerate when there is a lesion in the capsula interna as indicated.

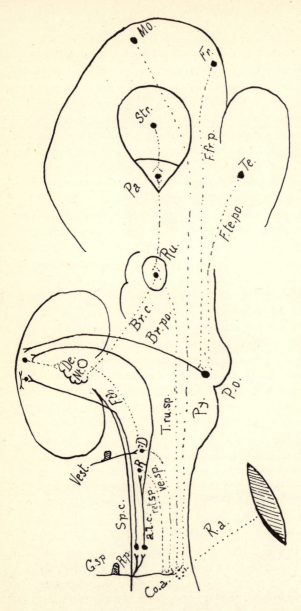

Fig. 6. Br.c.- brachium conjunctivum, Br.po.- brachium pontis, Co.a.- Cornu anterius, D.- Deiters nucleus, De.- nucleus dentatus, Fr.- Frontalbrain, F.fr.p.- frontopont.path, F.tb.- Fascic.tectobulbaris, F.te.po.- temporopontine path, G.sp.- Gangl.spinale, Sp.c.- spinocerebellar path, Mo.-Motor.region, N.t.-Nucl.tecti, Pa.- Pallidum, Py.-Pyramid, P.o - Pons, R.-Subst.reticularis, R.a.- Radix ant.,R.p.-Radix post.,Ru.-Nucl.rubcr, ret.sp.-reticulospinal path, Str.-Striatum, Te.-temporal lobe, T.ru.sp.-rubrospinal path, Vest.-N.vestibularis, a.l.c.-antero lateral column, ve.sp.- vestibulospinal path.

the thalamus opticus completely crossed. The thalamus opticus is the centre for all sensory impulses. The lesion of the thalamus opticus will provoke sensory disturbances of the contra-lateral side. Figs. 2 and 5 orient about the situation of these grey masses. The thalamus opticus is connected with the sensory part of the cortical region, especially the gyrus centralis posterior, but also with other parts of the parietal lobe. Lesion of the thalamus opticus provokes not only sensory disturbances but also hyper-algesias. The sensory impulses do not only provoke sensations, but there are continual interactions between the afferent impulses and the motor system, which is under the continual regulation of sensory and afferent impulses. Afferent impulses which do not lead to any sensations go through the lateral column of the spinal cord to the cerebellum.

Just as motor impulses are not due to a single apparatus but are the expression of activities of an individual who plans the actions, sensations also are sensations of a total personality. The final sensations and perceptions are always the result of the activity of the whole brain, or better, of the whole organism.

The so-called vestibular apparatus deserves a special interest among the senses. Under normal conditions we experience little of its functions. Under pathological conditions it provokes dizziness. Its peripheral apparatus is connected with the inner ear, which is called the labyrinth. It has two parts, one of which consists of the semi-circular canals, the other of the so-called vestibulum, which contains the otoliths. The semi-circular apparatus reacts especially to acceleration of circular movements. The otoliths are of importance for our orientation in relation to gravity. The vestibular apparatus is not only an organ for per-ception, but also gives rise to reflexes to circular and progressive movements. But there are also reflexes which act according to the position of the labyrinth in space. The vestibular nerve sends its impulses to nuclei in the medulla oblongata which are con-nected with the cerebellum, with the eye muscles, and probably also indirectly with a cortical region. They also have an influence on the vegetative system. As has been mentioned, the vestibular apparatus is also of importance for the distribution of tone.

Fig. 3 gives a schematic orientation about the configuration of the cortical region. The sulcus centralis divides the brain roughly into two parts; the anterior part of the brain is more closely related to the motility, the posterior part to sensations. Modern investigations have shown that there are a great number of anatomically different regions in the cortical grey. Cortical fields, as they are called, differ in the architecture and size of the cells, in the architecture of the myelin fibres, the glia, and the blood-vessels. The surface configuration in gyri and lobes has certainly some relation to the functions of the cortical region. But the modern point of view emphasizes the importance of the different fields of special microscopic structure. The study of the structure of the cell distribution (Cytoarchitectonic) has a special importance. The motor region of the brain where the pyramidal tract originates is as well characterized as the parts where the sensory fibres end and as the parts where tone and posture originate. There is no question that there exists a localization in the cortical region. The optic radiation ends in the calcarine fissure which lies on the median side of the occipital lobe (Fig. 2).

The cortical fields are very well characterized. Acoustic impulses have to do with the Heschl circumvolution which lies near the upper end of the first temporal circumvolution, covered by the adjacent part of the parietal lobe. The gyrus centralis posterior and the gyrus parietalis superior have to do with sensory impressions. From the gyrus centralis anterior originates the pyramidal tract. Postural and tonic impulses originate in the frontal lobe and in the upper parts of the temporal lobe. Parts on the borderline between the parietal and occipital lobes are of importance for postural attitudes (Brodmann's field 19). All these functions are represented in both sides of the brain. This part of the cortical region which serves sensations and motility is also called the peripheral part of the cortical activity.

Higher psychic functions can also be impaired by cortical lesions. Lesion of the Broca region at the foot of the gyrus frontalis inferior where it meets the gyrus centralis anterior impairs the faculty of articulate speech. The motor impulses, especially those for speech, are diminished. Lesions of the first temporal circumvolution impair the understanding of spoken language, hinder the right use of words (paraphasia), increase

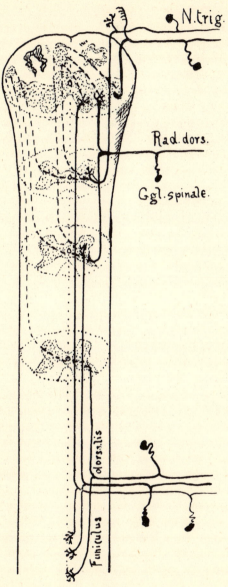

N.trig.

Rad. dors.

Ggl. spinale.

Funiculus dorsalis.

FIG. 7.

the impulses for speech, and in a minor degree, for other motor activities also. This syndrome is known as sensory aphasia. Lesion of the gyrus supramarginalis causes apraxia, the inability to act in a correct way. Mind-blindness follows the lesion of the occipital lobe, especially on its convexity. The final localization is still an object of controversy. Lesions of the parts of the gyrus supramarginalis which are near to the gyrus temporalis have something to do with the appreciation of pain impulses. The body-image has close relations to the functions of the parietal lobe. It is based upon the sensory impulses, optic impulses, and postural impulses from the parieto-occipital lobe. The apparatus which is necessary for action lies in the midst of this region. Whereas the more primitive sensory motor functions are represented in both hemispheres, the higher psychic functions such as speech, action, body-image, optic orientation, appreciation of pain, are especially based on the function of the left hemisphere. Lesion of this will be sufficient to disturb those functions. The actions of the left side of the body also need the guidance of the left hemisphere, and a slight degree of apraxia will occur on the left side whenever there is a lesion of the left side region for praxia. When there is a lesion of the corpus callosum which connects the two hemispheres, the impulses from the left hemisphere to the right hemisphere are interrupted and apraxia on the left side will appear (sympathetic apraxia).

The old neuro-pathology believed that the functions are localized in the parts of the brain, the lesion of which disturbs the function. We know to-day that this is not so. Particular parts of the brain are necessary for the function, but the psychic function does not have its seat in this part. It is even a matter of controversy whether an isolated impairment of a higher psychic function can occur in cortical lesions. Head, Goldstein, and Lashley believe that every cortical lesion impairs, more or less, every higher psychic activity. But there can be no question that the degree in which the functions are impaired varies according to the point of the lesion. Pötzl and I are convinced that isolated impairments of higher psychic functions such as speech or orientation are possible. Those who are deeply interested in this problem should study the works of Head on *Aphasia and Kindred*

Disorders of Speech, Goldstein, *Über Gehirn-Localisation*, and Pötzl, *Die Optisch-Agnostischen Störungen*. But there is no reason to believe in a rigid localization of function. Henschen is the most important figure among the moderns who still adhere to a strict and rigid localization. We should never forget that most of the symptoms we see in cortical lesions are not merely a defect but a changed activity, and this activity is the result of the parts of the brain which are still in function.

All my remarks so far have dealt with the sensory-motor system and its regulations, or, in other words, with the ' animalisch ' side of human existence. The voluntary functions and the conscious perception are connected with this part of the nervous system. But there exists a vegetative nervous apparatus in the organism, the afferent nerves of which supply the organs with unstriped muscles, for instance, the intestines, the vascular system, and the glands. In a physiological sense some organs with striped muscles belong to this group, especially the heart, but also some muscles of the oesophagus and of the phallus. Speaking generally, we may say that it is the intestines and the blood-vessels which are supplied by the nervous system which is not under the immediate influence of will; also all glands of the skin. It is characteristic of all these body-tissues that their functions can go on more or less independently of the central nervous system, although they can be influenced by it. Their nervous system has a limited independence of the central nervous system. Langley has therefore called it the autonomous nervous system. But Meyer and Gottlieb, whose description we follow, retain the name 'vegetative nervous system,' and call autonomous only that part of the vegetative nerves which is not furnished by the sympathicus. The part of the nervous system which Meyer and Gottlieb call autonomous is often called parasympathetic.

The efferent fibres of the vegetative system come to their organs, the muscles of the organs of circulation, digestion, sex organs, and glands, by passages which come from peripheral ganglia. But the fibres come out of the central nervous system, in different parts of which they originate. It is possible to differentiate between two different groups of the vegetative system according to their origin. One group consists of the sympathetic fibres which come from the median part of the spinal cord (the thoracic part and the lumbar part) and go through small white nerves (rami communicantes) to the so-called sympathetic string, which runs parallel to the spinal cord, to the cervical ganglia, and to the abdominal ganglion. From there, they go as grey rami communicantes to the spinal nerves. These sympathetic nerves supply blood-vessels, glands, and organs with unstriped muscles in the whole body. But almost all other organs are also supplied by the other type of vegetative nerves which originate in the mid-brain, the medulla oblongata, and the sacral spinal cord. We call these the cranial and sacral autonomous (parasympathetic) nerves. For us, those fibres have the greatest interest which leave the medulla oblongata and go into the intestines in the pathway of the vagus nerves. These are inhibitory fibres for the heart, constricting fibres for the bronchial muscles, motor nerves for the oeso-phagus, stomach, and intestines, and secretory for the stomach and for the pancreas. The sacral autonomous fibres innervate the rectum, the anus, the bladder and the genital organs.

The sympathetic nerves form a physiological unit, but all vegetative nerves never go, as do the fibres of the ' animalisch ' system, directly from the central nervous system to the end organ; but the fibres coming from the grey substance of the central nervous system first go to a ganglion. In this ganglion the central fibre ends; its end comes into connection with ganglion cells out of which the nerve fibre goes to the end organ. There is always an interruption in only one ganglion. Every vegetative organ has, therefore, one set of sympathetic and one set of para-sympathetic innervation.

In the spinal cord the lateral horn has the closest relation to the sympathetic and parasympathetic system. Further important centres lie around the fourth ventricle, at the basis of which are especially the important vegetative centres of the nervus vagus. There is no vegetative function which has not a representation around the fourth ventricle. There are centres for the heart and breathing, but also for metabolism and vasomotor functions. These vegetative centres at the basis of the fourth ventricle have an immediate importance for the maintenance of life. The same functions are also represented in the grey masses of the third ventricle, the posterior part of which has a close relation to the vegetative function of sleep. But at the basis of the third ventricle there are centres which regulate growth and sexuality. They also influence the glands of internal secretion, on the function of which they are on the other hand dependent. It is unknown, so far, in what way these vegetative centres are connected with the cortical region. But we know that emotions have an immediate influence upon them, and emotions are connected with pictures which are closely related to the cortical function. Since the picture of one's own body is closely related to the parieto-occipital lobe, it is reasonable to suppose that there are connections between the parieto-occipital lobe and the vegetative centres. But we have not sufficient knowledge about these connections.

BIBLIOGRAPHY

ABRAHAM, K., "Über ejaculatio præcox," *Klin. Beitr. zur Psychoanal.*, X, Wien, 1921.
"A short Study of the Development of the Libido," *Selected Papers*, London, 1924.
Versuch einer Entwicklungsgeschichte der Libido, Leipzig, 1924.
Psychoanalytische Studien zur Charakterbildung, Wien, 1925.

ACH, N., *Über die Willenstätigkeit und das Denken*, Göttingen, 1905.

ACHELIS, J. D., "Der Schmerz," *Ztschr.f.Psychol.*, 2 Abt., 1925, *56*, 31.

ADLER, A., *Der nervöse Charakter*, Wiesbaden, 1912 (Trans.: *The Neurotic Constitution*).
Studie über Minderwertigkeit von Organen, 2te. Aufl., München, Bergmann, 1927.

ADLER, A. & HOFF, H., "Beitrag zur Lehre vom Phantomgliede," *Monatsschr. f. Psychiat.u.Neurol.*, 1930, *76*, 80.

ALEXANDER, F., *Psychoanalyse der Gesamtpersönlichkeit* (Trans.: *Analysis of the Total Personality*, New York, 1930).

ALBRECHT, O., "Drei Fälle mit Anton's Syndrom," *Arch.f.Psychiat.*, 1918, *59*, 883.

ALLERS, R., "Zur Pathologie des Tonuslabyrinths," *Monatsschr.f. Psychiat.u.Neurol.*, 1909, *26*, 116.

ALLERS, R. & SCHEMINSKY, F., "Über Aktionsströme bei Muskeln bei motorischen Vorstellungen," *Arch.f.d.ges.Physiol.*, 1926, *212*, 169.

ALLPORT, F. H., *Social Psychology*, Boston, 1924.

ALVERDES, F., "Über vergleichende Soziologie," *Ztschr.f.Volkspsychol. u.Soziol.*, 1925, *1*.
Tiersoziologie, Leipzig, 1925.

ANTON, G., "Über die Selbstwahrnehmung der Herderkrankungen des Gehirns durch den Kranken bei Rindenblindheit und Rindentaubheit," *Arch.f.Psychiat.*, 1900, *32*, 86.
"Beiderseitige Erkrankung der Scheitelgegend des Grosshirnes," *Wien.klin.Wchschr.*, 1899, *12*, 1193.

BAUER, J. & SCHILDER, P. F., "Über einige psychophysiologische Mechanismen funktioneller Neurosen," *Deutsche Ztschr. f.Nervenheilk*, 1919, *64*, 279.

BENARY, W., "Studien zur Untersuchung der Intelligenz bei einem Fall von Seelenblindheit," *Psychol.Forsch.*, 1922, *2*, 209.

BENDER, L. & SCHILDER, P. F., "Encephalopathia alcoholica," *Arch. Neurol. and Psychiat.*, 1933, *29*, 990.

BERINGER, K., *Der Meskalinrausch*, Berlin, 1927.

BERNFELD, S., *Psychologie des Säuglings*, 1925 (Trans.: *The Psychology of the Infant*, New York, 1929).

BETLHEIM, S., " Säuglingsreflexe bei Apraxie," *Jahrb.f.Psych.u.Neurol.*, 1924, *43*, 226.
"Zur Lehre vom Phantom," *Deutsche Ztschr.f.Nervenheilk.*, 1926, *90*, 271.

BETLHEIM, S. & HARTMANN, H., " Über Fehlreaktionen bei der Korsakoffschen Psychose," *Arch.f.Psychiat.*, 1924, *72*, 278.

BIBRING-LEHNER, G., " Über die Beeinflussung eidetischer Phänomene durch labyrinthäre Reizung," *Ztschr.f.d.ges.Neurol.*, 1928, *112*, 496.

BOGARDUS, E. S., *The New Social Research*, New York, 1926.

BONNHOEFFER, K., " Zur Klinik und Lokalisation des Agrammatismus und der Rechts-Links Desorientierung," *Monatsschr.f. Psychiat.u.* Neurol., 1923, *54*, 11.

BONNIER, P., " L'aschematie," *Revue Neurol.*, 1905, *13*, 605.

BOZIC, D. & VUJIC, V., " Die Zweiteilung des Körpers in der Wahnidee," *Monatsschr.f.Psychiat.u.Neurol.*, 1930, *77*, 114.

BREED, F. S. & SHEPARD, J. R., "Maturation and Use in the Development of an Instinct," *Journ. Animal Behavior*, 1913, *3*, 274.

BROMBERG, W. & SCHILDER, P. F., " On Tactile Imagination and Tactile After-effects," *J.Nerv. and Mental Dis.*, 1932, *76*, 133.

BROWN, T. G. & STEWART, R. M., " On Disturbances of Sensations in Cerebral Lesion," *Brain*, 1916, *39*, 348.

BRUNNER, H. & HOFF, H., " Das Nebelsehen bei Labyrinthreizung," *Ztschr.f.d.ges.Neurol.*, 1929, *120*, 796.

BÜRGER-PRINZ, H. & KAILA, M., " Über die Struktur des amnestischen Symptomenkomplexes," *Ztschr.f.d.ges.Neurol.*, 1930, *124*, 553.

BÜHLER, K., *Die geistige Entwicklung des Kindes*, 4te.Aufl., Jena, 1924.

CANNON, W. B., *Bodily Changes in Pain, Hunger, Fear and Rage*, 2nd ed., New York, 1929.

CLAPARÈDE, E., "Note sur la localisation du moi," *Arch.de Psychol.*, 1924, *19*, 172.

COMAR, G., " L'autoreprésentation des organes," *Rev.Neurol.*, 1901, *9*, 490.

CURSCHMANN, H., " Beiträge zur Physiologie und Pathologie der kontralateralen Mitbewegungen," *Deutsche Ztschr.f.Nervenheilk.*, 1906, *31*, 1.

DEUTSCH, F., " Der gesunde und der kranke Körper," *Internat. Ztschr. f. Psychoanal.*, 1926, *12*, 493.
"Biologie und Psychologie der Krankheitsgenese," *Internat.Ztschr.f.Psychoanal.*, 1933, *19*.

DEWEY, J., *Reconstruction in Philosophy*, New York, 1920.

DIX, W. K., *Körperliche und geistige Entwicklung eines Kindes*, 4 Bde., Leipzig, 1911-23.

DUSSER DE BARENNE, J. G., " Zur Kenntnis der Alloaesthesie," *Monats-schr.f.Psychiat.u.Neurol.*, 1913, *34*, 523.

EHRENWALD, H., " Anosognosie und Depersonalisation," *Nervenarzt*, 1931, *4*, 681.

" Störung der Selbstwahrnehmung der Menstruation und der Blasenfunktion bei einer Kranken mit Hirntumor," *Ztschr.f.d.ges.Neurol.*, 1928, *118*, 224.

" Verändertes Erleben des Körperbildes mit konsekutiver Wahnbildung bei linksseitiger Hemiplegie," *Monatsschr. f.Psychiat.u.Neurol.*, 1930, *75*, 89.

EIDELBERG, L., " Quantitative Untersuchungen der Lagebeharrung," *Monatsschr.f.Psychiat.u.Neurol.*, 1926, *61*, 101.

EISINGER, K. & SCHILDER, P. F., " Über Träume bei Labyrinthläsionen," *Monatsschr.f.Psychiat.u.Neurol.*, 1929, *73*, 314.

ENGERTH, G., " Zeichenstörungen bei Patienten mit Autotopagnosie," *Ztschr.f.d.ges.Neurol.*, 1933, *143*, 381.

FEDERN, P., " Narcissism in the Structure of the Ego," *Internat.J. Psychoanal.*, 1928, *9*, 401.

" Beiträge zur Analyse des Sadismus und Masochismus," I, " Die Quellen des männlichen Sadismus," *Internat. Ztschr.f.Psychoanal.*, 1913, *1*, 29.

" Ego Feelings in Dreams," *Psychoanal. Quarterly*, 1932, *1*, 511.

" The Reality of the Death Instinct," *Psychoanal.Rev.*, 1932, *19*, 129.

" Einige Variationen des Ichgefühls," *Internat.Ztschr.f. Psychoanal.*, 1926, *12*, 263.

" Das Ich als Object und Subject des Narzissismus," *Internat.Ztschr.f.Psychoanal.*, 1929, *15*, 393.

FENICHEL, O., *Perversionen, Psychosen, Charakterstörungen*, Vienna, 1931. *Hysterien und Zwangsneurosen*, Vienna, 1931.

FERENCZI, S., *Hysterie und Pathoneurosen*, Leipzig, 1919.

" Ein kleiner Hahnemann," *Internat.Ztschr.f.ärzt.Psycho-anal.*, 1913, *1*, 240.

FISCHER, M. H., *Die Regulationsfunktion des menschlichen Labyrinthes und die Zusammenhänge mit verwandten Funktionen*, München, 1928.

" Über Gleichgewicht und Gleichgewichtsstörungen," *Zbl.f.d.ges.Ophthalmol.*, 1926, *17*, 209.

FISCHER, M. H. & WODAK, E., " Beiträge zur Physiologie des mensch-lichen Vestibularapparates," *Arch.f.d.ges.Physiol.*, 1924, *202*, 523.

FLACH, A., " Zur Psychologie der Ausdrucksbewegung," *Internat. Tagung für angewandte Psychopath.*, Berlin, 1931, pp. 202-209.

FLÜGEL, J. C., " Symbolik und Ambivalenz in der Kleidung," *Internat. Ztschr.f.Psychoanal.*, 1929, *15*, 306.

FLÜGEL, J. C., *Psychology of Clothes*, London, 1930.

FÖRSTER, O., " Die Schussverletzungen der peripheren Nerven und ihre Behandlung," *Berlin.klin.Wchschr.*, 1915, *52*, 823.
" Die Leitungsbahnen des Schmerzgefühles, usw.," *Beitr. zur klin.Chir.*, 1926, 136, Sonderband., pp. 360.

FÖRSTER, O. & GAGEL, O., " Die Vorderseitenstrangdurchschneidung beim Menschen," *Ztschr.f.d.ges.Neurol.*, 1932, *138*, 1.

FOLSOM, J. K., *Social Psychology*, New York, 1931.

FORSTER, E., " Selbstversuch mit Meskalin," *Ztschr.f.d.ges.Neurol.*, 1930, *127*, 1.

FRAZER, SIR J. G., *Man, God and Immortality*, London, 1927.
The Golden Bough, 3rd. ed., 12 vol., London, 1913-5.
The Belief in Immortality and the Worship of the Dead, 3 vol., London, 1913-24.

FREUD, S., " Zur Einführung des Narzissismus," *Jahrb.der Psychoanal.u. Psychopath.Forsch.*, 1914, *6*, 1.
" On Narcissism," In : *Collected Papers*, Vol. IV, pp. 30-59, London, 1925.
Totem und Tabu, Leipzig, 1913.
Das Unbehagen in der Kultur (Trans. *Civilization and its Discontents*, London, 1930).
Hemmung, Symtom und Angst, Leipzig, 1926.
Inhibition, Symptom and Anxiety, Stamford, 1927.
Vorlesungen zur Einführung in die Psychoanalyse, 5te.Aufl., Leipzig, 1930.
Introductory Lectures on Psychoanalysis, London, 1929.
The Ego and the Id, London, 1927.
Three Contributions to the Theory of Sex, 2nd ed., New York, 1916.
(*Cf.* the eleven volumes which have appeared in Vienna, under the title " Gesammelte Schriften").

FREY, M. VON., *Cf.* Stein & Weizsäcker.

FRIEDLÄNDER, H. F., " Die Wahrnehmung der Schwere," *Ztschr.f. Psychol.u.Physiol.der Sinnesorgane*, 1920, *83*, 129.

FRÖBES, J., *Lehrbuch der experimentellen Psychologie*, Bd. 1., Freiburg, 1917.

GALLINEK, A., " Untersuchungen am Phantom," *Arch.f.Psychiat.*, 1931, *95*, 760.
" Über die Entstehung des Phantomgliedes," *Deutsche Ztschr.f.Nervenheilk.*, 1931, *122*, 38.

GAMPER, E., " Bau und Leistungen eines menschlichen Mittelhirnwesens (Beobachtungen auf einem Falle von Arrhinencephalie)," *Ztschr.f.d.ges.Neurol.*, 1926, *102*, 154 ; *104*, 49.
" Zur Frage der Polioencephalitis hæmorrhagica," *Deutsche Ztschr.f.Nervenheilk.*, 1928, *102*, 122.

GELB, A., "Die psychologische Bedeutung pathologischer Störungen der Raumwahrnehmung," *Bericht über den IX. Kongress für experimentelle Psychologie am* 21-25 *April,* 1925, *in München,* Leipzig, 1926. pp. 23-80.

GELB, A. & GOLDSTEIN, K., "Über Farbennamenamnesie, usw.," *Psychol. Forsch.,* 1925, *6,* 127.

"Über den Einfluss des vollständigen Verlustes des optischen Vorstellungsvermögens auf das taktile Erkennen," *Ztschr.f.Psychol.,* 1919, *83,* 1.

GERSTMANN, J., "Fingeragnosie und isolierte Agraphie," *Ztschr.f.d.ges. Neurol.,* 1927, *108,* 152.

"Zur Symptomatologie der Herderkrankungen in dei Übergangsregion der unteren Parietal- und mittleren Okzipitalhirnwindung," *Deutsche Ztschr.f.Nervenheilk.,* 1930, *116,* 46.

GERSTMANN, J., HOFF, H. & SCHILDER, P. F., "Optisch-motorisches Syndrom der Drehung um die Körperlängsachse," *Arch. f.Psychiat.,* 1925, *76,* 766.

GERSTMANN, J. & KESTENBAUM, A., "Monokuläres Doppeltsehen bei cerebralen Erkrankungen," *Ztschr.f.d.ges.Neurol.,* 1930, *128,* 42.

GESELL, A. L., "Maturation and Infant Behaviour Pattern," *Psychol. Rev.,* 1929, *36,* 307.

GESSLER, H. & HANSEN, K., "Über die suggestive Beeinflussbarkeit der Wärmregulation in der Hypnose," *Deutsches Archiv.f. klin. Medizin,* 1927, *156,* 352.

GOLDSTEIN, K., "Das Kleinhirn," Bethe's *Handbuch der normalen und pathologischen Physiologie,* 1927, Bd. 10, pp. 1-96.

"Über die gleichartige funktionelle Bedingtheit der Symptome bei organischen und psychischen Krankheiten," *Monatsschr.f.Psychiat.u.Neurol.,* 1925, *57,* 191.

"Über die Abhängigkeit der Bewegungen von optischen Vorgängen," *Monatsschr.f.Psychiat.u.Neurol.,* 1923, *54,* 141.

"Über den Einfluss unbewusster Bewegungen resp. Tendenzen zu Bewegungen auf die taktile und optische Raumwahrnehmung," *Klin.Wchschr.,* 1925, *4,* 294.

"Veränderungen über des Gesamtverhaltens bei Hirnschädigung," *Monatsschr.f.Psychiat.u.Neurol.,* 1928, *48,* 217.

"Über Störungen des Gewichtschätzens bei Kleinhirnkranken, usw.," *Deutsche Ztschr.f.Nervenheilk.,* 1924, *81,* 68.

GOLDSTEIN, K. & GELB, A., "Zur Psychologie des optischen Wahrnehmungs und Erkennungsvorganges," *Ztschr.f.d. ges.Neurol.,* 1918, *41,* 1.

GOODENOUGH, F. L., *Measurements of Intelligence by Drawings,* New York, 1926.

GRÜNBAUM, A. A., "Über Apraxie," *Zbl.f.d.ges.Neurol.,* 1930, *55,* 788.

GUREWITCH, M., "Über das interparietale Syndrom bei Geisteskrankheiten," *Ztschr.f.d.ges.Neurol.*, 1932, *140*, 593.

HANSEN, K. & GESSLER, H., "Über die suggestive Beeinflussbarkeit der Wärmregulation in der Hypnose," *Deutsch.Arch.f.klin. Med.*, 1927, *156*, 352.

HANSEN, K., *Berichte über den 1. und 2. Kongress f.Psychotherapie*, Leipzig,
HARTMANN, *Die Orientierung*, 1902.

HARTMANN, H., "Ein Fall von Depersonalisation," *Ztschr.f.d.ges.Neurol.*, 1922, *74*, 593.
"Halluzinierte Flächenfarben und Bewegungen," *Monatsschr.f.Psychiat.u.Neurol.*, 1924, *56*, 1.

HARTMANN, H. & SCHILDER, P. F., "Körperinneres und Körperschema," *Ztschr.f.d.ges.Neurol.*, 1927, *109*, 666.
"Zur Psychologie Schädelverletzter," *Arch.f.Psychiat.*, 1925, *75*, 287.

HAYWORTH, D., "The Social Origin and Function of Laughter," *Psychol. Review*, 1928, *35*, 367.

HEAD, SIR H., "On Disturbances of Sensation, with especial reference to the Pain of Visceral Disease," *Brain*, 1893, *16*, 1.
"Aphasia and Kindred Disorders of Speech," *Brain*, 1920, *43*, 87.
Studies in Neurology, 2 vol., London, 1920.

HEAD, SIR H. & HOLMES, G., "Sensory Disturbances from Cerebral Lesions," *Brain*, 1911-12, *34*, 102.

HEILBRONNER, K., "Zur Frage des motorischen Asymbolie (Apraxie)," *Ztschr.f.Psychol.u.Physiol.d.Sinnesorgane*, 1905, *39*, 161.
"Die aphasischen, apraktischen und agnostischen Störungen," Lewandowsky's *Handbuch der Neurologie*, Berlin, 1910, *1*, 982.

HEILIG, R. & HOFF, H., "Psychische Beeinflussung der Organfunktion, insbesondere in der Hypnose," *Zbl.f.ärzt.Psychotherapie*, 1928.

HEMPELMANN, F., *Tierpsychologie*, Leipzig, 1926.

HENRI, V., *Über die Raumwahrnehmung des Tastsinnes*, Berlin, 1898.

HOEPLER, E. & SCHILDER, P. F., "Suggestion und Strafrechtswissenschaft," *Abhandlungen a.d. juristisch-medizinischen Grenzgebiete*, Wien, 1926.

HERRMANN, G., "Über eine besondere Projektions- und Raumsinnstörung bei Grosshirnläsionen," *Med.Klinik*, 1924, *24*, 9.
"Über eine eigenartige Projektionsstörung bei doppelseitiger Grosshirnläsion," *Monatsschr.f.Psychiat.u.Neurol.*, 1923-24, *55*, 99.

HERRMANN, G. & PÖTZL, O., Cf. Pötzl.

HESS, W. R., "Über die Wechselbeziehungen zwischen psychischen und vegetativen Funktionen," *Schweiz.Arch.f.Neurol.*, 1925, *16*, 32 ; 285.

HOFF, H., " Psychische Beeinflussung der Organfunktion," *Wien.med. Wochenschr.*, 1929, *79*, 932.

    Die zentrale Abstimmung der Sehsphäre, Berlin (*Abhandlung aus der Neurologie*, Heft *54*, 1930).

HOFF, H. & PÖTZL, O., " Experimentelle Nachbildung von Anosognosie," *Ztschr.f.d.ges.Neurol.*, 1931, *137*, 722.

HOFF, H. & SCHILDER, P. F., *Die Lagereflexe des Menschen* (with large Bibliography), Wien, 1927.

    " Über Drehbewegungen um die Längsachse," *Ztschr.f.d. ges.Neurol.*, 1925, *96*, 683.

    " Zur Kenntniss der Symptomatologie vestibulärer Erkrankungen," *Deutsche Ztschr.f.Nervenheilk.*, 1928, *103*, 145.

    " Verlauf der Lagebeharrung," *Monatsschr.f.Psychiat.u. Neurol.*, 1929, *60*.

HOLMES, G., " The Symptoms of Acute Cerebellar Injuries due to Gunshot Wounds," *Brain*, 1917, *40*, 461.

JAMES, W., *Principles of Psychology*, 2 vol., London, 1890.

    Pragmatism, London, 1907.

JANET, P. M. F., *L'automatisme psychologique*, Paris, 1889.

    Névroses et Idées fixes, Tom. 1., Paris, 1898.

JONES, E., " The precise Diagnostic Value of Allochiria," *Brain*, 1907, *30*, 490.

    " Die Pathologie der Dyschirie," *Journ.f.Psychol.u.Neurol.*, 1910, *15*, 144.

KANNER, L. & SCHILDER, P. F., " Über Bewegungen an Vorstellungsbildern und ihre Beziehungen zur Pathologie," *Nervenarzt*, 1930, *3*, 406.

    " Movements in Optic Images and the Optic Imagination of Movements," *J.Nerv. and Mental Dis.*, 1930, *72*, 489.

KANT, F. & KRAPF, E., " Über Selbstversuche mit Haschisch," *Arch.f. exper.Pathol.*, 1928, *129*, 319.

KATZ, D., " Psychologische Versuche mit Amputierten," *Ztschr.f.Psychol.*, 1920, *85*, 83.

    " Zur Psychologie des Amputierten und seiner Prothese," *Beihefte der Ztschr.f.angewandte Psychol.*, Heft 25, 1921.

KAUDERS, O., " Drehbewegungen um die Körperlängsachse, Halluzinationen im hemianopischen Gesichtsfeld als Folge eines Schädeltraumas," *Ztschr.f.d.ges.Neurol.*, 1925, *98*, 602.

    Zur Klinik und Analyse der psychomotorischen Störung, Berlin, 1931 (*Abhandlungen aus der Neurologie*, Heft 64, Sonderausgabe).

KLEIN, E. & SCHILDER, P. F., " The Japanese Illusion and the Postural Model of the Body," *J.Nerv. and Mental Dis.*, 1929, *70*, 241.

KLEIN, R., " Über Halluzinationen der Körpervergrösserung," *Monatsschr.f.Psychiat.u.Neurol.*, 1928, *67*, 78.

KLEIN, R., "Über die Empfindung der Körperlichkeit," *Ztschr.f.d. ges.Neurol.*, 1930, *126*, 453.

KOFFKA, K., *The Growth of the Mind*, 2nd ed., London and New York, 1928.
    "Some Problems of Space Perception," *Psychologies of 1930*, edited by C. Murchison, Worcester, Mass., 1930, pp. 161-187.

KOGERER, H., "Zur Psychologie des Phantomgliedes," *Ztschr.f.d.ges. Neurol.*, 1930, *126*, 381.

KÖHLER, W., "Ein altes Scheinproblem," *Naturwissenschaften*, 1929, *17*, 395.
    Die physischen Gestalten im Ruhe und im stationären Zustand, 1924.
    "Some Tasks of Gestalt Psychology," *Psychologies of 1930*, edited by C. Murchison, Worcester, Mass., 1930, pp. 143-160.
    The Mentality of Apes, 2nd ed., London, 1927.
    Gestalt Psychology, New York, 1929.

KORNILOW, K. H., "Psychology in the Light of Dialectic Materialism," *Psychologies of 1930*, edited by C. Murchison, Worcester, Mass., *1930*, pp. 243-278.

KRAMER, F., "Alloasthesie und fehlende Wahrnehmung der galähmten Körperhälfte," *Ztschr.f.d.ges.Neurol., Referate*, 1915, *11*, 379.
    "Bulbärapoplexie usw., mit. Alloästhesie," *Ztschr.f.d.ges. Neurol., Referate*, 1917, *14*, 58.

LANDIS, C., "Studies of Emotional Reactions, 5, Severe Emotional Upset," *Journ.Comp.Psychol.*, 1926, *6*, 221.

LANDIS, C. & GULLETTE, R., "Studies of Emotional Reactions, 3, Systolic Blood-pressure and Inspiration-expiration Ratios," *Journ. Comp.Psychol.*, 1925, *5*, 221.

LANDIS, C., GULLETTE, R. & JACOBSEN, C., "Criteria of Emotionality," *Pedagog.Seminar*, 1925, *32*, 209.

LANDIS, C. & SLIGHT, D., "Studies of Emotional Reactions, 6, Cardiac Responses," *Journ.Gen.Psychol.*, 1929, *2*, 413.

LANGE, J., "Fingeragnosie und Agraphie," *Monatsschr.f.Psychiat.*, 1930, *76*, 129.

LASHLEY, K. S., *Brain Mechanisms and Intelligence*, Chicago, 1929.

LE BON, G., *The Crowd : A Study of the Popular Mind*, London, 1924.

LEIBOWITZ, O., "Über einige kontralaterale Wirkungen des Fussohlenreizes," *Deuts.Ztschr.f.Nervenheilk.*, 1926, *95*, 123.

LEIDLER, R. & LOEWY, P., "Der Schwindel bei Neurosen," *Monatsschr.f. Ohrenheilk.*, 1923, *57*, 21, 103, 192, 278, 347.

LEVY, D. M., "A Method of Integrating Physical and Psychiatric Examination," *Amer.Journ. Psychiat.*, 1929, *9*, 121.
    "Body Interest in Children and Hypochondriasis," *Amer. Journ.Psychiat.*, 1932, *12*, 295.

LÉVY-BRUHL, L., *How Natives Think*, London, 1926.

LIEPMANN, H., " Das Krankheitsbild der Apraxie, usw.," *Monatsschr.f. Psychiat.u.Neurol.*, 1900, *8*, 15, 102, 182.
    Über Störungen des Handelns bei Gehirnkranken, Berlin, 1905.
    Drei Aufsätze aus dem Apraxiegebiet, Berlin, 1908.
    " Apraxie," *Ergeb.der.Med.* (von Brugsch), 1920, *1*, 516.

LOTMAR, F., " Zur Pathologie des Kleinhirns," *Monatsschr.f.Psychiat.u. Neurol.*, 1908, *24*, 217.

LOTZE, R. H., *Medizinische Psychologie*, Leipzig, 1852.

LUQUET, G. H., *Les Dessins d'un Enfant*, Paris, 1913.

LURIA, A. R., " Die moderne russische Physiologie und die Psychoanalyse," *Internat.Ztschr.f.Psychoanal.*, 1926, *12*, 40.

MACDOUGALL, W., *Social Psychology*, 22nd ed., London, 1931.
    " The Hormic Psychology," *Psychologies of 1930*, edited by C. Murchison, Worcester, Mass., 1930, pp. 3-36.

MAGNUS, R., *Körperstellung*, Berlin, 1924.

MALINOWSKI, B., *Sex and Repression in Savage Society*, London, 1926.

MANN, L., " Kriegsneurologische Fälle," *Berlin.klin.Wchschr.*, 1915, *52*, 823.

MARTIN, L. J., " Zur Lehre von den Bewegungsvorstellungen," *Ztschr. f.Psychol.*, 1910, *56*, 401.

MARKUSZEWICZ, R., " Beitrag zum autistischen Denken bei Kindern," *Internat.Ztschr.f.Psychoanal.*, 1920, *6*, 248.

MATTHAEI, R., " Nachbewegungen beim Menschen," *Arch.f.d.ges.Physiol.*, 1924, *204*, 587.

MAYER, C. & REISCH, O., " Über die Widerstandsbereitschaft des Bewegungsapparates," *Deuts.Ztschr.f.Nervenheilk.*, 1928, *102*, 28.

MAYER-GROSS, W., " Ein Fall von Phantomarm nach Plexuszerreissung," *Nervenarzt*, 1929, *2*, 65.

MAYER-GROSS, W. & STEIN, H., *Pathologie der Wahrnehmung*, Bumke's *Handbuch der Geisteskrankheiten*, I, Teil 1, Berlin, 1928.
    " Veränderte Sinnestätigkeit im Meskalinrausch," *Deuts. Ztschr.f.Nervenheilk.*, 1926, *88*, 112.

MEYER, E., " Empfindungstäuschungen im Bereiche amputierter Glieder," *Arch.f.Psychiat.*, 1923, *68*, 251.

MINKOWSKY, E., "Etude Psychologique," *Journ. de Psychol.*, 1923, *20*, 543.

MOHR, F., " Psychophysische Verursachung und Behandlung des Schmerzes," *Verhand.deutsch.Gesellsch.f.inn.Med.*, 1927, *39 Kongress*, 88.

MORGAN, C. LLOYD, *Emergent Evolution*, London, 1923.

MOTT, F. W., " Results of Hemisection of the Spinal Cord in Monkeys," *Phil.Trans.Roy.Soc.Lond.*, 1892, *183*, 1.

MÜLLER, G. E., " Zur Analyse der Gedächtnistätigkeit und des Vorstellungsverlaufes," *Ztschr.f.Sinnesphysiol.*, 1911, Ergänzungsband *5*, Teil 1.

MÜLLER, G. E., *Komplextheorie und Gestalttheorie*, Göttingen, 1923.

NEMLICHER, L. J., & SINEGUBKO, L. L., " Zum Bilde der subkortikalen (" vegetativen ") Epilepsie. Gleichzeitig zur Frage der Entstehung der Makroparästhesien," *Monatsschr.f.Psychiat. u.Neurol.* 1931, *79*, 165.

NUNBERG, H., " Über Depersonalisationszustände im Lichte der Libidotheorie," *Internat.Ztschr.f.Psychoanal.*, 1924, *10*, 17.

OBERSTEINER, H., " On Allochiria, a peculiar Sensory Disorder," *Brain*, 1882, *4*, 153.

OPPENHEIM, H., " Zur Kriegsneurologie," *Berlin.klin.Wchschr.*, 1914, *51*, 1853.
　" Bemerkung zur Alloparalgie," *Neurol.Zentralbl.*, 1916, *35*, 866.

OWRE, A., " Reflexes of Spinal Automatism," *Acta Psychiat. et Neurol.*, 1926, *1*, 260.

PARKER, S. & SCHILDER, P. F., " Das Körperschema im Lift," *Ztschr. f.d.ges.Neurol.*, 1930, *128*, 777.

PIAGET, J., *Judgment and Reasoning in the Child*, London, 1928.

PICK, A., *Beiträge zur Pathologie und pathologische Anatomie des Zentralnervensystems. XIV. Über Störungen der Tiefenlokalisation infolge cerebraler Erkrankungen*, Berlin, 1898.
　Hirnpathologische Untersuchungen, 1898.
　Über Störungen der Orientierung am eigenen Körper.-Arbeiten aus der deutschen psychiatrischen Klinik, Prag, Berlin, 1908.
　" Zur Pathologie des Bewusstseins vom eigenen Körper," *Neurol.Zentralblatt*, 1915, *34*, 257.
　Die neurologische Forschungsrichtung in der Psychopathologie, Berlin, 1921.
　" Störung der Orientierung am eigenen Körper," *Psychol. Forsch.*, 1922, *1*, 303.

PIKLER, J., " Über die Angriffspunkte des Willens am Körper," *Ztschr.f. Psychol.*, 1929, *110*, 288.

PINÉAS, H., " Mangel an Krankheitsbewusstsein und seine Variationen als Symptom organischer Erkrankungen," *Deutsch.Ztschr. f.Nervenheilk.*, 1926, *94*, 238.
　" Ein Fall von räumlicher Orientierung mit Dyschirie," *Ztschr.f.d.ges.Neurol.*, 1931, *133*, 180.

PÖTZL, O., " Experimentell erregte Traumbilder," *Ztschr.f.d.ges.Neurol.*, 1917, *37*, 278.
　" Über die Herderscheinungen bei Läsion des linken unteren Scheitellappens," *Med.Klinik*, 1923, *19*, 7.
　" Über die räumliche Anordnung der Zentren in der Sehsphäre des menschlichen Grosshirns," *Wien.klin. Wchschr.*, 1918, *31*, 745.
　Zur Klinik und Anatomie der Worttaubheit, Berlin, 1919.

PÖTZL, O., *Die Aphasielehre vom Standpunkt der klinischen Psychiatrie, I. Die optisch-agnostischen Störungen*, Wien, 1928.
"Über das Syndrom bei Herderkrankungen der Scheitel-hinterhauptslappen," *Med. Klinik*, 1924, *20*, 10.

PÖTZL, O. & HERRMANN, G., *Die optische Alloaesthesie*, Berlin, 1928 (*Abhandlungen aus der Neurologie*, Heft 46).

PÖTZL, O. & HERRMANN, G., *Über die Agraphie*, Berlin, 1926 (*Abhand. aus der Neurol., Bd. 35*).

PÖTZL, O. & REDLICH, E., "Demonstration eines Falles bilateraler Affection der Occipitallapen," *Wien.klin.Wchschr.*, 1911, *24*, 517.

PREUSS, K. Th., "Der Ursprung der Religion und Kunst," *Globus*, 1904-5, *86*; 87.

PREYER, T. W., *Die Seele des Kindes*, Leipzig, 1882.

REDLICH, E. & BONVICINI, G., *Über das Fehlen der Wahrnehmung der eigenen Blindheit bei Hirnkrankheiten*, Leipzig, 1908.
"Weitere klinische und anatomische Mitteilungen über das Fehlen der Wahrnehmung der eigenen Blindheit bei Hirnkrankheiten," *Neurol,Zentralb.*, 1911, *30*, 227.

REICH, W., *Die Funktion des Organismus*, Vienna, 1927. (*Neue Arbeiten über ärztliche Psychoanalyse*, Nr. 6.)

REIK, T., *Wie man Psychologe wird*, Vienna, 1927.

RIESE, W., "Über die sogenannte Phantomhand der Amputierten," *Deuts.Ztschr.f.Nervenheilk.*, 1928, *101*, 270.

ROHEIM, G., "Das Selbst," *Imago*, 7, 1, 142, 310, 348, 453.

ROMBERG, M. F., *Lehrbuch der Nervenkrankheiten*, Leipzig, 1857.

ROSENBERG, M., "Zur Pathologie der Orientierung nach rechts und links," *Ztschr.f.Psychol.*, 1912, *61*, 25.

ROSS, N., "The Postural Model of the Head and the Face," *Journ.Gen. Psychol.*, 1932, 7, 144.

ROTHSCHILD, F. S., "Über Links und Rechts," *Ztschr.f.d.ges.Neurol.*, 1930, *124*, 451.

SADGER, I., "Über Depersonalisation," *Internat.Ztschr.f.Psychoanal.*, 1928, *14*, 315.

SANDER, F., "Structure, Totality of Experience and Gestalt," *Psychologies of 1930*, ed. by C. Murchison, Worcester, Mass., 1930, pp. 118-204.

SCHELER, M., *Der Formalismus in der Ethik und die Materiale Wertethik*, 2 Bde., Halle, 1913-16.

SCHILDER, P. F., *Selbstbewusstsein und Persönlichkeitsbewusstsein*, Berlin, 1914.
Wahn und Erkenntnis, Berlin, 1918.
"Projektion eigener Körperdefekte in Trugwahrnehmungen," *Neurol.Zentralbl.*, 1919, *38*, 300.
"Über Halluzinationen," *Ztschr.f.d.ges.Neurol.*, 1920, *59*, 169.

SCHILDER, P. F., "Studien über Bewegungsstörungen, III," *Ztschr.f.d.ges. Neurol.*, 1920, *61*, 203.

" Über Identifizierung auf Grund der Analyse eines Falles von Homosexualität," *Ztschr.f.d.ges.Neurol.*, 1920, *59*, 217.

" Über Gedankenentwickelung," *Ztschr.f.d.ges.Neurol.*, 1920, *59*, 250.

" Über elementare Halluzinationen des Bewegungssehens," *Ztschr.f.d.ges.Neurol.*, 1923, *80*, 424.

" Einige Bemerkungen zu der Problemsphäre : Cortex, Stamganglien—Psyche, Neurose," *Ztschr.f.d.ges.Neurol.*, 1922, *74*, 1.

Seele und Leben, Berlin, 1923.

Medizinische Psychologie, Berlin, 1924.

" Zur Lehre von der Hypochrondrie," *Monatsschr.f. Psychiat.und Neurol.*, 1924, *56*, 142.

" Probleme der klinischen Psychiatrie," *Med.Klinik*, 1925, *21*, 77.

Psychiatrie auf psychoanalytischer Grundlage (Trans : *Psychoanalytic Psychiatry*, Washington, 1928, *Nervous and Mental Disease Monographs*, 50).

" Notiz über Gewichtsschätzungen," *Ztschr.f.d.ges.Neurol.*, 1927, *109*, 676.

" Zerstückelungsmotiv," *Allgem.ärztl.Ztschr.f.Psychotherap*, 1928, *1*, 23.

" Kurze Bemerkung über die Mittellinie," *Nervenarzt*, 1928, *1*, 23.

" Psychische Symptome bei Mittel- und Zwischenhirnerkrankung," *Wien.klin.Wchschr.*, 1927, *40*, 1147.

" Eine neue Tasttäuschung und ihre Beziehung zum Körperschema," *Ztschr.f.Sinnesphysiol.*, 1929, *60*, 284.

" Posture, with Special Reference to the Cerebellum," *Arch. Neurol. and.Psychiat.*, 1929, *22*, 1116.

" Zur Kenntnis der Psychosen bei chronischer Encephalitis epidemica," *Ztschr.f.d.ges.Neurol.*, 1929, *118*, 327.

" Über Komplexe," *Berichte über d.XI.Kongr.f.exper.Psychol.*, 1930, pp. 136-150.

"The Somatic Basis of the Neurosis," *Journ. Nerv. and Ment. Dis.*, 1929, *70*, 502.

" Vestibulo-Optik und Körperschema in der Alkoholhalluzinose," *Ztschr.f.d.ges.Neurol.*, 1930, *128*, 784.

"The Unity of the Body, Sadism and Dizziness," *Psychoanal. Rev.*, 1930, *17*, 1

" Organic Problems in Child Guidance," *Mental Hygiene*, 1931, *15*, 480.

" Über Neurasthenie," *Internat.Ztschr.f.Psychoanal.*, 1931, *17*, 368.

SCHILDER, P. F., " Fingeragnosie, Fingerapraxie, Fingeraphasie," *Nerven-arzt*, 1931, *4*, 625.
    " Notes on the Psychopathology of Pain in Neurosis and Psychosis," *Psychoanal.Rev.*, 1931, *18*, 1.

SCHILDER, P. F. & KAUDERS, O., *Hypnosis*, Washington, 1927 (*Nervous and Mental Disease Monographs*, 46).
    Lehrbuch der Hypnose, Berlin, 1926 (Trans.: *Hypnosis*, New York, 1927).

SCHILDER, P. F. & STENGEL, E., " Schmerzasymbolie," *Ztschr.f.d.ges. Neurol.*, 1928, *113*, 143.
    " Das Krankheitsbild der Schmerzasymbolie," *Ztschr.f.d. ges.Neurol.*, 1930, *129*, 250.

SCHLESINGER, B., " Zur Auffassung der optischen und konstruktiven Apraxie," *Ztschr.f.d.ges.Neurol.*, 1928, *117*, 649.

SCHOLL, K., " Das räumliche Zusammenarbeiten von Auge und Hand," *Deuts.Ztschr.f.Nervenheilk.*, 1926, *92*, 280.
    " Sensomotorische Einstellungen," *Deuts.Ztschr.f.Nerven-heilk.*, 1924, *83*, 318.
    " Vom Zielen und Zeigen," *Ztschr.f.d.ges.Neurol.*, 1925, *87*, 217.

SCHULTE, H., " Versuch einer Theorie der paranoischen Eigenbeziehung und Wahnbildung," *Psychol.Forsch.*, 1924, *5*, 1.

SCHULTZ, J. H., *Das autogene Training*, Leipzig, 1932.

SEARL, M. N., " A Note on Depersonalisation," *Internat.J.Psychoanal.*, 1932, *12*, 329.

SELLING, L. S., " An Experimental Investigation of the Phenomenon of Postural Persistence," *Arch.Psychology*, 18, No. 118.

SHERRINGTON, C. S., *Integrative Action of the Nervous System*, New York, 1906.

SKRAMLIK, E. VON., " Lebensgewohnheiten als Grundlage von Sinnes-täuschungen," *Naturwissenschaften*, 1925, *117*, 134.
    " Varianten zur aristotelischen Täuschung," *Arch.f.d.ges. Physiol.*, 1923, *201*, 250.
    " Über die Beeinflussung der Tastwahrnehmungen durch Innervationsantriebe," *Klin.Wchschr.*, 1923, *3*, 967.
    " Über Tastwahrnehmungen," *Ztschr.f.Sinnesphysiol.*, 1925, *56*, 256.

SKWORRZOFF, K., " Doppelgänger-Halluzinationen bei Kranken mit Funktionsstörungen des Labyrinths," *Ztschr.f.d.ges.Neurol.*, 1931, *133*, 762.

SMITH, W. ROBERTSON, *Kinship and Marriage in Early Arabia*, Cambridge, 1885.

SOLLIER, P., *Les Phénomènes d'Autoscopie*," Paris, 1905.

SPIEGEL, E., " Hirnrinden-Erregung (Auslösung epileptiformer Krämpfe) durch Labyrinthreizung," *Klin.Wchschr.*, 1931, *10*, 1723.

STÄRCKE, A., *Psychoanalyse und Psychiatrie*, Vienna, 1921 (Beihefte 4, *Internat.Ztschr.f.Psychoanal.*).

STEIN, H., *Cf.* Mayer-Gross, W.

STEIN, H. & WEIZSÄCKER, V. VON., "Zur Pathologie der Sensibilität," *Ergeb.der.Physiol.*, 1928, 27, 657.

STENGEL, E., "Zur Klinik und Pathophysiologie des postenzephalitischen Blickkrampfes," *Monatsschr.f.Psychiat.u.Neurol.*, 1928, 70, 305.
"Über taktile Bewegungs- und Scheinbewegungswahrnehmung bei Störung der Oberflächensensibilität," *Deuts. Ztschr.f.Nervenheilk.*, 1927, 99, 31.

STOCKERT, F. G. VON., "Klinik und Aetiologie der Kontaktneurosen," *Klin.Wchschr.*, 1929, 8, 76.

STRATTON, G. M., "Some Preliminary Experiments on Vision without Inversion of the Retinal Image," *Psychol.Rev.*, 1896, 3, 611.
"Vision without Inversion of the Retinal Image," *Psychol. Rev.*, 1897, 4, 314.

STRAUS, E., "Das Zeiterlebnis in der endogenen Depression und in der psychopathischen Verstimmung," *Monatsschr.f.Psychiat.u. Neurol.*, 1928, 68, 640.

STRÄUSSLER, E., "Über sensibile Störungen bei Schussverletzungen peripherer Nerven, die sogennante 'Alloparalgie,'" *Ztschr.f.d.ges.Neurol.*, 1919, 50, 1.

TARDE, J. G., "Les Lois d'Imitation," Paris, 1911.
"Les Lois Sociales," Paris, 1913.

TAUSK, V., "Über die Enstehung des Beeinflussungsapparates in der Schizophrenie," *Internat.Ztschr.f.Psychoanal.*, 1919, 5, 1.

TRÖMNER, E., "Reflexuntersuchungen an einem Anencephalus," *Journ. f.Psychol.u.Neurol.*, 1928, 35, 194.

TROTTER, W., *Instincts of the Herd in Peace and War*, London, 1916.

TYLOR, E. B., *Primitive Culture*, 6 ed., 2 vol., London, 1920.

UEXKÜLL, J. VON, *Theoretical Biology* (International Library of Psychology), 1927.

VIERKANDT, A., *Naturvölker und Kulturvölker*, Leipzig, 1896.
"Die Anfänge der Religion und Zauberei," *Globus*, 1910, 92.

VOLKMANN, A. W., "Über den Einfluss der Übung auf das Erkennen räumlicher Distanzen," *Ber.u.d.Verhand.der k.sächs.Akad. der Wiss. Leipzig*, 1858, 10, 38.

WATSON, J. B., *Behaviorism*, Revised ed., New York and London, 1930.

WEIZSÄCKER, V. VON., "Über einige Täuschungen in der Raumwahrnehmung bei Erkrankungen des Vestibularapparates," *Deuts.Ztschr.f.Nervenheilk.*, 1919, 64, 1.
"Über eine systematische Raumsinnstörung," *Deuts. Ztschr.f.Nervenheilk.*, 1924, 84, 179.

WEIZSÄCKER, V. VON., *Reflexgesetze*, Bethe's *Handbuch der norm.u.path. Physiol.*, Berlin, 1927, Bd. 10, pp. 35-102.

" *Einleitung zur Physiologie der Sinne*," Bethe's *Handbuch der norm.u.path.Physiol.*, Berlin, 1926, Bd. 11, pp. 1-67.

" Kasuistische Beiträge zur Lehre vom Funktionswandel, usw.," *Deuts.Ztschr.f.Nervenheilk.*, 1931, *117-9*, 716.

" Körpergeschehen und Neurose," *Internat.Ztschr.f.Psychoanal.*, 1933, *19*, 16.

" Über neurotischen Aufbau bei inneren Erkrankungen," *Verhand.Gesellsch.Deutsche Nervenarzt*, 1925, p. 168.

WERNICKE, C., *Grundriss der Psychiatrie*, 2 Aufl., Leipzig, 1906.

WERTHEIMER, M., " Experimentelle Studien über das Sehen von Bewegungen," *Ztschr.f.Psychol.u.Physiol.der Sinnesorgane*, 1912, *61*, 161.

" Untersuchungen zur Lehre von der Gestalt," I, *Psychol. Forsch.*, 1921, *1*, 47 ; II, *Psychol.Forsch.*, 1923, *4*, 301.

WHEELER, R. H., *The Laws of Human Nature*, London, 1931.

WILSON, S. A. K., " On Decerebrate Rigidity in Man and the Occurrence of Tonic Fits," *Brain*, 1923, *43*, 220.

WOOSTER, M., " Certain Factors in the Development of a new Spatial Co-ordination," *Psychol.Monographs*, 1923, *32*, No. 146.

WUNDT, W., *Physiologische Psychologie*, 2. Aufl., Bd. 2, Berlin, 1910.

ZÁDOR, J., " Meskalinwirkung bei Störungen des optischen Systems," *Ztschr.f.d.ges.Neurol.*, 1930, *127*, 30.

" Meskalinwirkung auf das Phantomglied," *Monatsschr.f. Psychiat.u.Neurol.*, 1930, *77*, 71.

ZUCKER, K. & ZÁDOR, J., " Zur Analyse der Meskalinwirkung am Normalen," *Ztschr.f.d.ges.Neurol.*, 1930, *127*, 15.

I. SUBJECT INDEX

II. INDEX OF NAMES